J. Walter

PHARMACEUTICAL
DOSAGE FORMS

PHARMACEUTICAL DOSAGE FORMS

Tablets

In Three Volumes

VOLUME 2

EDITED BY

Herbert A. Lieberman
Warner-Lambert Company, Inc.
Morris Plains, New Jersey

Leon Lachman
United Laboratories, Inc.
Makati, Metro Manila
The Philippines

MARCEL DEKKER, INC.   New York and Basel

Library of Congress Cataloging in Publication Data

Main entry under title:

Pharmaceutical dosage forms, tablets

   Includes bibliographies and indexes.
   CONTENTS: v.   Tablets.
   1. Drugs--Dosage forms. I. Lieberman,
Herbert A., [date]. II. Lachman, Leon,
[date]. [DNLM: 1. Dosage forms. 2. Drugs--
Administration and dosage. QV785 P535]
RS201.A2P48   615'191   80-12751
ISBN 0-8247-1269-2 (v. 2)   AACR1

MARCEL DEKKER, INC.
270 Madison Avenue, New York, New York 10016

Current printing (last digit):
10 9 8 7 6 5 4 3 2

PRINTED IN THE UNITED STATES OF AMERICA

Preface

The most widely used dosage form in medicine today is the tablet. Yet despite this popularity, books describing the technology involved in developing, producing, and testing this dosage form are limited. Chapters concerned with tablets have appeared in various pharmaceutical texts. However, no comprehensive volume has been prepared that fully describes all facets of the technology related to the formulation of various tablet dosage forms.

The United States Pharmacopeia defines tablets as "solid dosage forms containing medicinal substances with or without suitable diluents. They may be classed according to the method of manufacture, such as molded or compressed tablets."

The compacted solid dosage form exists in many shapes and forms stressing convenience for the patient, ease of identification, and drug availability. There are tablets which are chewable, sublingual, or buccal, or are meant to be sucked, such as certain compressed tablets or molded sugar tablets, referred to as troches, in the former case, and lozenges in the latter. Most tablets are meant to be swallowed with the aid of water, and others are meant to be palatable when dropped in water—effervescent tablets. Some tablets, when swallowed, readily dissolve in the stomach; others are formulated as enteric, coated tablets, to dissolve in the intestine, or to slowly release the medicament throughout the gastrointestinal tract—sustained-release tablets. Some tablets are layered to keep chemically reactive materials apart, and other tablets are coated to help cover the bad taste of the medicines, and also to keep medicines in the coating away from the chemically reactive materials in the tablets or atmosphere.

Each of these tablet forms requires special formulation techniques. Knowing how to make one type does not mean that one can make another. Expertise in each tablet form requires specialized experience. The editors have chosen the authors of chapters describing particular types of tablets on the basis of their experience and training and of their high degree of knowledge of their subject. Since considerable expertise is required for the myriad tablet dosage forms, a multiauthored text seemed to the editors to be the only way to accomplish their goal of a text which provides a knowledgable coverage of subject matter in an applicable fashion. The purpose of this multivolume treatise is to fully describe the technology used today in formulating, producing, and controlling the many compacted and molded solid dosage forms that are part of modern medicine.

The authors chosen for the various chapters were charged with the task of covering their technology so that their material would teach and not be presented as a review of the literature. Each chapter begins by assuming the reader is not very familiar with the subject matter. Gradually, as each chapter develops, the discussion becomes more advanced and specific. By writing in this fashion, the text is intended as a teaching source for undergraduate and graduate students, as well as experienced and unexperienced industrial pharmaceutical scientists. The book can also act as a ready reference to all those interested in tablet technology, namely, students, product development pharmacists, hospital pharmacists, drug patent attorneys, governmental and regulatory scientists, quality control personnel, pharmaceutical production personnel, and those concerned with production equipment for making tablets.

Three volumes are the result of the in-depth treatment given this subject. The first discusses the various solid dosage forms; the second is concerned with the processes involved in producing tablets, bioavailability, and pharmacokinetics; and in the third and final volume additional processes in tablet production are discussed, as well as sustained drug release, stability-kinetics, automation, pilot plant, and quality assurance.

The authors are to be commended for the manner in which they covered their subject matter and their patience with the editors' continued comments concerning their manuscripts. The editors wish to express their special thanks to the contributors for the excellence of their works, as well as their continued forebearance with our attempts to achieve this level of accomplishment. In many instances no previous pharmaceutical literature existed to which the authors could refer to facilitate the writing of their chapters. Since this book is the first complete coverage of tablets, many technological descriptions appear for the first time. Although there has been a great deal written about various types of tablets, no particular type has been as completely described in one chapter as appears in this multivolume text. The acceptability and usefulness of these volumes will be attributable to the efforts and skills of each of the contributing authors.

The subject matter, format, and choice of authors are the responsibilities of the editors. Any multiauthor book has problems of coordination and minimizing repetition. Some repetition was purposly left in the text because in the editors' opinions it helped the authors in developing their theme, and because each treatment is sufficiently different to be a valuable teaching aid. It is our hope that the labors of the contributors and the judgments of the editors have resulted in a text on tablets that will facilitate the work of the many people who refer to it.

Herbert A. Lieberman
Leon Lachman

Contents

1. Mixing 1

Russell J. Lantz, Jr. and Joseph B. Schwartz

2. Drying 55

Michael A. Zoglio and Jens T. Carstensen

Contents

7. Pharmaceutical Tablet Compression Tooling 451

George F. Loeffler

Contributors

Neil R. Anderson, Ph.D., Assistant Professor of Industrial Pharmacy, Department of Industrial and Physical Pharmacy, Purdue University School of Pharmacy and Pharmacal Sciences, West Lafayette, Indiana

Gilbert S. Banker, M.S., Ph.D., Head, Department of Industrial and Physical Pharmacy, Purdue University School of Pharmacy and Pharmacal Sciences, West Lafayette, Indiana

Jens T. Carstensen, M.S., Ph.D., Professor, University of Wisconsin School of Pharmacy, Madison, Wisconsin

Dale E. Fonner, M.S., Ph.D., Manager, Production and Technical Support, The Upjohn Company, Kalamazoo, Michigan

Russell J. Lantz, Jr., B.S., Manager, Process Improvement, Department of Pharmaceutical Manufacturing, Smith Kline Corporation, Philadelphia, Pennsylvania

George F. Loeffler, B.S.M.E., Director of Engineering, Thomas Engineering Incorporated, Hoffman Estates, Illinois

James W. McGinity, Ph.D., Assistant Director, Drug Dynamics Institute, and Associate Professor, Department of Pharmacy, University of Texas College of Pharmacy, Austin, Texas

Alfred Martin, M.S., Ph.D., Coulter R. Sublett Professor, Drug Dynamics Institute, University of Texas College of Pharmacy, Austin, Texas

Eugene L. Parrott, Ph.D., Professor of Industrial Pharmacy and Head, Division of Pharmaceutics, University of Iowa, Iowa City, Iowa

Joseph B. Schwartz, M.S., Ph.D., Research Fellow, Department of Pharmaceutical Research and Development, Merck Sharp and Dohme Research Laboratories, West Point, Pennsylvania

Salomon A. Stavchansky, Ph.D., Associate Professor of Pharmacy, College of Pharmacy, Drug Dynamics Institute, Department of Pharmaceutics, The University of Texas at Austin, Austin, Texas

Michael A. Zoglio, Ph.D., Director, Department of Pharmaceutical Research and Development, Merrell Research Center, Cincinnati, Ohio

Contents of Volume 1

Contents of Volume 3

PHARMACEUTICAL DOSAGE FORMS

1

Mixing

Russell J. Lantz, Jr.

Smith Kline Corporation
Philadelphia, Pennsylvania

Joseph B. Schwartz

Merck Sharp and Dohme Research
  Laboratories
West Point, Pennsylvania

I. Introduction

Almost every industry depends in some way on a blending or mixing operation at some stage of manufacture. Figure 1 is a tabulation of some typical dry-blending operations. Mixing is a process used in all walks of life by people who are totally unaware of the principles and theory of this unit operation; for example, the housewife blends the dry salt, flour, baking powder, and so on, for a cake; the mason's helper realizes the importance of preblending the sand, gravel, and cement before adding the water; and the gardener mixes loams with peat moss and fertilizer to obtain a uniform potting soil. Although each of these examples does not have stringent specifications for completeness (uniformity) of mix, there is some point of mixing below which the outcome of the final product is affected adversely. In pharmacy, however, the mixing objective is clear: one is attempting to obtain dosage units each of which will contain the same quantity of medicament. The most elementary approach to the mixing subject can be illustrated by the hand-mixing methods used not too long ago in pharmaceutical dispensing [2]:

Spatulation: mixing of small quantities of powders on paper or on a pill tile using a spatula.
Trituration: mixing powders using a mortar and pestle.
Sifting: passing ingredients through a sieve gives some mixing, but also aids the dispersion of agglomerated particles.
Tumbling: mixing ingredients by tumbling in a wide-mouth closed container. This method yields a minimum of mixture particle size reduction.
Geometric Dilution: each of the four methods described above may incorporate the process of geometric dilution to aid in the more thorough mixing of potent smaller quantities of active ingredients into the larger bulk of the mix by first mixing the active ingredient with an equal amount of diluent, then adding an amount of diluent equal to the original mix and mixing again, and so on, until the desired dilution and mixing has been obtained.

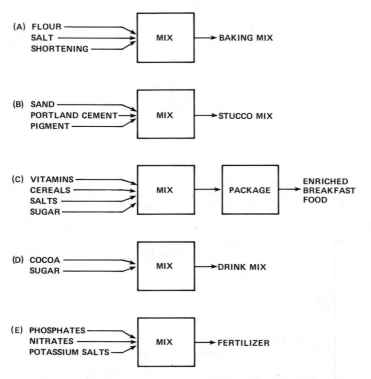

Figure 1. Examples of common dry mixing. [Adapted from Fisher, J. J., Chem. Eng., August: 107-128 (1962).]

For large-scale industrial pharmaceutical mixing, only the size of the batch is changed. The same objectives are present.

Assuming that a tablet formula has been developed which performs its function in the desired manner, the ultimate objective of pharmaceutical processing is to produce each batch of this product uniformly--not a small task.

It is the purpose of this chapter to discuss the unit operation of mixing or blending as related to the production of tablets. Although the principles and some of the problems will be discussed here, it must be noted at the outset that in a practical situation, common sense must prevail. It must be kept in mind that the objective is to obtain dosage units each of which contains the same ratio and amount of ingredients per batch.

II. The Mixing Process

A. Definition of Mixing

The American College Dictionary [3] differentiates between the words "mix" and "blend" in that blending is a way of mixing. The definitions are as follows:

mix (verb): to put together (substances or things, or one substance or thing with another) in one mass or assemblage with more or less thorough diffusion of the constituent elements among one another.

blend (verb): to mix smoothly and inseparably together.

The terms are very close in definition and are commonly used interchangeably in the industry. However, in this chapter an attempt will be made to use these two terms properly as they apply to the mixing unit operation.

Therefore, mixing is the putting together of ingredients, and the mixing of solid particles is accomplished through three principal mechanisms [4, 5]:

1. Diffusion: the redistribution of particles by the random movement of particles relative one to the other
2. Convection: the movement of groups of adjacent particles from one place to another within the mixture
3. Shear: the change in the configuration of ingredients through the formation of slip planes in the mixture

Diffusion is sometimes referred to in the literature as micromixing [6], whereas convection is referred to as macromixing [6, 7]. These three principal mechanisms are illustrated in Figure 2.

B. Solid-Solid Mixing

The unit operation of solid-solid mixing can be separated into four principal steps [8].

1. Bed of solid particles expands.
2. Application of three-dimensional shear force to the powder bed.
3. Mix long enough to permit true randomization of particles.
4. Maintain randomization (no segregation) after mixing has stopped.

Initially, when dry materials or particles are loaded into a mixer, they form a static bed. Before mixing or interparticulate movement can take place, this static bed must expand as shown in Figure 3 [8], as a result of mixing forces. It must be noted that before a particle bed can expand for mixing, there must be room for it to expand; that is, there must be enough void space remaining in the mixer after it has been charged with the ingredients to be blended.

Once particle movement is possible with the expansion of the powder bed, shear forces are necessary to produce movement between particles. Tension and compression forces merely change the bed volume (Fig. 3). Induction of movement in all three directions requires adequate three-dimensional stress, resulting in the essential random and sometimes turbulent particle movement. Should these forces be inadequate, dead spaces in the form of particle agglomerates in the powder bed move together without mixing with adjacent particles, resulting in a poor mix.

Mixing is the process that produces a random distribution of particles, and it is dependent on the probability that an event happens in a given time. The law of mixing appears to follow a first-order decay [8]:

$$M = A(1 - e^{-kt}) \tag{1}$$

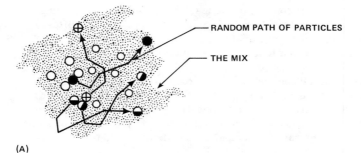

(A)

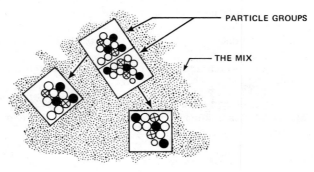

(B)

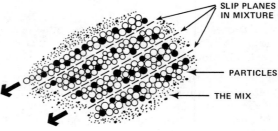

(C)

Figure 2. Principal mechanisms of mixing. (A) Diffusion: random action of individual particles in the mix; (B) convection: transfer of adjacent particle groups in the mix; (C) shear: configuration change through slip planes.

where

M	=	degree of mixing
t	=	time
A and k	=	constants that depend on mixer geometry, its use, and the physical characteristics and proportions of the materials being mixed

Therefore, mixing results are a function of time, and although the initial rate of mixing may be very rapid, the end point or perfect mixture is not attainable because of the asymptotic characteristic of Equation (1).

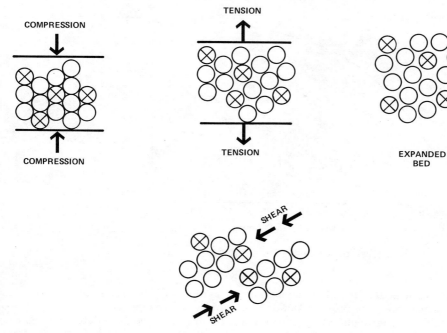

Figure 3. Mixing forces and bed expansion.

If we assign a value of 10 to the constant A and of 0.1 to the constant k, and select specific time intervals, the plot in Figure 4 is obtained. For this particular set of values for the A and k constants, it appears from the curve that the best mixing time would fall between 30 and 35 min. because the most rapid change in rate of the slope begins within this time period.

Once the desired mixing has been attained, it is essential that the particles in the mix cease movement such that the system may exist in a state of static equilibrium without segregation taking place [8]. This is an important point because each subsequent handling of the mixture jeopardizes the static equilibrium.

Although less significant effects as a result of unusual characteristics peculiar to specific particulate systems may create complications now and then, poor mixtures usually result from violating the four principal steps that should take place during mixing [8].

C. Liquid-Solid Mixing

In addition to solid-solid blending, the mechanics of liquid-solids blending must also be considered in the mixing process because it is also a major step in tablet wet granulating. The term "liquid-solid blending" is used because the liquid, which in most instances constitutes a minor ingredient as compared to the percentage of solids, is added to the solids, or powder bed.

During tablet wet granulating, the sequence of blending events is usually as follows:

1. Premixing of dry powders to be granulated: called internal ingredients (solid-solid mixing)

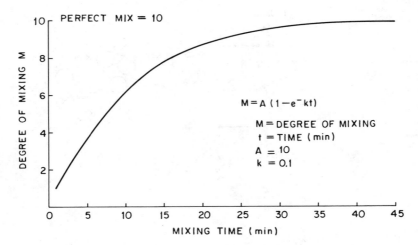

Figure 4. Plot of first-order decay for mixing.

2. Addition of liquids to solids during mixing to distribute the liquid uniformly
    throughout the premixed dry powders (liquid–solid mixing)
3. Mixing the nongranulated or external ingredients with the granulated portion
    of the formula (solid–solid mixing)

The solid–solid mixing in steps 1 and 3 in the foregoing sequence has been addressed earlier in this section.

A number of stages occur during the addition of a liquid to a powder bed being
mixed as shown in Figure 5 (a high-shear mixer is necessary for liquid–solid mixing).

1. Agglomeration: Droplets of solvent such as water or alcohol or binding solution (e.g., polyvinylpyrrolidone dissolved in water) contact the moving powder
particles that build up around the periphery of the droplet. As the powder is wetted
by the liquid, the liquid migrates in part by capillary action into the particle interstices, and forms large powder–liquid agglomerates. It is assumed that the interfacial tension between the liquid and solids in the mixture is low enough to permit
good wetting. If this is not the case, the addition of a surface-active agent may be
necessary.

2. Agglomeration Breakdown: After the initial large agglomerate formation,
mixing shear and tension forces break the large agglomerates down such that the
liquid is now carried throughout the mixture via smaller agglomerates which continue to diminish in size as the liquid is distributed over the powder particle surfaces. At this point no hard agglomerates are detectable, and the wet mass easily
crumbles to a powder if compacted by the grip of a hand.

3. Reagglomeration: As mixing proceeds and the liquid becomes completely
distributed throughout the mixture, the powder bed now becomes a wet mass acting similarly to a highly viscous slurry. This slurry resists shear forces and begins to generate heat as particle-to-particle contact increases, requiring more
mixer shear force for continued mixing. This is a result of the displacement of

1. AGGLOMERATION

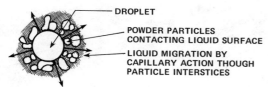
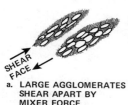

— DROPLET

POWDER PARTICLES
CONTACTING LIQUID SURFACE

LIQUID MIGRATION BY
CAPILLARY ACTION THOUGH
PARTICLE INTERSTICES

a. INITIAL LIQUID PARTICLE CONTACT   b. LIQUID MIGRATING TO FORM
                                             LARGE WET AGGLOMERATE

2. AGGLOMERATION BREAKDOWN

SHEAR FACE

a. LARGE AGGLOMERATES   b. MORE DRY   c. LESS LIQUID AT
   SHEAR APART BY   PARTICLES   PARTICLE SURFACE
   MIXER FORCE   CONTACTING   AS AGGLOMERATES
                                AGGLOMERATES   BREAKDOWN

3. REAGGLOMERATION   4. PASTE FORMATION

PARTICLE POINT CONTACT   WET MASS WITH MUCH
BRIDGED BY BINDER SOLUTION   LOSS OF DISCRETE
AND/OR SOLUBILIZED   PARTICLE UNITS
INGREDIENT

Figure 5. Stages of liquid–solid mixing.

air by liquid at the particle surface, liquid viscosity, and/or partial solubilization of some of the more-soluble ingredients that may be present in the formula. This solubilization creates even more resistance to the high shear mixing, because it usually increases the viscosity of the liquid phase of the mixture. A wide size range of agglomerates can be seen forming in the mixture as mixing proceeds, the end point of which has heretofore normally been gaged by how easily a wet compaction (which would not reduce back to a powder) could be formed in the grip of a hand. More recently, measurements of mixer shear force as seen in Figure 6 show the phases a granulation goes through while being wetted and mixed. This was accomplished with a special torque-sensing setup, since ammeters are not that accurate or reproducible [9] for indicating a granulation end point. A properly granulated formula may or may not require wet milling. It dries easily and forms granules which are easily milled to the desired size and yield a satisfactory compaction in the tablet machine.

4. Paste Formation: If mixing is continued beyond the normal granulating end point, which is different for each formula, a thick wet mass resembling a paste

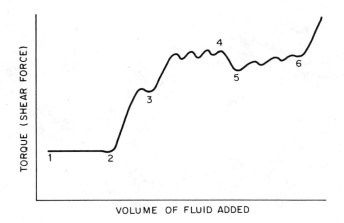

VOLUME OF FLUID ADDED

Figure 6. Shear force required during wet-down in wet granulating. 1-2, before liquid addition; 2, liquid added; 2-3, rapid increase in resistance to mixer shear; 4, wet mass resistance to shear; 5, end point of granulation; 6, mass becomes excessively wet, forming large agglomerates. [Adapted from Travers, D. N., et al., J. Pharm. Pharmacol., 27, Suppl. 3P (1975).]

begins to form as a result of solubilization, solvation, and so on. This paste, unlike the granulation at its end point, is difficult to break up for drying, will dry to extremely hard granules which will be difficult to mill, and usually forms a poor compaction in the tablet machine.

D. Perfect Mixture

As illustrated by Equation (1) (Fig. 4), the mixing process will never yield an ideal or perfect mixture, which is defined as that state in which any sample removed from the mixture will have exactly the same composition as all other samples taken from the mix. The perfect mixture is represented schematically in Figure 7A by a chessboard with the black and white squares representing two separate components [10]. If one samples two adjacent squares at each sampling, the composition will be identical throughout the lot (see also Sec. IV).

E. Alternatives to the Perfect Mixture

Since the perfect mix cannot be achieved, consideration must be given to the other two alternatives for obtaining an acceptable mix of a particular formula. First, there is randomization or random mixing, which is that state in which the probability of finding a particle of a given component is the same at all points in the mixture [10] and is in the same ratio of components in the entire mixture. A chessboard randomization is shown in Figure 7B for two components.

   For illustration purposes, Lacey [4] takes a binary system of ingredients a and b and expresses the theoretical standard deviation (see Sec. IV) of the unmixed components as

$$\sigma_0 = \sqrt{ab} \qquad (2)$$

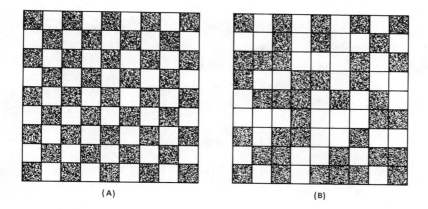

Figure 7. Types of binary mixtures. (A) Perfect mix; (B) randomized mix.

where a and b are proportions of the two ingredients. Lacey then shows the theoretical standard deviation for the totally randomized mixture to be

$$\sigma_t = \sqrt{\frac{ab}{n}} \qquad\qquad (3)$$

where n represents the total number of particles in the blend.

Therefore, if one has a particulate system with 20,000 total particles and a
fraction of the lower concentration ingredient a at 2%, the totally randomized at
best attainable is calculated to be

$$\sigma_t = \sqrt{\frac{98 \times 2}{20,000}\%} = 0.099\% \qquad\qquad (4)$$

There is a constraint on this mixing study in that the particle size and density of
components a and b were identical. Empirically, degree of randomness is determined by taking a series of samples. Referring again to the chessboard in Figure 7B, it can be seen that if two adjacent squares are samples in the random mix
as they were in the perfect mix (Fig. 7A), the composition of this sample will not
always be the same; that is, there is a probability that two black squares or two
white squares will be sampled instead of a black square and a white square. This
is the reason that accurately evaluating the quality of a random mix is dependent
on the number and size of samples rather than a single sample.

The degree of randomization must also be considered for the purposes of economics. Referring to the first-order decay plot in Figure 4, one determines when
a particular mixture has been mixed long enough to yield an acceptable randomization of the ingredients without using excessive time and energy.

The second alternative to the perfect mixture is ordered mixing, the theory of
which was developed by Hersey [11]. Ordered mixing is described as the use of
mechanical, adhesional, or coating forces or methods to prepare ordered units in
the mix such that the ordered unit will be the smallest possible sample of the mix
and will be nearly identical in composition to all other ordered units in the mix
[12] (e.g., a dry granule made by wet granulation or a coated particle).

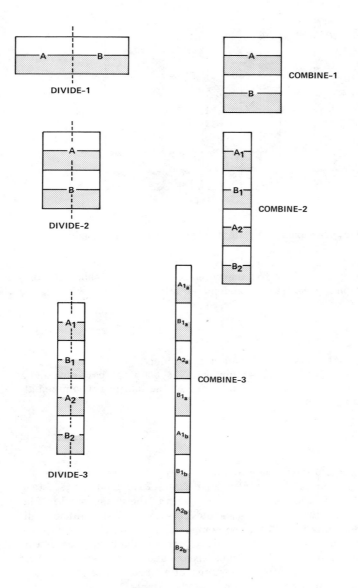

Figure 8. Ordered mechanical mixing. (From Hersey, J. A., Seminar on Bulk Solids Handling; Powder Mixing, presented May 1979, Philadelphia, Pennsylvania.)

Ordered mixing probably comes the closest to yielding the perfect mix and may be obtained in a number of ways [12].

1. Mechanical Means: dividing and recombining the powder bed any number of times until the desired subdivision unit is obtained, as illustrated in Figure 8. The smaller the units, the more uniform the mix. However, if no particulate adhesion is present, segregation of the mix easily takes place on further handling.

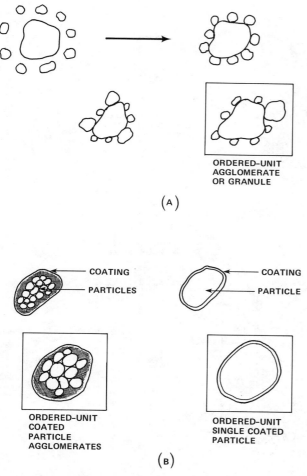

(A)

ORDERED-UNIT
AGGLOMERATE
OR GRANULE

COATING

PARTICLES

COATING

PARTICLE

ORDERED-UNIT
COATED
PARTICLE
AGGLOMERATES

ORDERED-UNIT
SINGLE COATED
PARTICLE

(B)

Figure 9. Ordered mixing: adhesion and coating. (A) Adhesional or binding forces, (B) coated particles. (From Hersey, J. A., Seminar on Bulk Solids Handling; Powder Mixing, presented May 1979, Philadelphia, Pennsylvania.)

2. Adhesion: adhesional forces of particles may create ordered units of nearly identical composition, depending on the process. Partial solubilization or the use of a binding agent during wet granulating approximates the same effect as that shown in Figure 9A.
3. Coating: Figure 9B shows that particles in an assemblage may also be coated with other ingredients to give an ordered mix either as individual or coated-particle agglomerates.

The major difference between the mechanically and the adhesional and coating ordered mixing is the inseparability of the ingredients in the ordered units of the latter two.

Ordered mixing is not only beneficial in approaching a perfect mixture, but it minimizes the possibility of segregation of a mixture by holding the ingredient

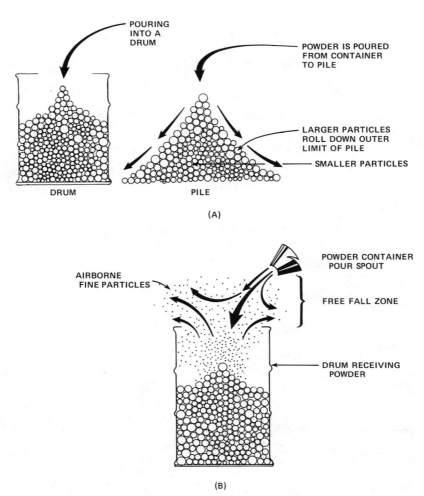

Figure 10. Segregation by pouring. (A) Segregation by rolling, (B) segregation by dusting.

ratio constant via the intact ordered units. Segregation occurs primarily as a result of wide differences in particle size in a dry mixture. Segregation may be produced by pouring a powder from one container to the next, as is done by emptying the contents of a blender into another hopper or into drums. This is shown in Figure 10A. Note that the larger particles, because of their mass, have a tendency to roll down the outside of the powder pile, segregating the coarse and fine particles. A second means of segregation, dusting, may also take place during pouring of a powder, particularly if there is considerable free fall of the particles as shown in Figure 10B. In this case the fine particles become airborne and separate from the bulk of the powder. Segregation may also take place inside the blender when the powder bed does not have mass flow characteristics; that is,

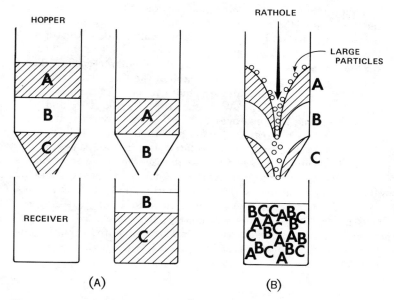

Figure 11. Segregation by flow from a hopper or blender. (A) In mass flow, coarse and fine particles flow as a mass and yield minimum segregation; (B) in ratholing or nonmass flow, coarse particles move more rapidly and separate from fine particles.

the powder does not flow from a hopper or mixer in the order in which it is situated in the container. This is illustrated in Figure 11, which shows the difference between mass flow and "ratholing," where again the large particles move as the powder structure breaks down because of their larger mass, leaving the smaller structured particles behind.

III. Homogeneity

It is necessary that one be able to describe the degree of mixing obtained in a given mixing operation. Much of the available mixing literature is devoted to discussions and proposals to measure and compare homogeneity or "degree of mixedness" by some mixing index. These mixing indices are then used to follow a mixing process with time, to compare mixers, to compare the mixing operation as it is scaled up, and to investigate the mechanism of mixing in a given piece of equipment. For the most part, these mixing indices are derived or empirically modified from binary systems which contain monosized particles having the same density. In the opinion of the authors, these are of little, if any, utility in practical pharmaceutical problems, although they serve to illustrate some basic mixing theory. For practical purposes, the authors suggest that the guidelines in Section IV will be adequate. An investigator must keep his or her particular objective in mind when selecting the parameter to be used.

The majority of mixing indices involve some comparison of the measured standard deviation S of the samples of the mixture under study with the estimated standard deviation of a completely random mixture σ_r. The standard deviation of a completely unmixed system σ_0 is included by some authors [13]. For this reason, these mixing indices are mentioned here for the sake of completeness. The use of the associated equations will not be demonstrated. The interested reader is referred to the following references for further study: Lacey [14], Stange [15], Poole et al. [16], Ashton and Valentin [17], Williams [18], Buslik [19], and Harnby [20]. The various mixing indices, over 30 in all, were reviewed and tabulated by Fan et al. [21]. In a separate report [22] Fan and Wang selected the nine most frequently used mixing indices and related them to each another. Several of these are listed in Table 1. Several other parameters have been suggested as methods of determining degree of mixedness, including Hersey's mixing margin and Buslik's homogeneity index [23]. In addition, Lai et al. have suggested the use of nonparametric statistics to sampling in solid mixing [24].

Unless one is investigating the mechanism of mixing, the authors recommend that the method used to determine homogeneity in a mixture be suited to the objective at hand. Other primary considerations include the effort (including the analytical support available) and the accuracy required.

IV. Sampling and Statistics of Mixing

Sampling is an integral part of the statistics of mixing because, at any time, spot samples generate the data necessary to evaluate the quality of the mixture (i.e., the data necessary to estimate the true mean and standard deviation of the mixture). This is accomplished in two stages [25]:

1. The estimation of the arithmetic mean and the standard deviation
2. An accuracy and precision assessment of these estimates

Precision is normally expressed in terms of the confidence with which these estimates will fall within specified limits [25]. These limits assume that the assay distribution of the samples will have a normal or bell-type curve.

The data for the statistics are developed by assaying, or in some manner identifying, the active ingredient(s) in a number of random samples taken from the blend at a specified time. The mean assay value of a group of random samples taken from a mixture is a measure of the central tendency of the batch population (active ingredient content). The arithmetic mean value is given by

$$\bar{y} = \sum_i^n \frac{y_i}{n} \tag{5}$$

where y_i = the value of a given sample and n = the number of samples.

Since it is impractical to sample and assay the entire batch to obtain a true mean μ, a limited number of samples are taken and an estimate of the true mean $\bar{y}$ is calculated from these samples.

In addition to the estimated mean $\bar{y}$ of the true mean μ, an additional statistic is calculated to describe or characterize the spread or dispersion of individual

Table 1

Mixing Indices

Mixing index[a]	Comment	Reference
$M = \dfrac{\sigma_R}{\sigma}$	Ratio less than 1	Lacey [14]
$M = \dfrac{\sigma_0 - \sigma}{\sigma_0 - \sigma_R}$	Ratio less than 1	Lacey [4]
$M = \dfrac{\sigma_0{}^2 - \sigma^2}{\sigma_0{}^2 - \sigma_R{}^2}$	Ratio less than 1	Lacey [4]
$M = \dfrac{\sigma}{\sigma_R}$	Ratio greater than 1; better differentiation between mixtures	Poole [16]
$M^2 = \dfrac{\log \sigma_0{}^2 - \log \sigma^2}{\log \sigma_R{}^2 - \log \sigma_0{}^2}$		Ashton and Valentin [17]

[a] M = degree of mixedness; σ_0 = standard deviation of unmixed xystem; σ_R = standard deviation of completely randomized mixture.

samples about the mean $\bar{y}$. This is the standard deviation S for n number of random samples, which is given by

$$S = \sqrt{\frac{\sum\limits_{i}^{n} (y_i - \bar{y})^2}{n - 1}} \qquad (6)$$

Based on the numbers of samples used to obtain the $\bar{y}$ estimate of the true mean μ, the standard deviation S is an estimate of the total population standard deviation σ of the total mixture.

For computational purposes the standard deviation may also be expressed as

$$S = \sqrt{\frac{\sum\limits_{i}^{n} y^2 - \dfrac{1}{n} \left(\sum\limits_{i}^{n} y \right)^2}{n - 1}} \qquad (7)$$

Table 2

Five- and 10-Minute-Mix-Time Assay Data

Sample number	5-Minute mix time	10-Minute mix time
1	4.90	5.20
2	5.10	5.00
3	5.10	5.00
4	5.10	5.10
5	4.80	5.00
6	4.90	4.90
7	5.30	5.10
8	5.00	5.00
9	5.20	5.00
10	4.90	5.00
11	4.90	4.90
12	4.70	4.90
13	5.10	4.80
14	5.00	5.00
15	4.80	5.20
16	5.00	5.10
17	5.00	4.80
18	5.00	5.10
19	5.20	4.90
20	5.00	5.00

The square of the standard deviation S^2, called the variance, is also used to characterize a mixture because of its additive properties.

$$S^2 = \frac{\sum\limits_{i}^{n} (y_i - \bar{y})^2}{n - 1} \tag{8}$$

Again, this value is an estimate of the true variance σ^2 of the mixture. It is logical that the simple course is to take samples from different parts of the mixer and analyze them for the component of interest.

An example of tabulated assay data from a mixture mixed for 5 and 10 min is shown in Table 2. These data are put into frequency distribution curves in Figure 12. Each sample has a mean assay $\bar{y}$ of 5.00. However, note that the scatter about the mean or standard deviation S is greater at the shorter mixing time. The high standard deviation indicates less uniformity of the mixture assuming no variation in the assay method.

One may also follow the mixing operation in a given process by plotting the standard deviation as a function of time, as shown in Figure 13.

If one wishes to compare the efficiency of two or more mixing operations and has different sample sizes or different compositions, the relative standard

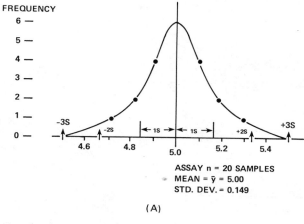

(A)

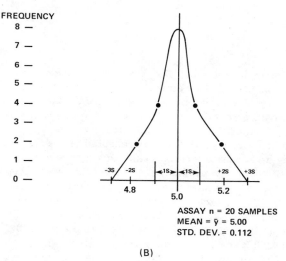

(B)

Figure 12. Frequency distribution curves. (A) Five-minute mix assay samples plot (Table 2); (B) 10-min mix assay samples plot (Table 2).

deviation (RSD) should replace the standard deviation as a measure of sample uniformity. The relative standard deviation is the standard deviation divided by the mean, that is,

$$RSD = \frac{\sigma}{\overline{x}}$$
(9)

This value is usually expressed as a percent, by multiplying the values by 100.

It is important to note at this point that differences in the assay mean from the assay theory may indicate not only homogeneity problems, but may also be the result of poor or inadequate sampling, improper handling of the powder for assay in

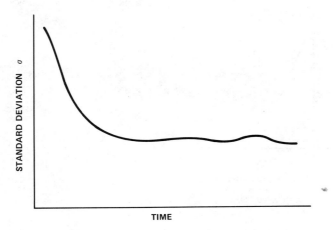

Figure 13. Standard deviation of a mixture as a function of time. [Adapted from Wang, R. H., et al., Chem. Eng., May, 27:88-94 (1974)].

the lab, or may point up an assay method problem. The same is true when considering the standard deviation of a mixture. Therefore, it is essential that each variable that may contribute to differences in the mean and standard deviation of a mixture be investigated thoroughly to determine the extent to which they contribute to the overall mean and standard deviation of the mixture.

A mixture begins with the unmixed dry ingredients, represented in Figure 14A as a binary mixture. After mixing an adequate length of time, a randomized mixture results, as seen in Figure 14B. For comparison, the perfect mixture is represented in Figure 7. The problem is how to differentiate among the three mixtures (i.e., how to determine the quality of each mixture). To illustrate the problems one may encounter, both the unmixed and randomized mixture have several possible sample sizes shown (sample through X for 1/2 the mix; sample through Y for 1/8 the mix, and sample through Z for 1/32 of the mix). Each sample when assayed will show 50% white and 50% black squares. This indicates a perfect mix for each example. It is obvious that these are erroneous results because the two samples have not been distinguished from the perfect mix, or from each other, and all three examples are different mixtures.

The solution to the problem lies within certain statistical guidelines, including:

1. The number of samples required should be no less than 20, preferably 30, and more ideally 100. The larger the number of samples obtained and assayed per granulation sampling time, the greater the confidence in estimating the true mean and standard deviation of the mixture at that time. Since economics plays a major role in limiting the number of sample assays in a production atmosphere, many of the examples shown will be composed of 20 samples.
2. Random sampling is the method of choice for the statistics.
3. The sample size, in most cases, should approximate the unit dose size of the final product.

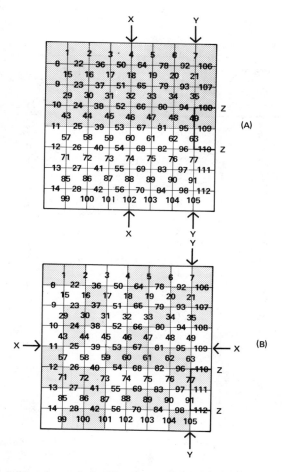

Figure 14. Unmixed (A) and random-mixed (B) binary systems.

4. Comparison between the mean value of the sample analysis and the target value gives the first estimate of the degree of mixing.
5. If the mean value of the sample analysis is on or near the target value, calculation of the standard deviation (and/or variance) will give an indication of the uniformity of the samples.

Applying these guidelines to the examples in Figure 14A and B, the unit sample or smallest unit dose is two adjacent squares, since the example is a binary mixture.
   To illustrate the random sampling of each of these examples, the units of all two adjacent square possibilities in Figure 14A and B have been numbered on each chessboard. Both examples have been randomly samples for 20 samples using a table of random numbers. This sampling has been repeated three times, as shown

Table 3

Random Sampling of Unmixed Binary System

Sample number	Assay group 1			Assay group 2			Assay group 3		
	Random number	B[a]	W[a]	Random number	B	W	Random number	B	W
1	42	0	1	9	1	0	39	1/2	1/2
2	6	1	0	102	0	1	37	1	0
3	56	0	1	83	0	1	112	0	1
4	101	0	1	32	1	0	110	0	1
5	51	1	0	77	0	1	45	1	0
6	74	0	1	80	1	0	54	0	1
7	42	0	1	38	1	0	75	0	1
8	77	0	1	47	1	0	7	1	0
9	86	0	1	64	1	0	94	1	0
10	64	1	0	41	0	1	108	1	0
11	7	1	0	54	0	1	107	1	0
12	29	1	0	98	0	1	102	0	1
13	110	0	1	88	0	1	73	0	1
14	4	1	0	34	1	0	74	0	1
15	46	1	0	72	0	1	53	1/2	1/2
16	70	0	1	37	1	0	47	1	0
17	87	0	1	19	1	0	35	1	0
18	55	0	1	108	1	0	52	1	0
19	83	0	1	55	0	1	5	1	0
20	76	0	1	43	1	0	18	1	0
		7	13		11	9		12	8

Percent active (B):   7/20 = 35%   11/20 = 55%   12/20 = 60%
Theoretical mean = 50%

[a] B, black; W, white.

in Tables 3 and 4. Note the difference in assays of each table. There is one over-lap at 55%, but the unmixed system shows a much wider spread from the theoreti-cal mean in the three assay groups than does the random mixed sample. Note that the random mixed sample shows some variation, as it should when compared to the perfect mixture, which will show no spread in the assay if sampled in the same manner.

Statistically, one may sample using one of two approaches: (1) by not return-ing the sample to the mixture after evaluating it, or (2) by returning the sample to the mixture after its evaluation. Destructive testing such as putting the sample into solution for assay will not permit the second sampling approach. Therefore, it is necessary in most cases to use destructive sampling when checking for dis-tribution of ingredients in a mixed formula.

Table 4

Random Sampling of Random Mixture of Binary System

Sample number	Assay 1			Assay 2			Assay 3		
	Random number	B[a]	W[a]	Random number	B	W	Random number	B	W
1	100	1	0	55	0	1	91	0	1
2	84	1/2	1/2	53	1/2	1/2	83	1/2	1/2
3	98	1/2	1/2	22	1/2	1/2	76	1/2	1/2
4	44	1/2	1/2	74	0	1	108	1/2	1/2
5	5	1	0	102	0	1	69	1/2	1/2
6	10	0	1	24	1	0	104	1/2	1/2
7	17	1/2	1/2	17	1/2	1/2	86	1/2	1/2
8	99	1/2	1/2	30	1	0	102	0	1
9	73	1/2	1/2	15	0	1	62	1	0
10	93	1/2	1/2	54	1/2	1/2	98	1/2	1/2
11	20	1/2	1/2	99	1/2	1/2	6	1/2	1/2
12	53	1/2	1/2	105	1/2	1/2	12	1	0
13	35	1/2	1/2	93	1/2	1/2	18	1/2	1/2
14	62	1	0	89	1	0	3	0	1
15	111	1/2	1/2	33	1/2	1/2	13	1/2	1/2
16	13	1/2	1/2	40	1/2	1/2	30	1	0
17	17	1/2	1/2	42	1	0	79	1/2	1/2
18	36	1/2	1/2	83	1/2	1/2	75	0	1
19	2	1/2	1/2	35	1/2	1/2	33	1/2	1/2
20	79	1/2	1/2	8	1/2	1/2	37	1	0
		11	9		10	10		10	10

Percent active (B):   11/20 = 55%   10/20 = 50%   10/20 = 50%
Theoretical mean = 50%

[a]B, black; W, white.

There are two golden rules of sampling [26]:

1. "A powder should be sampled when it is in motion."
2. "The whole of the stream of powder should be taken for many short increments of time, in preference to part of the stream being taken for the whole time."

Although these rules are the ultimate in sampling, from a practical point of view one must be satisfied with less than the ultimate. This is usually not the choice of the experimenter; rather, it results from limitations of the system. For example: a number of ingredients are placed in a blender for mixing. The mixer is activated for various lengths of time and after each time interval a number of samples are removed to determine homogeneity of the mixture. The object: to determine the optimum blending time. How is each sample removed from a mixer to follow the golden rule of sampling? The powder mixture usually cannot be sampled from a moving stream because of (1) the configuration of the mixer (i.e., bowl shape)--does not lend itself to dumping; (2) the size of the batch--large volumes are not conducive to routine transfer from the blender to drums or into large hopper-type collectors; and (3) the possibility of mixture segregation biasing the sample. Therefore, one is left with several less than desirable options, including:

1. Scoop sampling of the bulk mixture
2. Thief probing of the bulk mixture

Each of these sampling options has limitations, and although they are discussed at length in Chapter 3, comment must also be made here.

Scoop sampling has two basic drawbacks:

1. Scooping from the top of a container of powder may produce a sample that has segregated on standing; that is, smaller particles have sifted down through the interstices of the larger particles, biasing the sample to the larger particles.
2. Scooping cannot remove a sample from the middle or bottom of a blender or container without considerable disturbance of the mixture.

The thief probe also has drawbacks:

1. As the thief is inserted into the powder bed, some compaction takes place around the thief and flow into the thief is poor.
2. As the thief is inserted in the powder bed, it carries material from the surface of the mixture down into the mixture. This puts a portion of top sample down at the lower portion of the thief, and if a compartmentalized thief is used, the lower samples are biased or contaminated with top sample.

However, from a practical point of view, the thief probe sample is preferred over the scoop because samples can be taken from deep within the powder bed, and a fair degree of random sampling can be achieved.

Probably the most significant measure of quality of a mixture is how the blend actually performs, and the sampling approach used is dependent on whether the mixer or the mixture is being evaluated [1].

V. Material Properties

A. Basic Concepts of Dry Blending--The Unit Particle

Since mixing plays such an important role in tableting, an understanding of the characteristics of the materials being mixed is paramount. Many of the studies presented in the literature, and used previously in examples, deal with binary mixtures of physically and chemically similar materials which can easily be differentiated for the study by color, size, or assay. However, pharmaceutical, binary, particulate systems in tableting are the exception, and results dealing with binary systems have limited applicability in industrial practice.

PURE SUBSTANCES DIFFERENT SHAPE CONFIGURATIONS INDIVIDUAL PARTICLES

PURE SUBSTANCES AGGLOMERATED BY FREE SURFACE ENERGY, ELECTROSTATIC FORCES, ETC.

PURE SUBSTANCES AGGREGATED WITH A BINDER

PURE SUBSTANCE COMPACTED AND MILLED

BINARY MIXTURE AGGLOMERATED BY FREE SURFACE ENERGY, ELECTROSTATIC FORCES, ETC.

BINARY MIXTURE AGGREGATED WITH A BINDER

MULTICOMPONENT MIXTURE

WET-GRANULATED MULTICOMPONENT MIXTURE— MILLED

Figure 15. Several different types of particles encountered in tablet granulation dry blending.

Each component in a mixture has distinct physical characteristics that contribute to, or detract from, the completeness (uniformity) of a mixture. Therefore, it is important to define and characterize the unit particles that make up a mixture, whether it is a premix of a wet granulation, a direct-compression formula, or the addition of lubricants or other components to a granulation. Figure 15 is an illustration of several different types of particles handled in tablet granulation mixing.

The unit particles in a system may range in size from a pure-substance raw material particle of <1 μm to a multicomponent granule of 8 to 12 mesh held together by a binder. Since dry mixing is a dynamic state of an assemblage of particles, the properties of the unit particle must be discussed in terms that affect these dynamics.

Table 5

Effect of Particle Size on Powder Flow

Particle size (μm)	Type of flow[a]	Reason
2000-250 (10 mesh[b]- 60 mesh)	Flow is usually good if shape is not interfering	Mass of individual particles is relatively large
250-75 (60 mesh to 200 μm)	Flow properties may be a problem with many pure substances and mixtures	Mass of individual particles is small and increased surface area amplifies effects of surface forces
100-75	Flow becomes a problem with most substances	Cohesive forces or free-surface-energy forces, as well as static electrical forces, are large relative to particle size

[a]Assume that particle shape is constant and does not interfere with flow.
[b]U.S. Standard mesh size.

There are three properties intrinsic to each component in the mixture [27]:

Composition (physicochemical structure)
Size (and size distribution)
Shape

The composition of each particle is "its qualitative and quantitative makeup" [28]. Each unit of pure substance has a molecular composition and arrangement that distinguishes it from all other materials, and dictates its behavior as a powder per se, or in combination with other tablet-mixture ingredients. Chemical composition is important, because chemical reactivity limits a material's use with other tableting components; for example, acids and bases such as aspirin and phenylpropanolamine would not be blended together because of their potential to react. The same applies to components that may affect the stability of a mixture, such as the potential Schiff base reaction between certain sugars and amines when in contact even in the dry state.

Physically, the molecular makeup determines crystallinity manifested as color, hardness, tackiness, general appearance, and so on.

Particle size and size distribution of the unit particles have considerable impact on the flow properties of powders and, therefore, the dynamics of mixing. Table 5 shows, in general, the effect of particle size on the flow properties of powders. Table 6 is a list of some common substances used in the pharmaceutical industry, and their flow characteristics.

Large (sieve size range >60 mesh) dry particles tend to flow better than smaller dry particles because they have greater mass. Smaller particles (<100 mesh) may create mixing problems because the very large surface area may give rise to strong electrostatic forces as a result of processing and/or interparticle friction from

Table 6

Flow Characteristics of Some Common Substances

Material	Working bulk density (g cm^{-3})	Type of powder	General comments on flow
Acrawax C	0.46	Very fluid powder	Dusty, slippery material
Ammonium chloride	0.75	Nonuniform powdered granules	May form hard lumps, as a result of hygroscopicity
Calcium carbonate	0.92 0.36	Fluid cohesive powder Cohesive powder	Flow becomes very poor if powder is packed
Dicalcium phosphate	0.99 1.31	Uniform granules Very fluid granules and powder	Powder form is very dusty Material is hygroscopic, which reduces flowability
Cellulose	0.09	Fibrous not free-flowing; crystalline free-flowing	Flow depends on size of fibers or crystals
Kaolin	0.48	Fluid powder	Dusty material which has poor flow when powder is packed excessively
Magnesium hydroxide	0.56	Fluid powder	Dusty material which is hygroscopic; flowability is reduced considerably when powder is packed excessively
Sodium chloride	1.10	Uniform granule or fluid granules and powder	Material is very hygroscopic and cakes at room relative humidity (40–50%)
Sodium bicarbonate	0.96 1.08	Fluid cohesive powder Uniform powdered granules	Very little dustiness Material is hygroscopic, which decreases flowability
Cornstarch	0.56	Very fluid powder	Very dusty; material is hygroscopic, which decreases flowability
Talc	0.67 0.19	Fluid powder Fluid cohesive powder	The two density powders are slippery and very dusty Material is hygroscopic, which decreases flowability
Titanium dioxide	0.56	Cohesive powder	Flow becomes extremely poor if packed
Zinc oxide	0.45 0.74	Fluid cohesive powder Cohesive powder	Dusty, tends to lump; flow becomes poorer when packed Some dustiness; tends to lump; flow becomes poorer when packed

Source: Ref. 29, pp. 69–72.

NEUTRAL PARTICLE
(electrical charge evenly
distributed over particle)

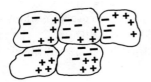

PROCESSING AND OR DRY
PARTICLE MOVEMENT CAUSES
POLARIZATION OF FINE
PARTICLES (static electric forces)

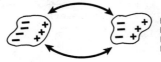

POLARIZATION CAUSES
AGGLOMERATION OF FINE
PARTICLES (electrical charges
inducted by one particle on
another van der Waals forces)

Figure 16.   Effect of electrical forces on fine particles.

movement. These forces may prevent the desired distribution of these smaller
particles throughout a mixture because of fine-particle agglomeration.

As the particle size approaches 10 μm and below, weak polarizing electrical
forces called van der Waals forces or cohesive forces also begin to affect the flow
of the powder. Both van der Waals and electrostatic forces usually inhibit powder
flow through particle agglomeration, as mentioned above. However, in some instances, improved flow results because the agglomerated particles behave as a
single large-mass particle (Fig. 16). Flow may be better in this case, but the
dynamics of distributing these small particles during mixing is very poor.

Increased surface exposure of fine particles to the atmosphere may present
oxidation and/or moisture adsorption/absorption problems which should be avoided
if possible. Fine-powder particles also create potential dust conditions, which may
require operators to wear respirators for safe handling and may also create potentially dangerous dust-explosion hazards.

Particle size distribution of unit particles, as suggested in the discussion above,
may also have an effect on the flow of a powder: too large a parcentage of fine particles with cohesive forces, or free surface energy, may inhibit flow. Although it
has been stated that cohesive forces are strong in powders composed of particles
10 μm or less in size, each powder has a "critical size" at which cohesive forces
begin to affect the powder flow properties. An example of this is shown in Table 7.

The angle of repose , or angle of slip, is a relative measure of the friction between powder particles but is also a measure, for the most part, of the cohesiveness of fine particles. The angle of repose may be measured in several ways, as
shown in Figure 17. Methods 1 and 2 are both dynamic angle-of-repose measurements: the powder in method 1 flows from a filled powder funnel onto a smooth
surface where the angle is measured as illustrated; in method 2 the powder is
moving in a rotating drum while the angle is measured as shown. Method 3 gives

Table 7

Critical Particle Size of Raw Materials

Raw material	Critical particle size (μm)[a]
Wheat starch	20–25
Boric acid	150–170

[a]Cohesive forces diminish at this particle size range and have little affect on raw material flow properties as the particle size increases above this range.
Source: Revised from data provided by Dr. P. L. Madan.

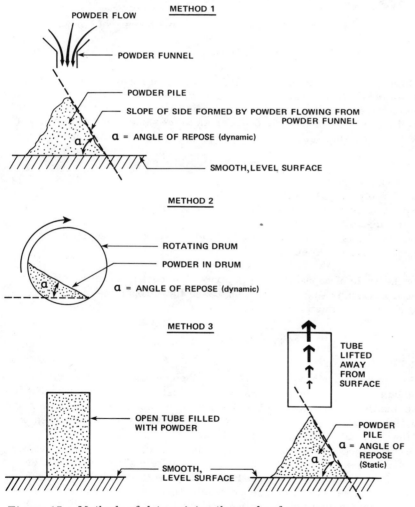

Figure 17.   Methods of determining the angle of repose.

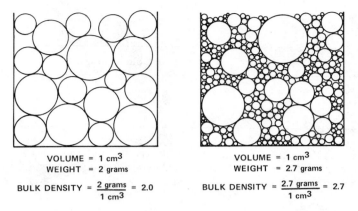

VOLUME   = 1 cm³   VOLUME   = 1 cm³
WEIGHT = 2 grams   WEIGHT = 2.7 grams

BULK DENSITY = $\frac{2 \text{ grams}}{1 \text{ cm}^3}$ = 2.0   BULK DENSITY = $\frac{2.7 \text{ grams}}{1 \text{ cm}^3}$ = 2.7

Figure 18. Effect of particle size distribution on the bulk density of a powder.

the static angle of repose, because the powder container is removed and the powder does not flow, or is not flowing before measurement.

Since many factors, such as particle size, shape, and moisture content, enter into the angle of repose, there is some question as to its value in characterizing a powder. However, certain generalizations can be made regarding the angle of repose:

1. $\alpha > 60°$ for cohesive powders.
2. $\alpha < 25°$ for noncohesive particles.
3. High α usually means poor powder flow and the particles are usually less than 75 to 100 μm in size.
4. Low α usually means good powder flow and the particles are usually greater than 60 mesh or 250 μm in size.

The tangent of the angle of repose (tan α) is termed the coefficient of friction of a powder and is preferred by some in referring to the flow properties of a powder. For example, a powder with an angle of repose of 65° will have a coefficient of friction of

tan 65° = 2.14

Size distribution of a powder also has an effect on the packing characteristics and, therefore, the bulk density of the powder. This is illustrated in Figure 18, which shows how the smaller particles of a size distribution occupies interstices between the larger particles, creating a more densely packed powder. Densely packed powders usually flow with difficulty.

Particle shape affects powder interparticle friction and, consequently, the flow properties of the powder. Figure 19 shows general particle shapes and their effects on powder flow. Materials composed of particles with rounded edges such as those in Figure 19A and B will flow more readily than those with sharper edges (C), and than two-dimensional flat, flakelike particles (E). Poor flow is usually

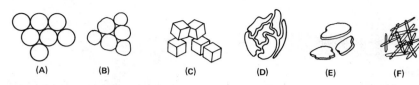

(A) SPHERICAL PARTICLES — NORMALLY FLOWS EASILY

(B) OBLONG SHAPES WITH SMOOTH EDGES — NORMALLY FLOWS EASILY

(C) EQUIDIMENSIONALLY SHAPED SHARP EDGES SUCH AS CUBES — DOES NOT FLOW AS READILY AS (A) OR (B)

(D) IRREGULARLY SHAPED INTERLOCKING PARTICLES — NORMALLY SHOWS POOR FLOW, AND BRIDGES EASILY

(E) IRREGULARLY SHAPED TWO-DIMENSIONAL PARTICLES SUCH AS FLAKES — NORMALLY SHOWS FAIR FLOW AND MAY BRIDGE

(F) FIBROUS PARTICLES — VERY POOR FLOW AND BRIDGES EASILY

Figure 19. General particle shapes and their effects on powder flow. Bridging refers to the stoppage of powder flow as a result of particles that form a semirigid or rigid structure within the powder bulk.

encountered with particles having an interlocking shape or of a fibrous configuration, illustrated respectively in Figure 19D and F.

It is apparent that particle shape affects the angle of repose of a powder, particularly of powders with low-magnitude surface forces (for example, particles larger than 100 μm), and some low-free-surface-energy fine powders, such as talc (hydrous magnesium silicate) and cornstarch [29]. It must be remembered that all the properties discussed above are intimately interrelated, and although each must be considered individually, they must also be considered as an entire group of variables when evaluating powder flow properties.

VI. Mixing Equipment

A general classification of mixers is shown in Table 8. Types of mixers can be divided first into two broad categories: batch type and continuous. By far the most prevalent type used in the pharmaceutical industry today is the batch type, which mixes a sublot or total lot of a formula at one time (i.e., all ingredients are placed in the mixer, the materials are mixed, and the mixture is removed as one unit lot or sublot). The continuous mixer, on the other hand, is usually dedicated to a single high-volume product. Ingredients are continuously proportioned into the mixer and collected from the continuous discharge. The lot size is usually determined by a specified length of mixing time, which may range from 8 to 24 hr or longer, depending on the process.

A. Batch-Type Mixers

The first general class of mixers are those which create particle movement by rotation of the entire mixer shell or body. A schematic of the four types listed in Table 8 is seen in Figure 20. Neither barrel nor cube mixers are used to any great extent in industry at present. However, V-shaped (Fig. 21) and double-cone (Fig. 22)

Table 8

General Mixer Classification

A. Batch type

    1. Rotation of the entire mixer shell or body with no agitator or mixing blade
        a. Barrel
        b. Cube
        c. V-shaped
        d. Double cone

    2. Rotation of the entire mixer shell or body with a rotating high-shear agitator blade
        a. V-shaped
        b. Double cone

    3. Stationary shell or body with a rotating mixing blade
        a. Ribbon
        b. Sigma blade
        c. Planetary
        d. Conical screw

    4. High-speed granulations (stationary shell or body with a rotating mixing blade and high-speed agitator blade)
        a. Barrel
        b. Bowl

    5. Air mixer (stationary shell or body using moving air as agitator)
        a. Fluid-bed granulator
        b. Fluid-bed drier

B. Continuous type

        a. Barrel
        b. "Zigzag"

blenders, in sizes from 10 to 150 ft^3 or larger, are used extensively for blending. The term "blending" is used in relation to these pieces of equipment because they mix the dry powders with a minimum of energy imparted to the powder bed. The rotating shell blenders are used only for dry mixes and have no packing glands (seals) around shafts entering the chamber to cause potential problems. Modifications such as the addition of baffles to increase mixing shear have been made to these types of blenders. The advantages of using V-shaped and double-cone blenders include:

1. Minimal attrition when blending fragile granules
2. Large-capacity equipment available
3. Easy to load and unload
4. Easy to clean
5. Minimal maintenance

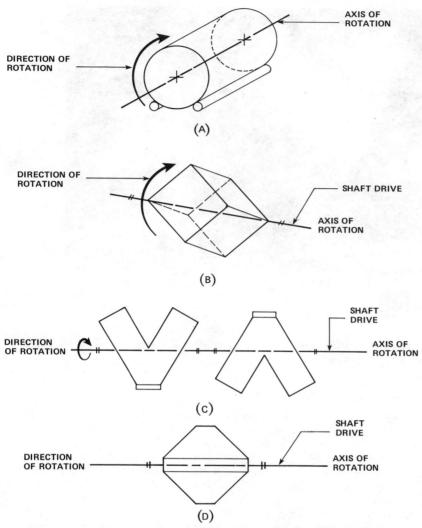

Figure 20. Schematics of rotating shell blenders. (A) Barrel blender, (B) cube blender, (C) V-shaped blender, (D) double-cone blender.

The primary disadvantages are:

1. High head space needed for installation.
2. Segregation problems with mixtures having wide particle size distribution and large differences in particle densities.
3. The tumbling-type blenders are not suitable for fine-particulate systems because there is not enough shear to reduce particle agglomeration.
4. If powders are free-flowing, serial dilution is required for the addition of low-dose active ingredients.

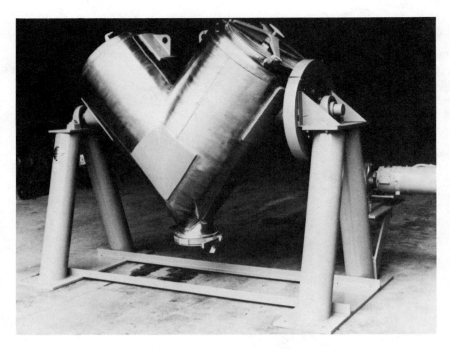

Figure 21. Twin Shell V-blender. (Courtesy Patterson-Kelley Company, Division HARSCO Corporation, East Stroudsburg, Pa. 18301.)

These blenders are operated by adding material to be blended to a volume of ap-proximately 50 to 60% of the blender's total volume. Blending efficiency is af-fected by the load volume factor, as shown in Table 9.

Blender speed may also be a key to mixing efficiency, because the slower the blender, the lower the shear forces. Although higher blending speeds provide more shear, they may also result in more dusting, causing segregation of fines; that is, as the blend is tumbling, the fines become airborne and settle on top of the powder bed after blending has ceased. There is also a critical speed which, if approached, will diminish blending efficiency of the mixer considerably. As the revolutions per minute (rpm) increase, the centrifugal forces at the extreme points of the mixing chamber will exceed the gravitation forces required for blend-ing, and the powder will gravitate to the outer walls of the blender shell. It should be noted that bench scale blenders turn at much higher rpm than the larger blend-ers, usually in proportion to the peripheral velocity of blender extremes.

Both V-shaped and the double-cone blenders usually have a variable-speed drive for adjusting the mixing speed of the shell. The double-cone blender is usually charged and discharged through the same port, whereas the V-shaped blender may be loaded through either of the shell hatches or the apex port. Emp-tying the V-shaped blender is normally done through the apex port.

The second general class of mixers is a modification of the tumbling blenders shown schematically in Figure 23 with the addition of a high-speed (1200-3000 rpm)

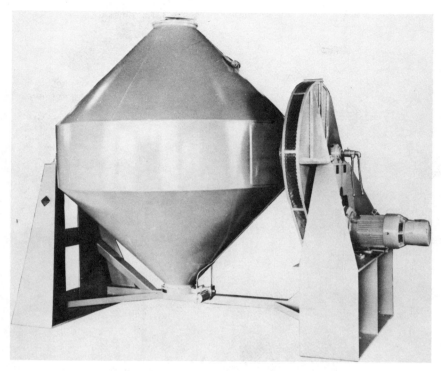

Figure 22. Double-cone blender. (Courtesy Patterson-Kelley Company, Division HARSCO Corporation, East Stroudsburg, Pa.)

Table 9

Effect of Powder Fill on Blending Time of Double-Cone Blenders[a]

Volume % of blender filled with powder charge	Approximate blend time (min) in production-size blenders
50	10
65	14
70	18
75	24
80[b]	40[b]

[a]Blending done in double-cone blenders and times measured to obtain comparable blends.
[b]Uniform blend not attainable with this fill level.
Source: G. R. Sweitzer, Blending and Drying Efficiency Double Cone vs. V-Shape, GEMCO, Newark, N.J.

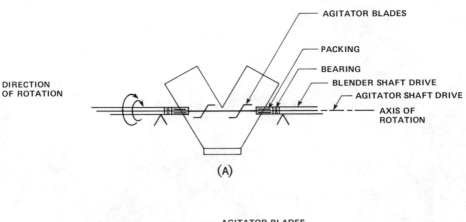

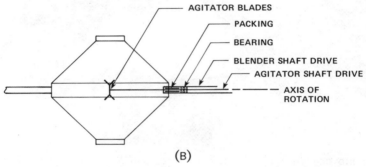

Figure 23. Schematics of rotating shell blenders with agitator mixers. (A) V-shaped mixer, (B) double-cone mixer.

agitator mixing blade. This agitator blade is situated as shown in Figure 24, and gives added versatility to the tumbling blenders by virtue of the high shear attainable. The advantages with the addition of the agitator bar to the tumbling blender include:

1. Good versatility, in that both wet and dry mixing can be accomplished in the blender.
2. A wide range of shearing force may be obtained, with the agitator bar design permitting the intimate mixing of very fine as well as coarse powder compositions.
3. Serial dilution not needed when incorporating low-dose active ingredients.

The disadvantages include:

1. Possible attrition of large, more friable particles or granules in a mixture as a result of the high-speed agitator mixer.
2. Scale-up can prove to be a problem, in that direct scale-up based on geometry, size, and peripheral velocity often does not work. Experimental work is advised, when possible, on the size of mixer planned for the process.

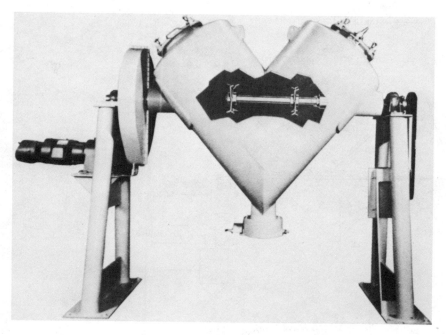

Figure 24. V-shaped blender with agitator mixing assembly. (Courtesy Gemco, Newark, N.J. 07114.)

3. Cleaning may be a problem, because the agitator assembly must be removed and the packings changed for a product changeover.
4. Potential packing (seal) problems (packings are used to prevent leakage through the shaft entrance into the mixing chamber and to prevent the blender contents from contaminating the bearings).

Most mixers with agitator bars are also available with a liquid-dispensing system separate, or incorporated into the agitator bar, so that a solid-liquid blend can be easily prepared without stopping the mixer for the addition of the granulating liquid. These units, known as processors, have a steam jacket around the shell of the blender for heating the wet granulation, and a vacuum system to remove the granulating liquid vapors during drying. In essence, the entire granulating and drying step is accomplished in one piece of equipment. A schematic of this operation is shown in Figure 25.

A typical sequence of operating steps for the processor would read as follows:

1. Prepare the granulating solution and adjust the feed rate through the pump.
2. Charge the blender with the ingredients to be granulated.
3. Turn on the vacuum to 15 in. Hg and start the condenser unit.
4. Premix the dry solids at normal processor-shell rpm and run the agitator mixer during blending.
5. Pump granulating solution into the processor and turn on full vacuum (30 in. Hg).

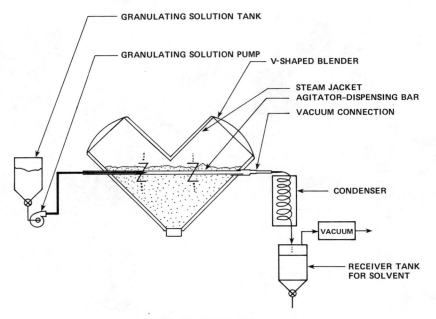

Figure 25. Schematic of V-shaped blender, processor.

6. Mix until granulation is properly set up (stop the processor), relieve the vacu-
    um, and open to examine granulation).
7. Shut off the agitator mixer and reduce the blender-shell speed to a minimum.
8. Dry until the solvent collector contains the specified quantity of solvent to be
    removed from the granulation.
9. Check the loss on drying (LOD) after drying is completed. Empty the granula-
    tion into a hopper or drums for further processing.

The problems encountered with the operation include packing gland (seal) leakage
under vacuum, and the granulation sticking to the sides of the blender shell. These
problems can often be overcome by careful packing of the agitator mixer packing
gland(s), optimizing the shell temperature and granulation composition, optimizing
the rate of addition of granulating solution, and developing the proper sequence of
steps during granulating. The processors are loaded and unloaded the same way
as are V-shaped and double-cone blenders.
     The third general category of mixer is mechanically different from the tumbling-
shell type of blender; that is, the mixing forces are transferred to the powder bed
by moving blades moving in a fixed (nonmovable) shell which confines the ingredients. The blades naturally have different configurations for each design, and
move the solid-solid or liquid-solid mixtures by the force exerted through a motor-driven drive shaft. Schematics for the more commonly used designs are shown
in Figure 26.

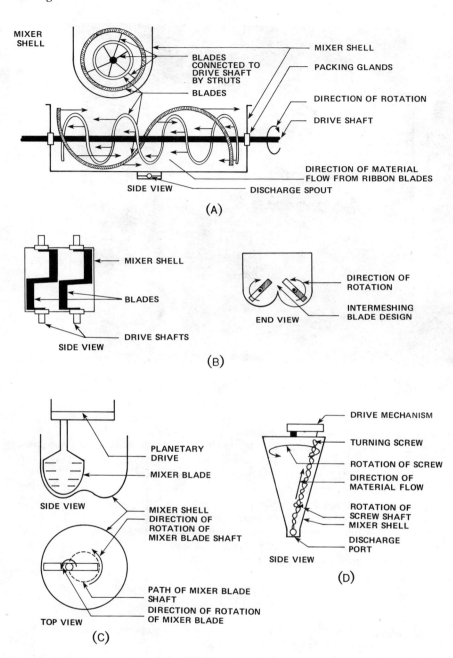

Figure 26. Schematics of fixed-shell, moving-blade mixers. (A) Ribbon mixer, (B) sigma blade mixer, (C) planetary mixer, (D) conical-screw mixer.

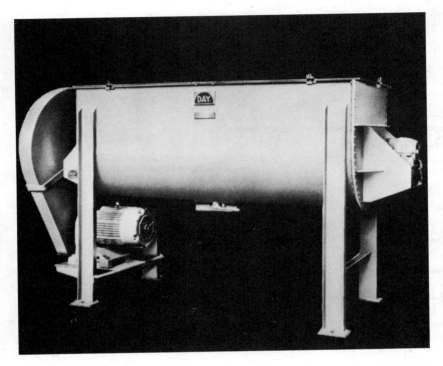

Figure 27. Ribbon mixer. (Courtesy Day Mixing, Cincinnati, Ohio.)

The ribbon mixer derives its name from ribbon-shaped blades that traverse the entire length of the U trough and are attached to the drive shaft by struts (not shown in the side view of the Figure 26A schematic). The ribbon mixer (Fig. 27) can be used for either solid-solid or liquid-solid mixing and gives somewhat less shearing action than the sigma or planetary mixer. The body of the mixer is covered during mixing because considerable dust may be created during dry blending, and granulating solution may evaporate during wet granulating. The normal procedure is to open the discharge spout several times during mixing, returning the discharged material to the mixer. This eliminates unmixed material trapped in this spout. This is a good all-purpose mixer, but has a major disadvantage--the possibility of dead spots (areas that remain unmixed) at the ends and in the corners of the mixer. For the same mixer volume, head-room requirements are less for the ribbon mixer. The ribbon mixer is top-loading, with a bottom discharge port.

The sigma blade mixer (Fig. 26B) is commonly used for dough mixing in the baking industry because of its high shear and kneading action, created by the intermeshing blades. The mixer is therefore an excellent choice for wet granulating, where heavy wetted powders require kneading for good liquid-solid distribution. This mixer, probably the most heavily constructed of the mixers, has close tolerances between the side walls and bottom of the mixer shell. This creates a minimum of dead space during mixing. The sigma blade mixer is used primarily for

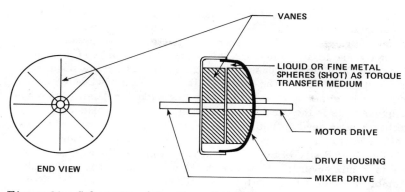

Figure 28. Schematic of liquid or shot drive.

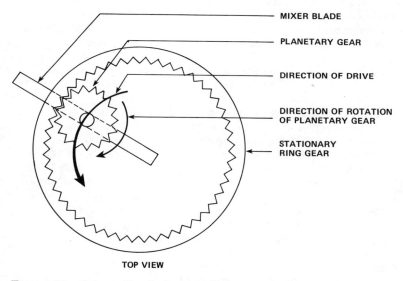

Figure 29. Schematic of planetary gear.

liquid-solid blending, although it can be used for solid-solid blending. The mixer is top-loading and is emptied by tilting the entire shell by means of a rack-and-pinion drive.

Both the ribbon and sigma blade mixers have a fixed-speed drive, and on large units the motor drive is usually connected to the blade shaft through a fluid drive or a shot drive (Fig. 28). This prevents the high torque developed by the drive motor from breaking gears or twisting drive shafts if the mixer is turned on while loaded with a wet granulation. Each of these drives absorbs the initial torque while the blades begin to move against the granulation.

The planetary mixer (Fig. 26C) is so named because the mixing shaft is driven by a planetary gear train, shown in Figure 29. As the small planetary gear, attached to the mixing blade, is driven in the indicated direction around the ring gear, it rotates the mixer blade. Therefore, both the mixer blade and the mixer blade shaft position are rotational. This mixer is also a high shear mixer and is normally built with a variable-speed drive. This allows slow blade speed for pre-mixing dry powder (which minimizes dusting) and faster speeds for the kneading action required in wet granulating. The mixer shell is a mixing bowl which is re-moved from the mixer by either lowering it beneath the blade, or raising the blade above the bowl, or both, as is the case with the larger (340-quart) planetary mix-ers. There are literally no dead spaces in the mixing bowl, and extra bowls per-mit the mixing of one sublot after another if so desired. The big disadvantage with this equipment is the limited size of the batch that can be made at one time. The common practice is to mix several sublots and then make a final blend of the sub-lots in a large tumbling mixer. For small batch work this may fit the need very well, but the granulation of large lots may be more easily done in large-volume granulating equpiment, such as that found with the processor and the ribbon and sigma blade mixers. It must be noted that since the mixer blade is mounted from above the mixer bowl, there are no packing glands in contact with the product, eliminating the need for repacking between lots and product changes. Emptying the bowls may be done by hand scooping or by obtaining a dumping mechanism that lifts and dumps.

The last of the more commonly used stationary shell mixers is the conical-screw type (Fig. 30). Again, as with the planetary mixer, the screw shaft ro-tates around the periphery of the cone and the screw turns such that the pitch transfers the material from the bottom of the mixer to the top, as illustrated in Figure 26D. This mixer provides a very mild shearing action and was, at one time, used only for solid-solid blending. However, with several modifications, the mixer may also be used for liquid-solid blending in wet granulating. Prob-ably the biggest drawback to the conical screw mixer is the high head space re-quired for installation of commercial-size (30-100 ft^3) units. The big advantage of such units is that when filled to any height, the same mixing action is obtained. For example, if a 10-ft^3 lot of material is to be scaled up to 50 ft^3, the 10-ft^3 lot may be blended in the 50-ft^3 blender and the same mixing action that a 50-ft^3 lot receives will be obtained. The conical-screw mixer is top-loading, with a bottom discharge port.

The fourth category of mixers is the high-speed granulator. These are stationary-shell mixers with a large mixer-scraper blade which mixes the in-gredients, eliminates dead spots in the mixer container, and presents the mixer contents to a high-speed chopper blade that intimately mixes the ingredients. The high-speed chopper is driven by a motor separate from that driving the larger, more slowly rotating mixer-scraper blade, and is located at the side of the mix-ing bowl or chamber. Schematics of the barrel type and bowl type are illustrated in Figure 31. The advantage of this equipment is extremely rapid, intimate solid-solid or liquid-solid mixing. Granulating times may be only 6-10 min long, which includes dry blending and wet granulating. The product usually has a fairly uni-form wet granule size of 14-8 mesh (1400-2400 μm) which needs no further wet milling or screening. The granules are usually emptied directly into a fluid-bed drier.

Disadvantages may include product contamination from the packing gland where the shaft passes through the mixer shell. This has been remedied some-what by the use of mechanical seals or air-flushed packing glands: air at a low

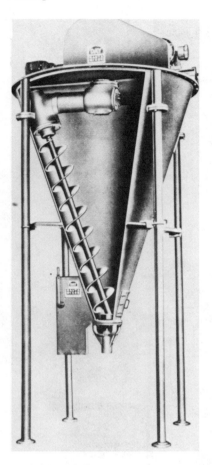

Figure 30. Conical-screw mixer. (Courtesy Day Mixing, Cincinnati, Ohio.)

positive pressure is continually flushed through the glands into the mixer to prevent
contamination of the bearings with the product and contamination of the product
from bearing grease and other substances. A second disadvantage may be the
limited batch size, because there is some expense limit in purchasing larger
models of the equipment. As with bowl mixers, this may necessitate the use of
a second larger tumbling blender when sublots made in the high-speed granulator are to be blended.

The barrel-type mixers are top-loading and have bottom discharge doors,
whereas the bowl types are top-loaded and may have a special rapid discharge
port located at the bottom of the mixer shell. The high-speed granulators are
made from small (2 ft^3) to production sizes (1000+ kg), depending on production needs. Because mixing is so rapid, it is almost standard procedure to
time the mixing accurately or put an ammeter or wattmeter on the high chopper motor to determine the end point of wet mixing. Care must be taken during

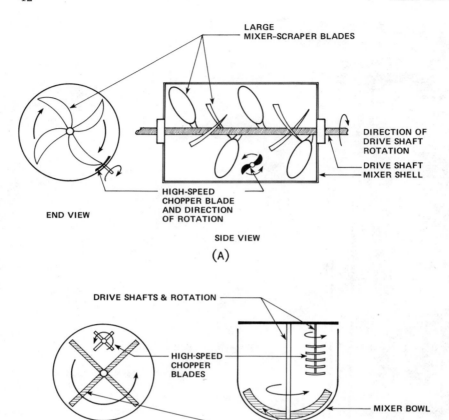

Figure 31. Schematics of high-speed granulators. (A) Barrel type, (B) bowl type.

dry mixing because too long a mixing time may cause unwanted particle size reduction, which could change the characteristics of the final granulation.

The last general category of mixer is the air mixer, which has a stationary
shell or body using moving air as the agitator. Figure 32 shows a general schematic of the fluid-bed granulator, which mixes very intimately and efficiently. By
fluidizing the powder bed, enough shear is developed to mix beds of some of the
smallest particles with very gentle action. The action is so gentle that even soft
granules mix with little or no attrition. The equipment is used in its mixing capacity, usually in the case where a wet granulation is made in the granulator. A
material that must be mixed and not granulated in the fluid-bed granulator normally is not mixed in the granulator. The same mixing action may be obtained
with fluid-bed driers, but this equipment is also usually reserved for the drying
of premade wet granules.

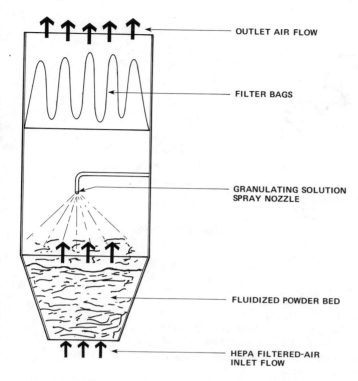

OUTLET AIR FLOW

FILTER BAGS

GRANULATING SOLUTION
SPRAY NOZZLE

FLUIDIZED POWDER BED

HEPA FILTERED-AIR
INLET FLOW

Figure 32. Schematic of fluid-bed granulator-mixer.

B. Continuous Mixers

Continuous mixing in the pharmaceutical industry is reserved for large-volume product that requires 8-24 hr day^{-1} mixing year-round to meet marketing demands. In all cases of continuous mixing, the ingredients to be mixed are carefully and accurately metered into the mixer at one end and are discharged at the other end as a homogeneous mix ready for further processing. The batch size is determined by a specific period of mixing time, so that lot numbers of raw materials and weighing records can be traced to reflect the composition of the final product from day to day.

The primary problems associated with continuous mixing are associated with materials-handling technology and raw material properties. Materials-handling technology problems are merely planning and selecting the auxiliary equipment to be used with a particular continuous-mixing process. Such equipment as storage hoppers, automatic weighing units, conveying methods, and metering equipment must be selected to handle the formula ingredients and scheduled volumes. There must also be enough flexibility to enable the producer to increase or reduce the process throughput to meet the market demands. The materials-handling system must be continuously monitored for accuracy of blend composition, and accurate operating records must be maintained.

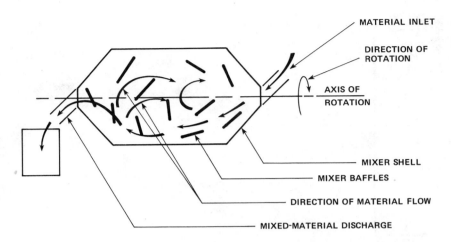

Figure 33. Barrel-type continuous mixer.

   All of this work in design and planning may be of little use if an effective raw
material control is not put into play. As discussed in Section V, there are many
variables that may cause problems with powder flow, density, and so on, and
these must be tested for and controlled as closely as possible to make and keep
a continuous-mixing operation working.
   There are several continuous mixers which may be used in the pharmaceutical
industry. The first is the barrel type, which resembles a large cement mixer
and is shown schematically in Figure 33. The shell of this mixer is fitted with
baffles along the interior surface. The baffles are so designed and arranged
that as the mixer shell rotates, the incoming ingredients begin moving toward
the opposite end of the blender. Mixing begins at this point because of the baffled
tumbling action. As the material approaches the midpoint of the mixer shell, the
baffles are so positioned to cause a foldback of the granulation over itself in the
direction of the inlet end. This foldback action continues up to the discharge end,
where, in addition to another set of baffles, designed to move the material out
the discharge port, overflow also causes the blended dry solids to discharge.
After startup, equilibrium blending is reached and the process becomes continuous.
   The next continuous mixer is also a rotating-shell type, but in this mixer the
shell takes the shape of several V-shaped blenders in series, with lower cone
angles (Fig. 34); Figure 35 is a photograph of the mixer. As the material is
metered into the rotating mixer, the throughput rate is determined in part by
the angle of the axis of rotation, which can be varied (i.e., as the angle increases, the throughput increases). The blender works on the principle that a
single preweighed charge can be dumped into a charge chamber, and portions of
it will gravitate into the V-shaped tubular sections as the shell rotates. With
each rotation, one-half of the blend in each downward V recycles back to the preceding chamber and one-half moves forward to the next leg of the blender. Because of the inclined axis of rotation toward the discharge, material movement

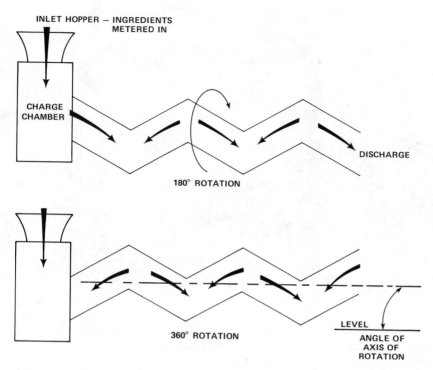

Figure 34. Schematic of "zigzag" continuous blender. (Courtesy Patterson-Kelley Company, Division of HARSCO Corporation, East Stroudsburg, Pa.)

is always forward. As the first charge clears the mixer, which may take only several minutes, the next charge is added. The mixer may also be operated using a continuous accurate metering of the feed materials, uniformity of blend depending on the flow properties of the ingredients. Although this equipment was originally designed for only solid-solid blending, a high-intensity chopper and liquid dispenser permit liquid-solid mixing on a continuous basis.

Depending on the size of the continuous blenders, very large quantities (500 tons hr^{-1}) of materials may be blended if required.

VII. Mixing Problems

From a practical point of view, it is necessary to learn how to use production equipment to achieve the same results obtained with a formula on both the development- and pilot-scale level. The scale-up to large mixers can be a very discouraging and frustrating step in putting a tablet formula into commercial production. This is primarily so because there are no hard and fast rules or equations that direct one to the use of a particular size and type of mixer during scale-up. Results are usually empirical, and the starting point depends

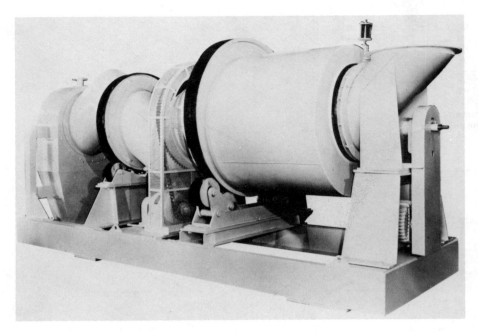

Figure 35. "Zigzag" continuous blender. (Courtesy Patterson-Kelley Company, Division HARSCO Corporation, East Stroudsburg, Pa.)

heavily on the experience of those responsible for the project. The frustration and problems in scale-up are further amplified by the fact that the tablet and/or granulation production department already has on hand specific sizes and types of mixers, and the mixing unit operation for a new formula must be adapted to this equipment. Unless the product has a large potential market and/or is a large-volume product necessitating expansion of facilities, one does not normally have the luxury of selecting and purchasing a new blender suited for a specific new product. In addition to these aspects of the commercial mixing unit operation, production scheduling often prefers, or requires, that a product have the potential of being mixed using several types of mixers.

All of these constraints are difficult to adhere to and still obtain the desired end product. However, several general approaches are used in industry today for dealing with potentially difficult mixing problems. Several of these potential mixing problems are listed in Table 10 with suggested approaches commonly used to overcome the difficulties. Note that the problems and suggested approaches in Table 10 are of a general nature and cannot be expected to cover all possibilities.

The first problem (A, Table 10) encountered is usually one of uniformly dispersing a low-dose, high-potency active ingredient in a diluent to make a tablet that is large enough to compress, and monitoring tablet weights with ease. Dilution of the active ingredient on a small scale may be done by serial dilution by hand. However, large-scale work can only approach the effectiveness of serial dilution method. In the dry state, where a direct compression tablet is desired

Table 10

Summary of Mixing Problems and Suggested Approaches

Problem		Suggested approaches		Suggested equipment
A.	Uniform dispersion of high-potency, low-dose active ingredient in a diluent for direct compression.	1.	Mill or pass active ingredient and equal amount of diluent through a small screen. Rinse screen with more diluent. Place in mixer with one-half of remaining diluent and mix. Add remaining diluent and additives (starch, microcrystalline cellulose, etc.) and mix to a final mixture.	1. Cutting or hammer mill with small screen or moisturized sifter. Use tumbling mixer: V-shaped or double cone. May use sigma, ribbon, or conical-screw mixers. Should create minimum dust.
		2.	Place active ingredient, all of diluent, and additives in mixer with high speed mixing bar or chopper. Mix to a final blend.	2. V-shaped or double-cone blender with high-speed agitator bar, or horizontal or vertical high-speed granulator (may have batch size restriction in these mixers).
B.	If uniform dispersion of active ingredient cannot be achieved.	1.	Dissolve active ingredient in a granulating solution solvent and wet granulate in preblended diluent and additives to uniformly disperse.	1. Sigma blade, ribbon, planetary, conical-screw, or high-speed mixer. The mixer must have high-enough shear to distribute granulating-active-ingredient solution in preblended diluent and additives. (May also use a fluid-bed granulator for this.) Fluid-bed drying is recommended to minimize active-ingredient migration during drying. A mill may also be necessary to bring to final granule size.

(continued)

Table 10 (continued)

Problem	Suggested approaches	Suggested equipment
C. Uniform dispersion of small quantities of dye lakes through-out diluent with low-dose, high-potency active ingredient for direct compression.	1. Use approach A1, milling active ingredient and dye lake together with diluent.	1. Same as A1.
	2. Use approach A1, milling active ingredient and dye lake separately with diluent. However, approach C1 is preferred, because material handling is minimized.	2. Same as A1.
	3. Use of high-speed mixer bar or chopper with all diluent and additives.	3. Same as A2.
D. Uniform dispersion of small quantities of dye lake through-out high-dose, large-volume product for direct compression.	1. Mill or pass dye lake and small quantity of additives through a small screen. Rinse screen with more additive. Place in mixer with one-half of remainder of ingredients and mix. Add remainder of ingredients and mix to final blend.	1. Same as A1.
E. Uniform dispersion of dyes in high- or low-dose products.	1. Use same wet granulation technique as B1.	1. Same as B1.

F. Poorly flowing cohesive powders in general.	1. Use high-shear equipment.	1. Sigma, ribbon, and planetary mixers; V-shaped and double-cone blenders with agitator bars or high-speed granulators.
	2. Use fluidized bed.	2. Fluid-bed granulators.
G. Overmixing of lubricants, yielding granulation or formula dry mixture with poor lubricating properties.	1. Cut blending time if it does not interfere with homogenicity of final blend.	1. Higher-shear mixing equipment (e.g., ribbon, sigma, high-speed granulators, and tumbling mixers with agitator blades).
	2. Use lower-shear mixer if it does not interfere with homogenicity of final blend.	2. Tumbling mixers.
	3. Leave lubricant out of final blend until last 5 to 10 min of mixing.	3. Both G1 and G2.

and can be made successfully with the proper combination and ratio of diluents, the active ingredient must be of a small enough particle size to allow relatively large numbers of particles to be distributed in each dosage unit. When this occurs, one often runs into surface electrical charge problems, as described in Section V. Assuming a minimum of surface and other problems, 10 kg of the active ingredient to be blended into 200 kg of final granulation, for example, is usually milled or passed through a small screen (20-40 mesh or smaller) with an equivalent amount of diluent, or enough diluent to obtain an amount of triturate that is easily handled (20-40 kg in this case). The mill may have knives or hammers at medium to high mill speeds, depending on the degree of dispersion required.

After the active ingredient has been passed through the mill, the mill is cleared of active ingredient by passing another portion of diluent through the mill, adding to the triturate. The triturate and "mill-cleaning" diluent are added to the mixer with about one-half of the remaining diluent and mixed for 10 to 15 min in any of the mixers without high-speed agitation, such as the tumbling mixers or the sigma blade, ribbon, or conical-screw mixers. The remainder of the diluent and additives, such as the disintegrating and lubricating agents, are then added to the mixer for the final mixing.

A second alternative may be used if high-speed agitation equipment is available, such as V-shaped or double-cone blenders with agitator blades, or high-speed granulating equipment, with a chopper blade. This type of equipment permits adding all the ingredients to the mixer at one time. No premixing is required because the mixing action is so intense. Mixing times are relatively short and must be watched carefully so that unwanted size reduction does not take place with the more friable materials, if present.

If the active ingredient cannot be successfully dispersed in a dry state (problem B, Table 10), and this is usually determined in the developmental stages of the product, it is dissolved in the granulating solution solvent and wet granulated in the premixed diluents and internal additives (additives that are granulated are called internal additives, and additives that are added to the dried granulation are called external additives).

Wet-granulating mixing equipment is used as listed in Table 10. It should be pointed out that slow drying of the wet granules may cause migration of the solubilized materials, possibly including the active ingredient, in the granulating solution. This could cause uniformity problems in the dry granulation which might show up in the final dosage unit if the granulation is not milled to a small enough particle size. This problem may be prevented by rapid drying in a fluid-bed drier or by granulating in a fluid-bed granulator.

The uniform dispersion of small quantities of dye lakes throughout the granulation, as in problems C and D in Table 10, follows very closely the approaches suggested for problem A. It should be noted that the mixing process must be optimized by reducing materials handling to a minimum. This includes premilling, premixing, and mixing times.

The uniform dispersions of dyes in high- or low-dose active-ingredient wet granulations follows closely the suggestions for problem B discussed above, as well as the equipment suggestions.

In general, poorly flowing cohesive powders can be mixed as suggested for problem F, Table 10, by using high-shear equipment, such as high-speed granulators or even the fluid-bed granulator. The use of this equipment for mixing poorly flowing ingredients will require some experimentation to determine the amount and type of shear required and the mixing time to yield a uniform mixture.

In some instances where new mixes are brought on-stream (put into production use) for established products and/or the efficiency of mixing is not anticipated for both established and new products, more mixing may take place than is needed. This is the case in problem G, Table 10, where very thorough mixing affects the lubricity of a granulation. Experience has shown that in many cases where poor lubrication is noted, it is the result of too intimate mixing of the lubricant (i.e., the lubricant is dispersed too well throughout the mixture). Usually, working directions call for the lubricant to be added initially in a direct compression mixture or added with the remaining external ingredients during the final blend of a dried, milled, wet granulation. If poor lubrication during compression of the granulation is noted, a number of steps may be taken other than increasing the concentration of the lubricant (the new drug application permitting). First, the mixing time may be decreased if it does not affect the homogeneity of the overall mixture. This is particularly useful if high-shear mixing equipment is used and the mixing time has not been optimized (the blend time may be too long initially). It may even be necessary to change mixers before the lubricant is added, as noted in the second suggestion, using a lower-shear mixer. The third suggestion, which also works well, consists of adding the lubricant for the last 5-10 min of mixing. The higher the mixing shear, the shorter the mixing time required to obtain satisfactory lubrication dispersion.

VIII. Scale-up and Mixer Selection

The biggest problem is scale-up from development to pilot to commercial production. As mentioned before, there are no set formulas for scaling up because each particulate system, dry or wet, has its own particle-particle interactions. In addition, there has been very little mixing data accumulated to provide a base for scale-up equations. Several recent references may give the reader more insight into both the practical and theoretical aspects of scale-up [5, 30, 31].

The best advice is to use common sense and, where possible, optimize mixing in the size of mixer intended for use in pilot or production. This may sound like an expensive approach, but in actuality it means working with mixers that a company's staff has considerable experience with and so can estimate with some certainty the results that will be obtained.

On the other hand, if a mixing process is to be upgraded by changing the mixer, or a new product requires a type of mixer that is not already available in the research, pilot or commercial production facility, a logical plan for mixer selection originally flowcharted by Miles, is shown in Figure 36. The chart is clear, self-explanatory, and covers most mixing pitfalls.

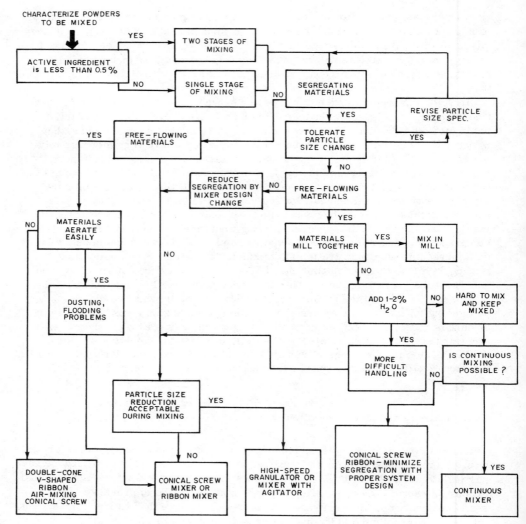

Figure 36. Flowchart for mixer selection. [Adapted from J. E. P. Miles and C. Schofield, Process Eng., p. 77 (Sept. 1968).]

References

1.   Fischer, J. J., Chem. Eng., 69:107–128 (Aug. 1962.)
2.   Martin, E. W., ed., Husa's Pharmaceutical Dispensing, 6th ed., Mack, Easton, Pa., 1966.
3.   Barnhart, C. L., ed., The American College Dictionary, Random House, New York, 1967.
4.   Lacey, P. M. C., J. Appl. Chem., 4:257 (1954).

5.   Wang, R. H., and Fan, L. T., Chem. Eng., 81:88 (May 27, 1974).
6.   Cahn, D. S., and Fuerstenau, D. W., Powder Technol., 2:215 (1968/1969).
7.   Cahn, D. S., and Fuerstenau, D. W., Powder Technol., 1:174 (1967).
8.   Train, D. J., J. Am. Pharm. Assoc., Sci. Ed., 49:265 (1960).
9.   Travers, D. N., Rogerson, A. G., and Jones, T. M., J. Pharm. Pharmacol., 27 (suppl.):3P (1975).
10. Williams, J. C., Powder Technol., 2:13 (1968/1969).
11. Hersey, J. A., Powder Technol., 11:41 (1975).
12. Hersey, J. A., Seminar on Bulk Solids Handling; Powder Mixing, presented May 1979, Philadelphia, Pa.
13. Hersey, J. A., J. Soc. Cosmet. Chem., 21:259 (1970).
14. Lacey, P. M. C., Trans. Inst. Chem. Engrs., 21:53 (1943).
15. Stang, K., Chem.-Ing.-Tech., 26:331 (1954).
16. Poole, K. R., Taylor, R. F., and Wall, G. P., Trans. Inst. Chem. Eng., 42:T305 (1964).
17. Ashton, M. D., and Valentin, F. H. H., Trans. Inst. Chem. Eng., 44:T166 (1966).
18. Williams, J. C., Powder Technol., 3:189 (1969/1970).
19. Buslik, D., Bull. Am. Soc. Test. Mater., 165:66 (1950.
20. Harnby, N., Trans. Inst. Chem. Eng., 45:CE270 (1967).
21. Fan, L. T., Chen, S. J., and Watson, C. A., Ind. Eng. Chem., 62:53 (1970).
22. Fan, L. T., and Wang, R. H., Powder Technol., 11:27 (1975).
23. Buslik, D., Powder Technol., 7:111 (1973).
24. Lai, F. S., Wang, R. H., and Fan, L. T., Powder Technol., 10:13 (1974).
25. Harnby, N., Powder Technol., 5:81 (1971/1972).
26. Allen, T., Particle Size Measurement, 2nd ed. Chapman & Hall, London, 1975, Chap. 1.
27. Lopper, C. E. J., Stanford Res. Inst., 5(3):95 (1961).
28. Woolf, H. B., ed., Webster's New Collegiate Dictionary, Merriam, Springfield, Mass., 1976.
29. Carr, R. L., Chem. Eng., 72:69 (Feb. 1, 1965).
30. Schofield, C., Chem. Ind., 3:105 (1977).
31. Yip, C. W., and Hersey, J. A., Drug Dev. Ind. Pharm., 3:429 (1977).

2

Drying

Michael A. Zoglio

Merrell Research Center
Cincinnati, Ohio

Jens T. Carstensen

University of Wisconsin
Madison, Wisconsin

I. Introduction

Drying in the process industries is usually carried out to remove solvent and produce pure substances, whereas drying in pharmaceutical operations generally deals with the drying of granulations. Wet granulation is a step in the production of many tablet products (and some capsule products) [1] and serves to enlarge the particle and to make it fairly spherical. This affords good flow rates [2-6], that is, good weight uniformity. It also supplies a binder to the formulation, thus ensuring good physical strength of the final tablet, and desirable compression characteristics during tableting. Finally, wet granulation methods frequently render hydrophobic surfaces hydrophilic, and in this manner dissolution rates and bioavailability of a drug may be improved [7]. Since most granulations are aqueous, the first part of this chapter will deal with the drying of water from aqueous granulations.

Wet granulations can be made by (1) mixing dry powders, (2) adding a paste (e.g., a starch paste) containing the binder, (3) continued mixing to form granules, and (4) drying the wet granules. If x_0 kg of water is added to 1 kg of dry weight, the drying curve (as defined here) will be a plot of x as a function of the time the granulation has been exposed to a stream of drying air.

II. The Psychrometric Chart

The term "dry air" is frequently used (loosely), but very rarely does an air sample contain 0% moisture. In order to have a basis of comparison, moisture contents in air are frequently expressed as absolute humidity Y, defined as the number of kilograms of water per kilogram of dry air. It follows that the lower the absolute humidity of an air sample at a given temperature, the more rapidly it will dry a given granulation.

Humidity can also be measured as the relative humidity RH, which is 100 x the partial water vapor pressure P (atm) of an air sample divided by the saturation water vapor pressure P' (atm) at the temperature in question.

In an air sample, the partial vapor pressures P_i of the air and the water add up to the total pressure (which, generally, is 1 atm); or

$$P_{water} + P_{air} = P_{total} \; (= 1 \text{ atm in most cases}) \tag{1}$$

The amount of water and of air can be estimated by the gas law:

$$n_{water} = \frac{P_{water} V}{RT} \tag{2}$$

where n denotes moles, V the volume, R the gas constant (0.083 liter-atm mol^{-1} deg^{-1}), and T the absolute temperature (K). It follows that if the total pressure is 1 atm, then $P_{air} = 1 - P_{water}$, so that

$$n_{air} = \frac{(1 - P_{water})V}{RT} \tag{3}$$

It is therefore possible to calculate the amount of each component in 1 m^3 (V = 10^3 liters) of moist air, simply from knowing the water vapor pressure. For instance, in saturated air at 50° C, given that P_{water} is 0.1217 atm, P_{air} = 0.8783 atm. The molecular weight of water is 0.018 kg mol^{-1}, and that of air is 0.029 kg mol^{-1}. The masses M (kg) of water and of air in a 1 m^3 sample of saturated air at 50° C are, therefore,

$$M_{water} = \frac{0.1217 \times 10^3 \times 0.018}{0.083 \times 323.15} = 0.0817 \text{ kg} \tag{4}$$

$$M_{air} = \frac{0.8783 \times 10^3 \times 0.029}{0.083 \times 323.15} = 0.9496 \text{ kg} \tag{5}$$

The absolute humidity is therefore 0.0817/0.9496 = 0.086 kg water per kilogram of dry air.

It is tempting to assume that for 50% relative humidity, the absolute humidity would be one-half of that found above. This is approximately correct, but to be exact, it is noted that P_{water} is one-half of saturation [i.e., P_{water} = 1/2(0.1217)= 0.06085 atm, P_{air} = 0.93915 atm], and a calculation similar to the one leading to Equations (4) and (5) now gives

$$M_{water} = 0.0408 \text{ kg}$$

$$M_{air} = 1.015 \text{ kg}$$

$$Y = \frac{0.0408}{1.015} = 0.0402 \text{ kg water/kg dry air}$$

Such figures can be found directly using a psychrometric chart (Fig. 1). In fact, the curves in the psychrometric chart are calculated in the manner described above.

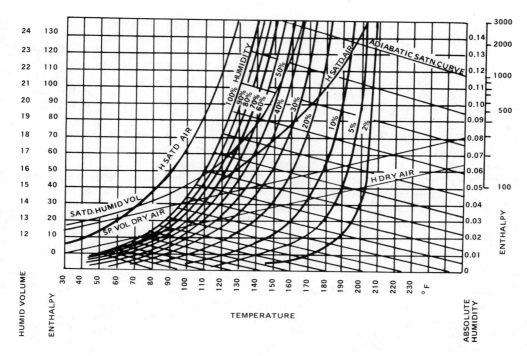

Figure 1. Psychrometric charts. The units given are °F, Btu, ft^3, and lb. These can be converted to new units (°C, joules, m^3, and kg) by the following conversion factors: to convert from °F to °C, subtract 32 from °F and divide by 1.8; to convert from ft^3 to m^3, multiply ft^3 by 0.027; to convert from Btu lb^{-1} to J kg^{-1}, multiply Btu lb^{-1} by 2324; to convert from lb to kg, divide lb by 2.2.

To use the chart, the temperature (50°C or 120°F) is first sought out on the x axis. A vertical line is drawn to the curve labeled 50%, and the ordinate value (on the y axis to the right) is read off (0.04 kg of water per kilogram of dry air).

The density of moist air at given temperature and relative humidity can also be of importance. Here one seeks out the lines indicating the specific volume of dry air (reading the ordinate on the V scale), finds the value indicated by the saturated humid volume curve, and then takes the prorated average between the two (in this case 50%, simply the average). The units in Figure 1 are typical of psychrometric charts: humid volume being expressed in ft^3 lb^{-1}, temperature in °F, enthalpy in Btu, and absolute humidity in kg kg^{-1}. New charts will replace °F by °C, ft^3 by m^3, lb by kg, and Btu by joules. The conversion factors are given in the legend for Figure 1. Using the conversions for this problem, the humid volumes are 0.89 and 1.0 m^3 kg^{-1} and the value for 50% is 0.95 m^3 kg^{-1}. The example worked out above gives M_{total} = 0.95 + 0.08 [from Eq. (5)] = 1.03 kg m^{-3} and 0.97 m^3 kg^{-1} is the density.

It should be noted that drying is actually evaporation of water (solvent), which is accomplished by supplying heat Q joules to the granulation. If the potential heat of vaporization of water is L^* (joules kg^{-1}), the amount that can be evaporated is Q/L^* (kg). It is thus important to know the heat content [the enthalpy H (joules kg^{-1}, of dry air] of the air. In this manner it is possible to calculate the heat Q (joules) given off to the granulation as the difference between the total enthalpy of the incoming (H_0) and the outgoing (H_1) air. The heat content of air samples can be determined by use of the psychrometric chart in the same manner as the humid volumes were determined. At 50% relative humidity and 50° C, for instance, a vertical line is drawn at 50° and the left ordinate of the intersection with the line denoting the humidity of dry air (22 Btu lb^{-1} or 51,000 J kg^{-1} of dry air) is found. Next, the right ordinate of the intersection with the line denoting the humidity of saturated air (130 Btu lb^{-1} or 302,000 J kg^{-1} of dry air) is found, and then the prorated average of the two figures. For example, for 50%, the heat content would be 51,000 + 50/100 (302,000 - 51,000) = 176,500 J kg^{-1} dry air.

It should be noted that the psychrometric chart can be used to determine relative humidities from knowledge of the wet- and dry-bulb temperatures (e.g., obtained by means of a sling psychrometer). If these are 40 and 50° C, respectively, for instance, a vertical line is drawn at 40° C. The intersection with the line denoted 100% RH is noted and a line is drawn parallel to the adiabatic saturation curve. This intersects a vertical line drawn through 50° C on the curve, denoting the actual percent relative humidity (50% in this example).

In a drying operation there is a certain rate of air going into the drier (W kilograms of dry air per second) and the same amount of dry air leaves the drier. On a moist basis, a larger amount leaves then enters the drier, because the outgoing air contains the amount of water evaporated during the residence time of the air. By means of psychrometric calculations as shown above, and knowledge of the flow rate of air and the drying time t (sec), it is possible to calculate the amount M_1 (kg) of water that can be evaporated. This should equal the amount of moisture lost by the granulation as determined by moisture assay before and after of the total amount of granulation M_2 (kg of water lost). In reality, M_1 never equals M_2 and the ratio M_2/M_1 is a measure of the efficiency of the drier.

Aside from the mass and heat balances discussed, the rate of drying is exceedingly important and is discussed next.

III. Kinetics of Drying

Aside from the thermodynamic efficiency of a drier, the speed with which it will dry a granulation is of importance. Drying rates are in general proportional to the surface A (m^2), the load L (kg dry weight), and the proportionality constant N, which is a type of effective heat-transfer coefficient. In the following discussion, a distinction will be made between moisture that is chemically bound (e.g., water of hydration of a hydrate) and moisture that is not chemically bound.

The following nomenclature will be used: dry solid includes the mass of bound moisture; L' denotes dry weight (kg) (i.e., the anhydrous weight); L denotes anhydrous weight (kg) plus the weight (kg) of bound water; X denotes kilograms of water per kilogram of dry solid; and m (kg) denotes the mass of the unbound water in the batch (i.e., m = LX).

Drying of granules can encompass three processes [8]. In general, the water is (1) partly on the surface of the granule, (2) partly in the porous void space of

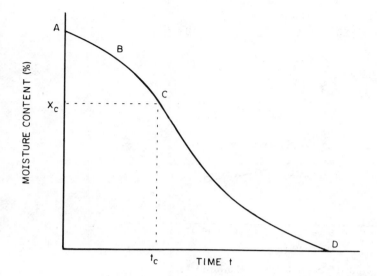

Figure 2. Drying curve expressed as moisture content as a function of time. The falling-rate period starts at point C. Moisture content is expressed as fraction or percentage moisture on a total weight basis.

the granule, and (3) chemically bound. Surface moisture dries first. This takes place at a constant rate; that is, during the constant rate period [9, 10],

$$\frac{dm}{dt} = L \frac{dX}{dt} = -NA \tag{6}$$

or

$$m = m_0 - (NA)t \tag{7}$$

where m_0 is the initial moisture content and N is a constant comparable to a heat-transmission coefficient. This part of the drying curve is denoted AB in Figure 2.

Once the surface moisture is removed, drying of the "internal" moisture starts. Since the granules are porous, moisture removal is a diffusional process giving rise to a falling-rate period, where the rate is linear in X (i.e., of the form bX + a) [11-14]:

$$\frac{dm}{dt} = L \frac{dX}{dt} = -AN(bX + a) \qquad (t_c < t < t_d; \ X_c > X > 0) \tag{8}$$

X_c and t_c (as shown in Fig. 2) are the moisture content and the time where the process changes from a constant to a falling rate, and are denoted critical moisture content and time. Equation (8) can be integrated to

$$\ln \frac{X + (a/b)}{X_c + (a/b)} = -\frac{NbA}{L} (t - t_c) \tag{9}$$

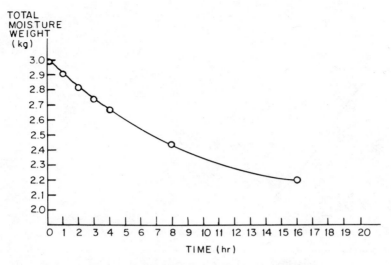

Figure 3. Drying curve utilizing data from Example 1.

Since X is unbound moisture, the curve will have the shape shown in Figure 3. Frequently, a is small, and if X^* denotes total moisture (i.e., as monitored by a total moisture assay), then Equation (9) becomes

$$\ln \frac{X^* - X_b}{X_c - X_b} = - \frac{NbA}{L} (t - t_c) \tag{10}$$

X_b, the bound moisture, can then be estimated as the asymptote toward which X^* tends in the falling-rate period (Fig. 3). Drying to moisture contents below X_b should never be carried out, and the practice of overdrying, and subsequent addition of moisture to get a granulation with specifications, is not advocated, because in overdrying the structure of the granule is frequently destroyed, which also affects the machinability of the granules.

The internal porosity is the principal factor that affects the falling-rate period, but there are other factors as well. All have in common that the rate-determining step in this period is diffusion-controlled [15-19].

Example 1. Determining Granulation Drying Time

The total moisture contents of a granulation at various drying times are as follows:

Time (hr)	Weight (kg)
0	3.000
1	2.905
2	2.819
3	2.740
4	2.670
8	2.449
16	2.202

Figure 3 shows that the weight levels off at 2.000 (i.e., X_b = 2 kg). $Q = (X^* - X_b)/(X_c - X_b)$ can now be calculated, and Q and ln Q are as follows:

Time (hr)	Q	ln Q
0	1.000	0
1	0.905	-0.1
2	0.819	-0.2
3	0.740	-0.3
4	0.670	-0.4
8	0.449	-0.8
16	0.202	-1.6

The log linearity starts at time zero, so that t_c = 0 and NbA/L is 0.1 hr^{-1} [Eq. (10)].

IV. Pharmaceutical Drying Methods

The three most common pharmaceutical drying methods are tray drying, fluid-bed drying, and vacuum drying. Somewhat less common is rotary current drying. Occasional operations call for truck drying and tunnel drying. Two methods very commonly used in the chemical industry, drum drying and spray drying, do not usually apply to drying of dosage-form granulations.

The descriptive approach used in this section is to first describe the process and then to outline the underlying theory, so that drying data can be interpreted in molecular or technological parameters. The least common processes are described first, then the three most common methods.

A. Truck Driers

A schematic of a truck drier is shown in Figure 4. Truck driers are, in essence, trucks upon which trays can be placed. They are placed in a room and the gentle movement of air across the trays (which contain the substance to be dried) causes the drying. One example of truck drying is the drying of soft-shell capsules. The drying air in this case is 37°C and the relative humidity is 10%; the air is dried by passing it over silica or through a saturated LiCl solution. In the former case the unit that dries the air consists of two towers (cylinders). One contains dry desiccant, and the air to be dried passes through this unit. The other contains "used" desiccant, and the redrying of this is accomplished by passing hot air through it. When the desiccant in use becomes too high in moisture content, the air stream is shifted to the regenerated tower, and the tower containing the moist desiccant is subjected to regeneration by hot air. The drying of soft-shell capsules is a diffusion process akin to diffusion out of a cylinder. The process has been treated in Ref. [20], and the drying equation is

$$\ln (c - c_\infty) = -\frac{t}{\alpha} + \ln (c_0 - c_\infty) \tag{11}$$

where

$$\alpha = \frac{h^2}{5.8D} \tag{12}$$

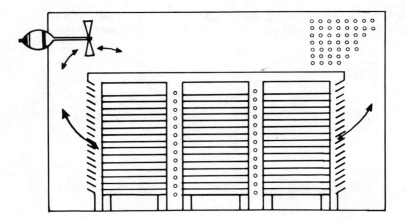

Figure 4. Tray/truck drying oven.

In these equations, c is the moisture content at time t, c_0 the initial moisture content and c_∞ the equilibrium moisture content of the capsule, h the thickness of the gelatin film, and D the diffusion coefficient of the gelatin film (assumed to be independent of moisture content). α is defined in Equation (12). Drying of soft-shell capsules generally does adhere well to a drying equation such as Equation (11). The drying end point (or end interval) is critical, because overdrying causes the capsules to be brittle, and insufficient drying gives rise to capsules that, owing to their excessive softness, will deform on storage.

Example 2. Determining Capsule Drying Time

A soft-shell capsule reaches the required moisture level (interval) after 24 hr of drying. If the capsule shell thickness is increased 20%, how long will it take to dry the capsule to the same moisture content, c^*?

Solution:

Making use of Equations (11) and (12), it is seen that if h is increased to h' = 1.2h (i.e., is increased by 20%), then α increases by a factor of $(1.2)^2 = 1.44$; for $(c^* - c_\infty)/(c_0 = c_\infty)$ to have the same value as for the thinner capsule shell, t must also be increased by a factor of 1.44 (i.e., increased so that t/α remains unaltered). The drying time for the thicker shell is, therefore, 1.44 × 24 = 35 hr.

B. Tunnel Drying

Tunnel drying is not a common pharmaceutical drying method in terms of the number of times it is encountered; however, some of the operations to be described produce a sizable number of products. Examples include hard-candy products

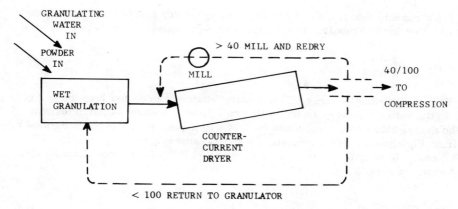

Figure 5. Schematic of semiautomated setup for granulation/drying in a counter-current drier.

(pharyngets), hard shells for hard-shell capsules, and filter-paper-carrier diag-nostic aids. In this type of drying operation the wet unit moves through a tunnel in which drying takes place gradually, so that the exiting unit has the desired (low) moisture content. The source of heat is either infrared light or hot air. The mechanism of drying, and the ensuing drying equations, are similar to those de-rived in the next section.

C. Countercurrent Drying

Countercurrent drying is carried out in rotary driers (Fig. 5). These are long cylinders with internal baffles (sometimes helical) that direct the product in the direction opposite to that of the air flow. Because of the rotation, the granules continuously cascade down through the airstream. The drier the product, the drier the air it encounters, because of the countercurrent nature of the flow. Countercurrent drying is usually applied only to large-volume products, and only in automated or semiautomated processes. In an automated setup, rotary and tunnel driers have the advantage of defining input and output points without man-ual operation (a point that does not hold for truck or tray driers, and holds only with modifications in fluid-bed or vacuum driers).

Pitkin and Carstensen [21] have shown that in rotary drying the rate-limit-ing step is the moisture movement within the granule. They showed that in this case

$$\frac{c - c_\infty}{c_0 - c_\infty} = \frac{6}{\pi^2} \sum_{j=1}^{\infty} \frac{1}{j^2} \exp\left(-\frac{j^2 t}{K}\right) \tag{13}$$

where

$$K = \frac{a^2}{4\pi^2 D} \tag{14}$$

where j is a running index, a the diameter of the granule, and D the diffusion coefficient of water in the granule. D is temperature–dependent by the relation

$$D = D_0 \exp\left(\frac{-E'}{RT}\right) \tag{15}$$

where E' is an activation energy, T the absolute temperature, and R is the gas constant. In the automatic setup shown in Figure 5, where a range of particles exit from the drier, note that the moisture content will depend on the particle diameter, since from Equation (13) the drying time t' is the same for all the particles. When t' is of a realistic magnitude, the terms in Equation (13) with j larger than 1 disappear, and we may write

$$\ln \frac{c - c_\infty}{c_0 - c_\infty} = - \frac{t' 4\pi^2 D}{a^2} \ln \frac{6}{\pi^2} \tag{16}$$

That is, $\ln (c - c_\infty)/(c_0 - c_\infty)$ should be linear in $1/a^2$, with an intercept of $\ln (6/\pi^2) = -0.5$. Figure 6 shows experimental data from a rotary drier run where t' = 3600 sec, and demonstrates the validity of Equation (16). D can be calculated from the slope and is of the correct order of magnitude, 3×10^{-11} cm^2 sec^{-1}.

Example 3. Determining Feedwater Amount

Suppose that the flow rate of the feed is 300 kg of powder per minute and that 10% of granulating water is needed (Fig. 5). The output is 250 kg of 40/100 mesh material, 30 kg of fines, and 20 kg of coarse material. What amount of feedwater should be used?

Solution:

The granulating vessel receives, in steady state, 300 kg + 30 kg of dry material per minute, so $0.1 \times 330 = 33$ kg of water is needed per minute.

Example 4. Determining Drying Time Based on Varying Kneading Times

The rate of diffusion of liquid within a granule is a function of the porosity (ϵ) of the granule. If it is assumed that D is proportional to ϵ, what effect will long kneading have on the drying rate for a wet granulated product? If a granulation is kneaded 5 min and has a porosity of 0.3 after drying, and if after 10 min of kneading it would have a porosity of 0.2 after drying, what is the difference in drying time of the two granulations?

Solution:

Increased kneading time causes a decrease in porosity, and hence an increase in drying time, because of the decrease in diffusion coefficient. In the following, subscripts denote kneading time. [Refer to Eqs. (13) and (15)]. For $(c - c_\infty)/(c_0 - c_\infty)$ to be the same, t/K must be the same (i.e., t_{10}/t_5 must equal K_{10}/K_5). Since $D_5 = (0.3/0.2)D_{10}$, it follows that $K_5 = (0.2/0.3)K_{10}$ [Eq. (14)]. Hence, $t_{10}/t_5 = K_{10}/K_5 = 1.5$, so that the drying time increases by 50%.

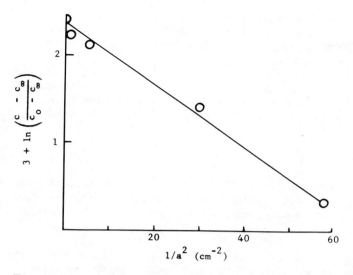

Figure 6. Moisture level as a function of reciprocal radius squared of granules dried in a countercurrent drier. (From Ref. 21; reproduced with permission of the copyright owner.)

Example 5. Determining Drying Time with a Change in Porosity

Since prolonged kneading is a squeezing process, suppose that a decrease in ϵ from 0.3 to 0.2 is a result of a decrease in the diameter by 10%. What is the new drying time?

Solution:

$$K_{10} = \frac{a_{10}^2}{4\pi^2 D_{10}}$$

$$K_5 = \frac{a_5^2}{4\pi^2 D_5} = \frac{1.11^2 a_{10}^2}{4\pi^2 1.5 D_{10}} = 0.82$$

So the drying time increases by a factor of $1/0.82 = 1.22$ (i.e., by 22%).

D. Tray Drying

In tray drying, wet granulation (or wet product) is placed on trays which are either placed in an oven, or placed on a truck which in turn is placed in an individual oven (as opposed to truck drying). The drying air enters from one wall of the oven, passes over the trays, and exits at the other wall. Although tray drying is not in the forefront of technology (being both slow and inefficient), it is still a widely used method of drying, and because of the considerable capital investment that would be required for an alternative, is not likely to be replaced by more efficient means in the near future. Tray drying has been widely reported in the pharmaceutical literature [22-27].

To illustrate the process, assume that a tray is filled with wet granulation to a depth of a (meters) and that the limiting step in drying is the transfer of moisture from the bed into the airstream. The rate of loss [20] will follow the equation

$$-D\left(\frac{\partial C}{\partial x}\right) = \alpha(C_0 - C_s) \tag{17}$$

where D is the diffusion coefficient (m^2 sec^{-1}) of water vapor, C the concentration (kg m^{-3}) of water (vapor) in the void space of the bed, $\partial C/\partial x$ (kg m^{-4}) the moisture (vapor) gradient over the interface between the bed and the airstream (where the subscripts 0 and s denote bed and airstream, respectively), and α is a proportionality constant.

The airstream is assumed to be dry; that is, $C_s = 0$ and C_0 will be denoted as simply C in the following. Initially, when the granules contain surface moisture, the vapor in the void space is of saturation pressure P_{sat} (N m^{-2}):

$$C = \frac{P_{sat}}{RT} 0.018 \text{ kg m}^{-3} \tag{18}$$

where R = 8.3143 Nm mol^{-1} deg^{-1}. C is therefore constant in this period, and application of Fick's law gives the drying rate dm/dt (kg sec^{-1}) as

$$-\frac{1}{\epsilon A}\frac{dm}{dt} = -D\left(\frac{\partial C}{\partial x}\right) = \alpha C \tag{19}$$

where A is the surface of the tray and ϵ the bed porosity (i.e., A ϵ is the cross-section through which diffusion occurs). Combining Equations (17) to (19) then gives the (zero-order) rate of evaporation as

$$-\frac{dm}{dt} = A\alpha\epsilon\frac{P_{sat}}{RT} 0.018 \tag{20}$$

Hence, α can be calculated from the slope of the initial drying curve if the granules contain surface moisture.

At a certain point during drying, the surface moisture will be exhausted and the vapor pressure in the void space will drop below P_{sat}. If in this period both the evaporation from the granule and the internal equilibration of vapor in the bed are rapid compared to the transfer of moisture over the bed-stream interface, then the diffusion equation can be solved. Introducing the dimensionless parameter

$$J = \frac{a\xi}{D} \tag{21}$$

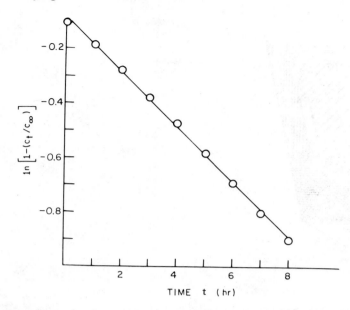

Figure 7. Drying curve according to Equation (22).

the first-order approximation of the solution will be

$$\ln\left[1 - \left(\frac{c_t}{c_\infty}\right)\right] = -\left(\frac{\beta^2 D}{a^2}\right)t + \ln\left[\frac{2J^2}{\beta^2(\beta^2 + J^2 + J)}\right] = -Gt + \ln K \tag{22}$$

where $-G$ and $\ln K$ denote slope and intercept, respectively, β is the smallest positive root of

$$J = \beta \tan \beta \tag{23}$$

c denotes mass (kg) of water in the granulation, and c_∞ is the final (equilibrium) amount of moisture in the granulation, usually that obtained by proper drying of the product.

Equation (22) shows that the amount of moisture left in the granulation, less the equilibrium moisture, is log-linear in time, and that β^2 can be calculated from the negative slope $(-G)$:

$$\beta^2 = \frac{Ga^2}{D} \tag{24}$$

Figure 7 shows a typical example of tray-drying data of a bed depth of a = 2.5 cm, treated according to Equation (22) [28]. The least-squares fitting slope is -0.102 hr^{-1} and the intercept is -0.021.

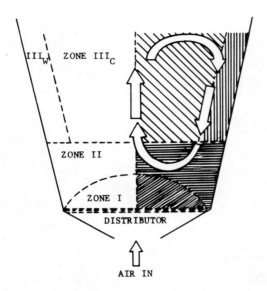

Figure 8. Schematic of flow patterns in a fluid-bed drier.

E. Fluid-Bed Drying

In fluid-bed drying, moist granules are placed in a slightly conical pot with a retaining screen on the bottom (Fig. 8), which is placed in an airstream (Fig. 9).
At low air velocities v (m sec^{-1}), the pressure drop experienced by the air by
passing through the bed of granules will simply adhere to the Kozeny-Carmen
equation:

$$\Delta P = \frac{q}{d^2} \frac{(\epsilon_b)^3}{(1 - \epsilon_b)^2}$$

(25)

where ϵ_b is the porosity of the granulation. This remains fairly constant at low
velocities [29-32].

At a certain air velocity, v' (m sec^{-1}), the implicit fluidization velocity, the
bed will become fluidized. Increasing the velocity will then expand the bed (i.e.,
increase the bed porosity). At a particular velocity v_e, the entrainment velocity,
air entrainment (air conveyance) will occur.

A plot of ϵ versus v is linear, as shown in Figure 10, and v_e can be obtained
from this by extrapolation; ϵ can be calculated from the bed thickness, which can
be observed directly. This is shown to be true by the following argument.

The drying chamber is assumed to be cylindrical with cross section A (m^2).
The height of the surface S (kg of granulation) [of particle density ζ (kg m^{-3}) and
bed porosity ϵ] is a (m); hence

$$S = Aa_0\zeta$$

(26)

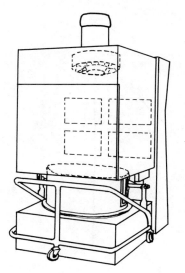

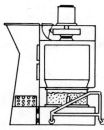

Figure 9. Schematic of fluid-bed drier for granulation drying. (Courtesy Fitz-patrick Co., Elmhurst, Illinois.)

where a_0 is the smallest bed thickness (at $\epsilon = 0$). At a bed porosity of ϵ, it follows that

$$\epsilon = 1 - \frac{S}{A\zeta a} \qquad \text{or} \qquad a = \frac{S}{A\zeta(1 - \epsilon)} \tag{27}$$

The entrainment velocity can be found from extrapolation of plots such as Figure 10, since at the entrainment velocity the porosity is essentially equal to unity.

Zoglio et al. [33] have described the time course of drying of pharmaceutical granulations. They established that the rate of the process is limited by moisture diffusion past the granule boundary. Figure 11 shows that the data follow the equation

$$\ln (RH - RH_0) = -\alpha t + \ln (100 - RH_0) \tag{28}$$

where RH is the relative humidity of the outlet air at time t and RH_0 is that of the inlet air.

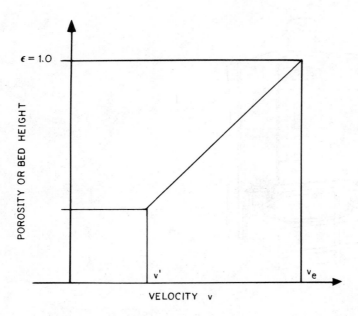

Figure 10.   Porosity or bed height as a function of air velocity in fluid-bed drying.

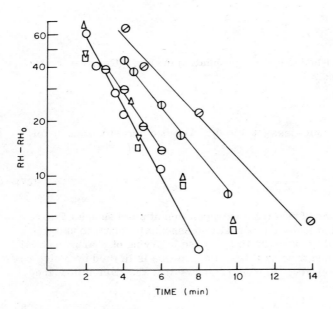

Figure 11.   Relative humidity of exit air during a drying experiment in a fluid-bed drier.

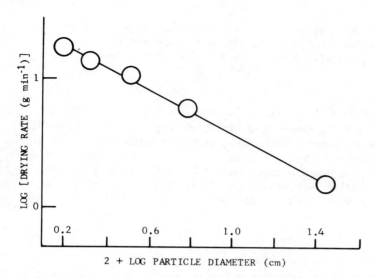

Figure 12. Logarithm of the drying rate (g min^{-1}) as a function of the log of particle diameter (cm) in a fluid-bed drying experiment.

The drying rate is a function of granule diameter, as shown in Figure 12. Particle size distributions do not change much on drying, so that in spite of the apparent vivid motion in the dryer, the relative velocities of the particles are small and the attrition is not great. It is of significance that the important parameter in the drying is the moisture content (not so much the temperature) of the incoming air. It is also interesting to note that the temperature falls very abruptly to the temperature of the bed as the incoming air crosses the distributor plate. Finally, it should be noted that fluid-bed driers are excellent mixers [34].

Example 6.   Determining the Entrainment Velocity

Assume the fluidization vessel in a fluid-bed dryer to be cylindrical with a cross section of 1 m^2. At an air flow rate of 4.5 m^3 sec^{-1}, the height of the bed is 0.5 m. The charge is 300 kg of material with a particle density of 1.5 g cm^{-3}. When the air flow rate is 5.4 m^3 sec^{-1}, the porosity of the bed is $\epsilon = 0.78$. What is the entrainment velocity in m sec^{-1}? (Assume that the porosity is linear with an air velocity above the incipient fluidization velocity, and that the latter is less than what corresponds to a flow rate of 4.5 m^3 sec^{-1}.)

Solution:

The flow rates are equal to linear velocity in m sec^{-1} because the cross section is 1 m^2. The porosity of the bed at a flow rate of 4.5 m^3 sec^{-1} can be calculated as follows. The weight of the bed is equal to the (particle) powder density times the solids volume fraction $(1 - \epsilon)$ times the volume. The particle density is $1.5 \cdot 10^3$ kg m^{-3}, so $1500(1 - \epsilon)$ $(0.5 \times 1) = 300$, from which $1 - \epsilon = 300/(1500 \times 0.5) = 0.4$ (i.e., $\epsilon = 0.6$). At $v = 4.5$, $\epsilon = 0.6$; and at v = 5.4, ϵ = 0.78. The slope of the ϵ versus v line is (0.78 - 0.6)/5.4 - 4.5) = 0.2, so that the equation for the line is ϵ - 0.6 = 0.2(v = 4.5), or ϵ = 0.2 v - 0.3. ϵ = 1 when 0.2 v = 1 + 0.3 or v = 6.5 m sec^{-1} (or m^3 sec^{-1}).

F. Vacuum Drying

In drying generally, the drying potential is [as shown, e.g., in Eqs. (17) and (18)] the difference between the vapor pressure in or at the wet particle P_0 and the vapor pressure P_1 in the airstream. The drying (at least in the constant-drying period) is also a function of A, the liquid surface area (or the surface area of the granules), and inversely proportional to the heat of evaporation of the wetting liquid [i.e., L^* (J/kg), since this is mostly water]. The rate may thus be written:

$$\text{Rate} = N \frac{A}{L^*} (P_0 - P_1) \tag{29}$$

The proportionality factor N is a transfer coefficient which is dependent on both heat and mass transfer; it depends, for example, on the interfacial energy γ between liquid and atmosphere.

Pure water has, at 25° C, a vapor pressure of 25 torr. If the pressure of the atmosphere in contact with the granulation is reduced to less than this figure, the water will boil. (Since the water initially present contains solutes, the vapor pressure will be somewhat less than 25 torr.) The formation of bubbles is, of course, related to γ, so when it occurs, it has the effect of greatly increasing A. Therefore, employing a vacuum to dry a granule should result in rapid drying and permit drying at low temperatures [35].

Vacuum drying is not widely used in the pharmaceutical industry. Nevertheless, it is a potentially useful method, as pointed out as early as 1961 by Cooper et al. [35], and a schematic layout is shown in Figure 13. A V-shaped blender can be substituted for the cylinder/double-cone blender.

As shown in Figure 14, placing wet granulation in a vacuum drier (or spray-granulating directly in the drier) may give rise to lumping and agglomeration. This can be overcome by the tubular principle shown.

The advantages of vacuum drying are that it allows for safe drying of heat-sensitive products. It is also more rapid than tray, truck, or countercurrent drying but is not as rapid as fluid-bed drying. The temperature effect in drying can be an overriding factor prompting consideration of a vacuum-drying system. Other advantages also exist, such as the fact that oxidation is minimized in vacuum drying. The potentially serious environmental problems of dust entrainment, although well minimized in other drying methods, gives vacuum drying an advantage, because the fact that air movement is minimized reduces the potential for particulate loss. Compliance with requirements of the Environmental Protection Agency and provisions of the Occupational Safety and Health Act, plus decreased overall energy consumption, provide vacuum drying with additional advantages.

As is evident in the figures, vacuum driers are usually jacketed, because of the considerable amount of heat that is required for vaporization. They can therefore also be used for drying at elevated temperatures should that be required.

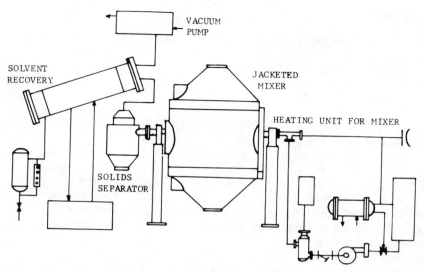

Figure 13. Schematic setup of vacuum drying. (Courtesy Patterson Kelley Co.,
East Stroudsburg, Pennsylvania.)

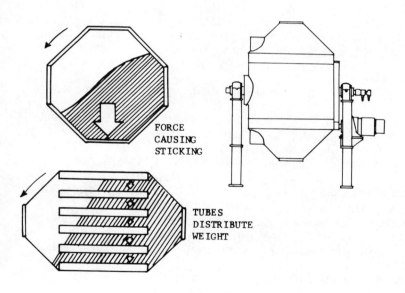

Figure 14. Baffle arrangement for breaking up lumps in vacuum drying. (Courtesy
Patterson Kelley Co., East Stroudsburg, Pennsylvania.)

Acknowledgments

The authors are indebted to Mrs. Donna J. McGue and Dr. William H. Streng for technical assistance.

References

1. Carstensen, J. T., in: Pharmaceutics of Solids and Solid Dosage Forms, Wiley, New York, 1977, pp. 210-213.
2. Jones, T. M., and Pilpel, N., J. Pharm. Pharmacol., 17:440 (1965).
3. Jones, T. M., and Pilpel, N., J. Pharm. Pharmacol., 18:81 (1966).
4. Jones, T. M., and Pilpel, N., J. Pharm. Pharmacol., 18:182S (1966).
5. Jones, T. M., and Pilpel, N., J. Pharm. Pharmacol., 18:429 (1966).
6. Ridgway, K., and Rupp, R., J. Pharm. Pharmacol., 21:30S (1969).
7. Finholt, P., in: Dissolution Technology (L. Leeson and J. Carstensen, eds.). Industrial Pharmaceutical Technology Section, the Academy of Pharmaceutical Sciences, Washington, D.G., 1974, p. 72.
8. Carstensen, J. T., in: Theory of Pharmaceutical Systems, Vol. 2. Academic Press, New York, 1973, pp. 224-238.
9. Shepherd, C., Hadlock, C., and Brewer, R., Ind. Eng. Chem., 30:388 (1938).
10. Lewis, W. K., Ind. Eng. Chem., 13:427 (1921).
11. Sherwood, T. K., Trans. AIChE, 27:190 (1931).
12. Newman, A. B., Trans. AIChE, 27:203 (1931).
13. Newman, A. B., Trans. AIChE, 27:310 (1931).
14. Sherwood, T. K., and Comings, E. W., Ind. Eng. Chem., 25:311 (1933).
15. Oliver, T. R., and Newitt, D. M., Trans. Inst. Chem. Eng., 27:1 (1949).
16. Pearse, J. F., Oliver, T. R., and Newitt, D. M., Trans. Inst. Chem. Eng., 27:9 (1949).
17. Nissan, A. H., George, H. H., and Bell, J. R., Am. Inst. Chem. Eng. J., 6:406 (1960).
18. Bell, J. R., and Nissan, A. H., Am. Inst. Chem. Eng. J., 5:344 (1959).
19. Adams, E. F., Ph.D. thesis, Rensselaer Polytechnic Institute, Troy, N.Y., (1962).
20. Jost, W., in: Diffusion. Academic Press, New York, 1960, p. 46.
21. Pitkin, C., and Carstensen, J. T., J. Pharm. Sci., 62:1215 (1973).
22. Ridgway, K., and Callow, J. A. B., J. Pharm. Pharmacol., 19:1555 (1967).
23. Luikov, A. V., Int. J. Heat Mass Transfer, 6:559 (1963).
24. Morgan, R. P., and Yerazunis, S., Am. Inst. Chem. Eng. J., 13:136 (1967).
25. Bhuthani, B. R., and Bhatia, V. N., J. Pharm. Sci., 64:135 (1975).
26. Opankunle, W. O., Bhutani, B. R., and Bhatia, V. N., J. Pharm. Sci., 64:1023 (1975).
27. Gilliland, E. R., Ind. Eng. Chem., 30:506 (1938).
28. Carstensen, J. T., and Zoglio, M. A., to be published.
29. Scott, M. W., Lieberman, H. A., Rankell, A. S., Chow, F. S., and Johnston, G. W., J. Pharm. Sci., 52:284 (1963).
30. Scott, M. W., Lieberman, H. A., Rankell, A. S., and Battista, J. V., J. Pharm. Sci., 53:314 (1964).

31. Mody, D. S., Scott, M. W., and Lieberman, H. A., J. Pharm. Sci., 53:949 (1964).
32. Rankell, A. S., Scott, M. W., Lieberman, H. A., Chow, F. S., and Battista, J. V., J. Pharm. Sci., 53:320 (1964).
33. Zoglio, M. A., Streng, W. H., and Carstensen, J. T., J. Pharm. Sci., 64:1869 (1975).
34. Mehta, A., Adams, K. A., Zoglio, M. A., and Carstensen, J. T., J. Pharm. Sci., 66:1462 (1977).
35. Cooper, M., Swartz, C. J., and Suydam, W., Jr., J. Pharm. Sci., 50:67 (1961).

3

Size Reduction

Russell J. Lantz, Jr.

Smith Kline Corporation
Philadelphia, Pennsylvania

I. Introduction

Size reduction is the process of reducing large solid unit masses to smaller unit masses by mechanical means. The complexity of the process has resulted in few theories of general applicability. Therefore, to a great extent, the subject is primarily a conglomeration of ideas and theories of limited scope, describing the size reduction of specific cases of single- and multiple-component particulate systems. A considerable amount of literature [1, 2] has accumulated over the past 15 to 20 years on the subject of size reduction, and this material will be used where applicable.

Size reduction is a rate process [3] that depends on the starting size of the feedstock, its orientation in the mill, and its mill residence time. The process may or may not follow a first-order equation, depending on the deviations that take place during milling; for example, (1) residual stresses within powder particles due to plastic deformation and/or changes in internal particle stresses from uneven thermal changes during size reduction [4]; (2) distribution of particle strengths [5]; and (3) caking or agglomeration of smaller particles to each other and/or to larger particles which occur simultaneously in the size reduction process [6].

The principal means of accomplishing size reduction are cutting or shearing, compression, impact, and attrition, and the design of most size reduction equipment is based on these four principles [7]. Because of the complexity of the operation, there are some differences of opinion as to exactly what takes place during the size reduction of powder particles or granules. However, the literature appears to agree, for the most part, on the following sequence of events.

Assume an assemblage of particles of uniform composition (which may or may not be irregular in shape), which are to be reduced in size. The particles may be subjected to one or a combination of three forces: compression, shear, or tension.

Compression is a crushing force, shear a cutting force, and tension a force that tends to elongate a particle or pull it apart.

Each particle in the assumed assemblage will have initial flaws of different degrees, and possible internal stress as a result of prior manufacturing operations [4]. A flaw in a unit particle, be it crystalline or amorphous, is a discontinuity or imperfection in the structure. This constitutes a weakness in the particle structure which may result in failure when the external milling forces applied exceed the cohesive forces of the particle flaw. This failure manifests itself as a crack or cracks, which eventually leads to particle cleavage at the crack upon the addition of greater force and/or repeated force. Cleavage yields two or more particles, hence additional surface area. During milling, cutting, compression, impact, or attrition initially produces a flexing or bending of the particle or granule, which returns to its original shape if it is not fractured. This results in the release of energy in the form of heat, a process known as plastic deformation. If the milling forces are great enough to overcome the inner or intraparticle cohesive forces, flaws or cracks are generated. Particles may cleave (Fig. 1) at various locations, such as through the mass of the particle itself as a result of impact, shear, or compression, and/or at the outermost edges as a result of attrition. This creates a distribution of smaller particles.

Comminution or milling is an extremely inefficient unit operation, with only 0.05 to 2% of the applied energy [8, 9] being utilized in the actual reduction of particle size. Milling efficiency is dependent upon the type of mill and the characteristics of the material (the feedstock) being milled. A large portion (10 to 50%) of the expended energy ends up as heat generated from:

1. Plastic deformation of particles that are not fractured
2. Friction of the particles contacting the mill
3. Friction of the particles colliding with each other
4. Friction of the mechanical parts of the mill

The situation is essentially the same for an assemblage of dried granules that are being reduced in size for proper flow and bulk density in tableting. Again, cleavage occurs at the weakest point or points in the granule:

1. The binder-particle interface
2. The bridge of binder between the individual ingredient particles being granulated
3. Flaws in the individual ingredient particles within the granule
4. A combination of any of the above

Granules held together with lower-strength binding agents such as polyvinylpyrrolidone will require less severe grinding conditions because the fractures take place primarily at the binder bridge and/or binder-particle interfaces.

There has been a continuing quest by researchers in the field to express or define size reduction in terms of a general mathematical model. However, this has not been very successful to date because of:

1. The lack of a generally accepted theory of comminution
2. The individuality of each size reduction case (i.e., each milling operation requires its own analysis)

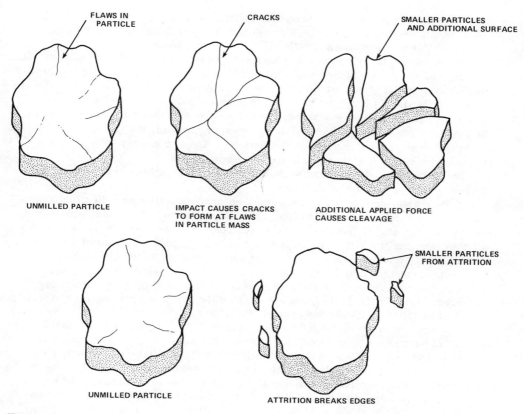

Figure 1. Particle cleavage.

3. The lack of a practical mathematical term to better represent the character-
    istics of a particle or an assemblage of particles in terms of size, shape, den-
    sity, fracturability, and so on [10]

A considerable amount of money has been spent in developing theoretical and practical approaches to improving efficiency and solving the problems of scale-up milling from the laboratory to production. This expenditure falls largely to "heavy industry"--the coal, coke, ore (steel included), cement, and paint industries. Because of the volume of materials handled in these industries (tons to thousands of
tons per hour), the scale-up, purchase, fabrication, and installation of equipment
that will handle these material volumes and withstand the loads and wear encountered constitute major investments for the corporations involved. With the exception of a number of continuous pharmaceutical manufacturing processes now in
operation, pharmaceutical production hardly approaches the production scale encountered in heavy industry. This is why the pharmaceutical industry is not oriented toward designing and testing new size reduction equipment. Although its
size reduction and scale-up problems are very similar to those of heavy industry,

these problems are more often solved empirically than through the theoretical route. Some mathematics has been developed for specific size reduction equipment, and this is discussed in Section II.

Size reduction is nothing new in pharmacy, as evidenced by the array of metal, wooden, and ceramic mortars and pestles that were used in the early apothecaries for the preparation of powder mixes, pills, and plant and animal extracts.

Size reduction as it applies to tablet production falls into three basic categories: (1) the reduction in size of oversize and/or agglomerated raw materials; (2) the reduction in size of wet and dry granular materials, usually of multiple-ingredient composition; and (3) the reduction in size of tablets or compactions that must be milled for dry granulating or reworking.

Size reduction and the use of size reduction equipment has certain advantages in tablet development and production:

1. Increased surface area, which may enhance an active ingredient's dissolution rate and hence its bioavailability. This is particularly important with compounds that are slightly soluble, such as phenacetin. The effect on phenacetin dissolution rate and bioavailability as a result of small particle size differences is illustrated in Figure 2. Improved bioavailability with improved dissolution rate has been demonstrated by Ullah et al. [12]. It must be noted, however, that active ingredients reduced in particle size to gain the advantage of increased surface area may not retain all of this advantage after being incorporated into a wet or dry granulation mix and compressed into tablets.

2. Improved tablet-to-tablet content uniformity by virtue of the increased number of particles per unit weight. A higher number of active-ingredient particles statistically diminishes the probability that a single tablet will contain too few or too many drug particles to place outside allowable assay limits. This is very important in formulas containing highly potent, low-dose medicaments.

3. Improved flow properties of raw materials that are needle-shaped or extremely irregular in shape and tend to form a structure that resists flow. This type of flow-resistant structure, when encountered in a hopper, storage bin, or silo is called "bridging."

4. Improved color and/or active-ingredient dispersion in the tablet excipient diluents by proper use of size reduction equipment to effect a more complete or intimate serial dilution of the ingredients.

5. Uniformly sized wet granules to promote uniform drying. This will tend to lend uniformity to dissolved color and active-ingredient migration to the surface of the uniformly sized granules during drying. Nonuniform color migration usually results in mottling, and nonuniform active-ingredient migration may yield content-uniformity problems in the final compressed tablet.

6. Controlled particle size distribution of a dry granulation or mix to promote better flow of the mixtures in tablet machine feed hoppers and into tablet dies. This ensures tablet weight uniformity when compressing on high-speed gravity- or force-feed rotary tablet machines.

7. Controlled particle size distribution of a dry granulation or dry mix to minimize segregation of fines and/or active ingredients while handling and tableting.

There are also disadvantages of size reduction, which may play an important part in the decision as to whether a powder component(s) should be milled, and to what extent. These disadvantages include:

1. A possible change in polymorphic form of the active ingredient, rendering it less or totally inactive, or unstable.

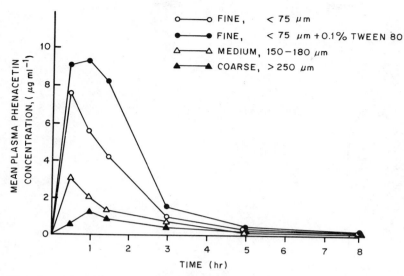

Figure 2. Mean plasma phenacetin concentration in six adult volunteers following administration of 1.5-g doses of phenacetin in different ranges of particle size. [From Prescott, L. F., Steel, R. F., and Ferrier, W. R., The effects of particle size on the absorption of phenacetin in man, Clin. Pharmacol. Therap., 11:496–504 (1970).]

2. Possible degradation of the drug as a result of heat buildup during milling by oxidation or adsorption of unwanted moisture due to the increased surface area.
3. A decrease in bulk density of the active compounds and/or excipients, which may cause flow problems and segregation in the mix. Often, a wet or dry granulation is used in lieu of a direct compression formula because of the bulk density differences between formula components.
4. A decrease in raw material particle size may create static charge problems, causing the small drug particles to agglomerate, thereby effectively decreasing surface area. This may diminish the solid-liquid interface, which, in turn, may decrease the dissolution rate.
5. An increase in surface area from size reduction may promote the adsorption of air, which may inhibit wettability of the drug to the extent that it becomes the limiting factor in the dissolution rate.

The milling process, whether used to reduce size or distribute coloring or active ingredients, is an important [13, 14], integral part of the successful development and mass production of a formula for particulates which yields tablets that are uniform and reproducible and physically and chemically stable.

II. Size Reduction Equipment

All milling or comminution equipment has three basic components (Fig. 3): (1) a structure for feeding material to the mill, (2) the milling chamber and its working

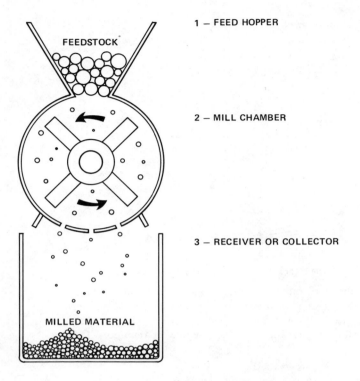

FEEDSTOCK

1 — FEED HOPPER

2 — MILL CHAMBER

3 — RECEIVER OR COLLECTOR

MILLED MATERIAL

Figure 3.   Three basic mill components.

parts, and (3) a take-off to a receiver or collector in which the milled product is deposited.   One exception to this are the small-batch ball mills, which do not have means for continuous feed or milled product removal.

Some mills are also fitted with means such as cyclones or centrifugation for classifying the particles by size, so that the larger and/or unmilled particles may be separated from the smaller milled material and/or recycled through the system for remilling.   Each of these basic components is discussed in detail below in connection with each mill type.

Table 1 is a general characterization of milling equipment commonly used in tableting.   The mills are listed roughly in the order of the milled product they may yield, starting from the smallest to the largest particle sizes.   The speeds of the mills listed in the table are approximations, as are the screen sizes, because each milling process (operation) is usually an individual case and must be treated according to the individually defined parameters (which are discussed later).   Table 2 provides examples of the hard, abrasive, moderately hard, and so on, raw materials mentioned in Table 1.

A.   Fluid Energy Mill

The fluid energy mill, which has no moving parts, is a rapid and relatively efficient method of reducing powders to 30 μm and less with a relatively narrow

Table 1

General Characteristics of Milling Equipment Used Commonly in Tablet Production and Powder Raw Material Processing

Mill action and setup	Use	Type and size of feedstock	Expected results	Materials not recommended for mill
1. Fluid energy mill: attrition and impact (compressed gases 80–150 psig)	Ultrafine grinding	20–200 mesh, moderately hard materials	30–5 μm or less with narrow size range	Soft, tacky, fibrous
2. Ball mill or rod mill: attrition and impact				
a. Wet	Fine grinding, closed system	4–100 mesh, moderately hard, abrasive materials	100–5 μm or less	Soft, tacky, fibrous
b. Dry	Fine grinding, closed system	4–100 mesh, moderately hard, abrasive materials	200–10 μm or less	Soft, tacky, fibrous
3. Hammer mill: impact, some attrition				
a. High speed: peripheral speed at 20,000 ft min^{-1}				
(1) Small screen	Fine grinding, depending on screen size	2–20 mesh, nonabrasive to moderately abrasive, brittley, dry material	100–325 mesh, depending on material; narrow size distribution	Sticky, fibrous material, low melting point
(2) Large screen	Moderate grinding	2–20 mesh, nonabrasive, soft, dry materials	40–100 mesh, depending on material; wide size distribution	Sticky, fibrous materials, low melting point; hard, abrasive material
(3) No screen				

(continued)

Table 1 (continued)

Mill action and setup	Use	Type and size of feedstock	Expected results	Materials not recommended for mill
b. Low speed: peripheral speed at 1500–300 ft min^{-1}				
(1) Small screen	Dispersion of dry powder blends and some size reduction of soft granules	Coarsely blended powders less than screen size used: 10–40 mesh	Dispersion of powders 80–100 mesh granules	Sticky, fibrous materials and hard, abrasive materials
(2) Large screen	Coarse dispersion of powder blends and size reduction of wet granulations	Coarsely blended powders 100 mesh and wet granulations	Dispersion of powders 10 to 40 mesh wet granules	Sticky, fibrous materials and hard, abrasive materials
(3) No screen				
4. Cutting mill: cutting or shear and some attrition				
a. High speed: peripheral speed at 20,000 ft min^{-1}				
(1) Small screen	Usually, do not use these milling conditions			
(2) Large screen	Coarse dispersion of powders and wet granulation size reduction	Dry powders, fibrous materials, wet granulation regarding compressed tablets	Dispersion of dry powders, chopping of fibrous materials, and reduced wet granule size	Hard, abrasive materials
(3) No screen				
b. Low speed: peripheral speed at 1500–3000 ft min^{-1}				
(1) Small screen	Usually, do not use these milling conditions			

(2) Large screen	Size reduction of large dry and wet granulations	Wet and dry granulation tablet reworks, slugged or chilsenated granulations, and wet granulation	4–80 mesh	Hard, abrasive materials
(3) No screen				
5. Oscillating granulator: attrition and shear				
a. Small screen (20 mesh)	Dry granulation size reduction, rework of tablets	Tablet reworks and dried granulation	20–60 mesh	Wet granulation
b. Large screen (4 mesh)	Stepwise size reduction	Tablet reworks, dry and wet granulations	20–40 mesh	
6. Extruder: shear large and small openings in head	Primarily for continuous preparation of wet granulations	Wet granulations formulated for continuous extrusion; batch work may also be done	Granular and spaghetti-like wet granules	Dry material
7. Hand screens: shear and attrition	Dispersion and delumping of powders; small-scale size reduction of wet and dry granulations	Raw materials, small-batch wet and dry granulations	Powder dispersion, delumped, narrow size distribution with both wet and dry granulations	Hard, abrasive materials

Table 2

Examples of Pharmaceutical Raw Materials of Different Hardness

Material	General hardness classification
Talc	Soft; abrasiveness varies
Chalk	Soft to brittle
Boric acid	Soft
Cellulose	Soft but plastic (resiliency)
Aspirin	Moderately hard to brittle
Lactose	Moderately hard to brittle
Ammonium chloride	Moderately hard to brittle
Sucrose	Moderately hard to brittle
Dextrin	Hard to brittle
Sorbitol	Hard
Kaolin	Hard
Magnesium oxide	Hard, abrasive
Calcium lactate	Hard, abrasive
Amobarbital	Very hard, abrasive

particle size distribution [15]. Figure 4 is a schematic of such a mill. The mill operates on the principle of attrition and impact. A high-velocity airstream introduces the powder to the milling chamber, usually by way of a venturi tube (a high-velocity airstream passing an opening containing the powder produces a vacuum in the opening and draws the powder into the airstream). Larger feedstock sizes must be reduced in size before they can be fed to, and milled by, fluid energy (prereduction in size is usually accomplished in a hammer mill). Milling takes place immediately because of the high-velocity collisions between particles suspended within the airstream (see Fig. 5). A limitation of this mill relates to how fast material can be fed to the mill, because effective grinding depends to a large extent on the particle mean free path (the distance a particle travels before colliding with another particle) and the energy gained for collision in a longer mean free path. Higher feed rates diminish the length of the mean free path and may reduce milling effectiveness and efficiency.

Grinding nozzles (usually two to six, depending on the size of the mill) may be placed tangential and/or opposed to the initial powder flow path (Fig. 6) to increase the particle velocity, resulting in higher impact energy. Grinding appears to depend on the number of particle collisions, the probability of breakage on collision, and whether attrition or impact is the principal mechanism [16]. The air from the grinding nozzles acts to transport the powder in the elliptical or circular track of the mill to the classifier, which removes the smaller particles by entrainment

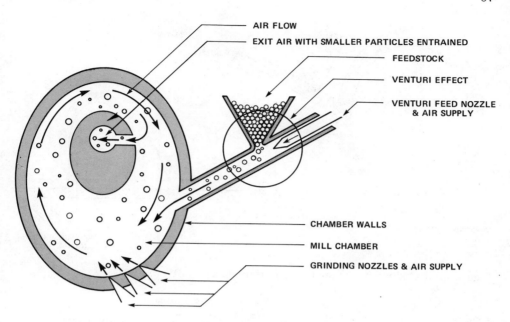

Figure 4. Schematic of fluid energy mill.

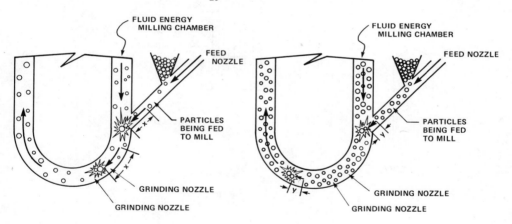

Figure 5. Effect of the mean free path of particles on the impact in fluid energy milling. x, long mean free path resulting in higher particle impact velocity and smaller particles (low feed rate of powder particles; y, short mean free path resulting in lower particle impact velocity and larger particles (high feed rates of powder particles).

The entrained particles are removed by cyclone and bag filters (Figs. 7 and 8). Because of the mass of the larger particles and the opposing drag and centrifugal forces, they recirculate, colliding again with the new incoming feedstock particles, and remain in the mill until they are reduced sufficiently in size to exit via the

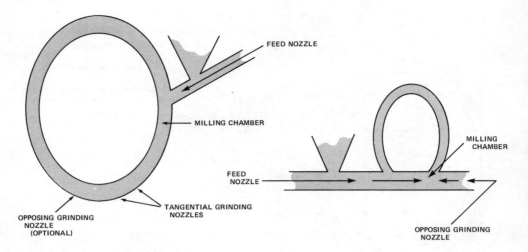

Figure 6. Grinding nozzle positions in fluid energy mill.

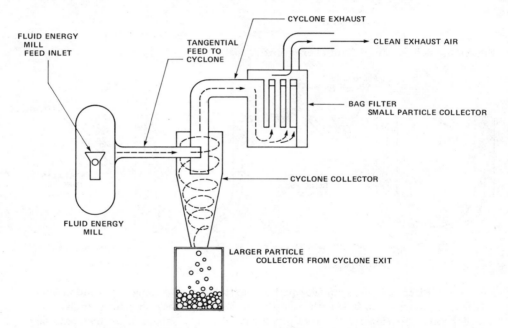

Figure 7. Schematic of fluid energy mill and particle collection system.

classifier--hence the narrow particle size distribution. The mean particle size and distribution appear to be dependent not on only the size, distribution, hardness, and elastic properties of the feedstock, but also on the configuration of the mill, placement of the nozzles, design of the classifier, and energy input to the mill.

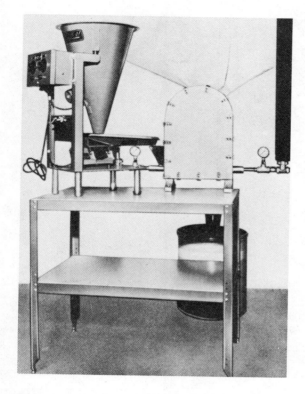

Figure 8. Trost fluid energy mill. (Courtesy Plastomer Products, Newtown, Pennsylvania 18940.)

The effects of feed rate and grinding nozzle pressure on the milling of $CaCO_3$ (99.4%) are shown in Figures 9 and 10, respectively. Figure 9 shows that as feed rate decreases, particle size also decreases. Figure 10 indicates that at a constant feed rate, product particle size decreases with increased grinding pressure.

The mill surfaces that contact the product may be made from a variety of materials, ranging from the softer stainless steels to the tough ceramics used for exceptionally abrasive materials such as barium sulfate and amobarbital. Usually, the mills are constructed such that the contact surfaces are merely linings, which can be removed and replaced if excessively eroded after use.

Size reduction using the fluid energy mill has the advantage that heat-labile substances can be milled with little danger of thermal degradation. This is a result of the cooling effect of the expanding gases and the rapid heat exchange between particle and milling gases. Inert gases can also be used to minimize or eliminate the oxidation of susceptible compounds which may occur with compressed air. Soft materials such as waxes may be milled by prechilling in liquid nitrogen to make them brittle.

Fluid energy milling is usually used to reduce the particle size of active ingredients that require a very small particle size to assure both maximum surface

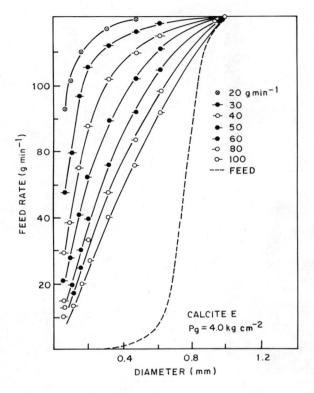

Figure 9. Effect of feed rate on product size distribution. [From Rumanujam, M., et al., Powder Technol., 3:92-101 (1969/1970).]

area for solubilization and bioavailibility, and for tablet content uniformity, particularly in dry granulations. Although not used in tablet granulating per se, fluid energy milling may be used as a means of intimately dispersing a coarse mixture of powders. However, one must be careful that classification does not segregate the various mixture ingredients by virtue of their differences in particle size, hardness, and absolute density.

B. Ball Mill

Ball milling is used to obtain extremely small particles but is not used in tablet granulating per se. Ball milling has been studied extensively [17] in an attempt to predict its action and to express the "dynamic characteristics" in mathematical terms. Potentially, these terms may then be used in the control of this process by computer. Scale-up and mill design are also areas that have benefited from the research that has been done on the ball mill. Since the theory cannot be dealt with adequately within the space of this chapter, the reader is referred to the wealth of literature [18, 19] dealing with various theoretical aspects of ball

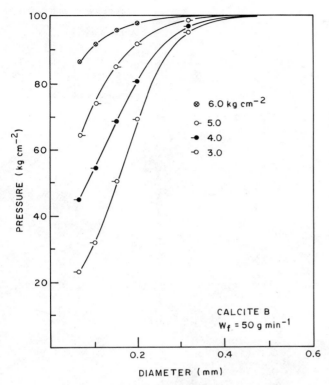

Figure 10. Effect of grinding nozzle pressure on particle size distribution. [From Rumanujam, M., et al., Powder Technol., 3:92-101 (1969/1970).]

milling. The discussion to follow takes a more practical point of view for those who will be, or are presently involved in the milling of raw materials in tablet making.

The ball mill* (Figs. 11 and 12) is a cylindrical or conical shell usually filled to about half its volume with grinding media, which can be varied in size (1/4 in. or smaller to 3 in. in diameter), size distribution, shape (balls, cylinders, cubes, etc.), and composition (Fig. 13). The shell rotates on its central axis by means of motor-driven rollers on which it rests. The drive may also be through a "bull gear," which follows the circumference of the outer shell. Ball mills designed for batch milling usually have removable end plates or side entrance covers, depending on the size of the installation, where the grinding media and unmilled material can be loaded, and then unloaded when milling is complete.

---

*Paul O. Abbe, Inc., Little Falls, N.J.

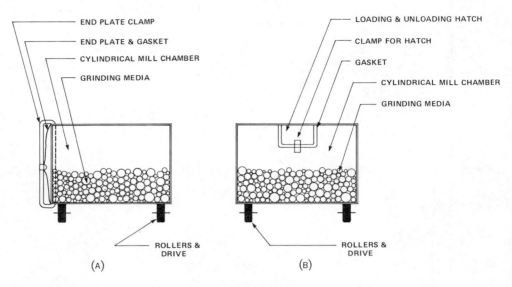

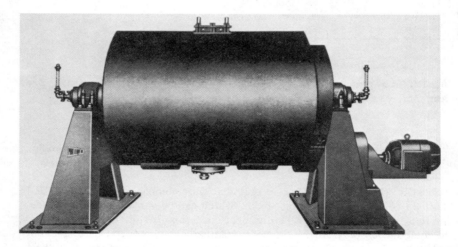

Figure 11. Schematic of ball mill. (A) Lab model design, (B) large-scale design.

Figure 12. Ball or pebble mill. (Courtesy Paul O. Abbe, Inc., Little Falls, New Jersey 97424.)

The continuous-milling design (Fig. 14) is usually a conical shell with grinding media of equal or varied sizes. The feedstock enters through the hollow trunion at one end of the mill, and milled material exits through a grating or small ports at the opposite end of the chamber. Continuous closed-circuit milling (Fig. 15) is arranged using the continuous mill with a gas or liquid classifying system. In this arrangement, the air-swept dry milling introduces the gas (in most cases

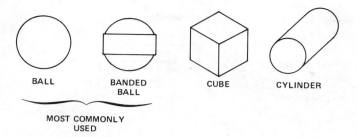

Figure 13. Grinding-media shapes.

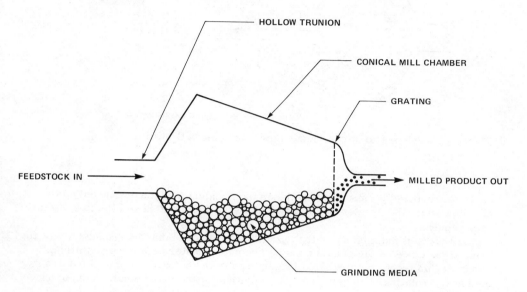

Figure 14. Schematic of continuous ball mixing.

air) and feed through the hollow trunion at one end of the mill. The large feedstock drops into the milling zone and the smaller particles become entrained in the airstream flowing through the mill and exiting through the opposite end to a particle classifier. The classifier removes the smallest particles, or the fraction of particles it is designed to remove, while the larger particles are recycled to the mill inlet for further size reduction. With certain mill and classifier modifications, wet milling with a liquid can also be carried out, in a very similar manner.

In general terms, milling takes place as the charged cylindrical or conical chamber rotates. The grinding media (balls, cubes, etc.) are made to climb the chamber walls (Fig. 16) as a result of the chamber rotation, and drop from their elevated position to the bed of media below, resulting in the primary means of

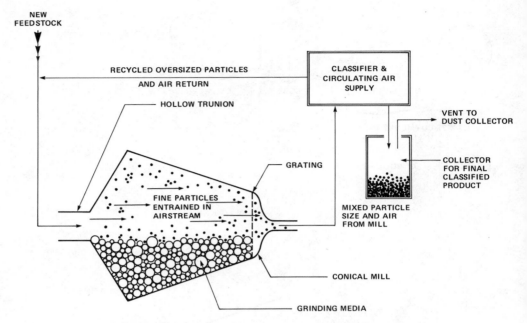

Figure 15. Schematic of continuous closed–circuit ball milling.

particle fracture by impact. The higher the grinding media are carried up the
chamber wall, the greater the capacity of the mill and the more effective the impact grinding.

However, it must be noted that a critical mill speed may be reached where the
centrifugal force on the grinding media becomes greater than the gravitational
force; at this point, the media no longer drop to the bottom of the mill but are
held at the rotating chamber wall. This critical speed may be calculated using
the following equation:

$$N_c = \frac{76.6}{\sqrt{D}}$$

where

N_c = critical speed, rpm
D = inside mill diameter, ft

For example, the critical speed of a 6-in.-diameter mill would be

$$N_c = \frac{76.6}{\sqrt{0.5}} = 108 \text{ rpm}$$

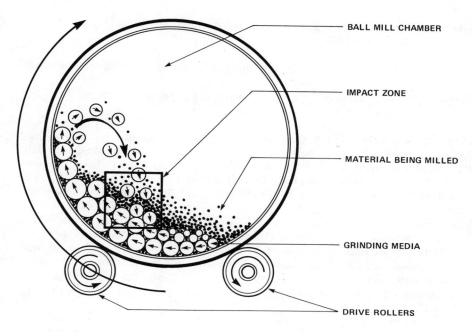

Figure 16. Schematic of ball mill and grinding media action.

In comparison, the critical speed of a 24-in.-diameter mill would be

$$N_c = \frac{76.6}{\sqrt{2.0}} = 54 \text{ rpm}$$

At and above the critical speed the mill is said to be "centrifuging," and milling all but ceases. Therefore, milling must be carried out below the critical speed of the mill--at some optimum speed where the grinding media are carried to the highest point in the chamber without centrifuging. This speed is dependent on the chamber size; grinding-media size; material size distribution, shape, and density; and the amount of material used in the mill. The optimum speed may range from 60 to 85% of the critical speed, and may be calculated from the following empirically derived equation:

$$N_o = 57 - 40(\log D)$$

where

N_o = optimum speed, rpm
D = inside diameter of the mill, ft

Calculating the optimum speeds for the examples above, the percentages of the critical speeds are:

6-in.-diameter mill: $N_O = 57 - 40(\log 0.5) = 69$ rpm $= 64\%$ of the critical speed

24-in.-diameter mill: $N_O = 57 - 40(\log 2) = 45$ rpm $= 83\%$ of the critical speed

Grinding also takes place by attrition as the media move against one another and against the walls of the mill. Slower-than-optimum speeds may be used such that attrition is the primary type of milling taking place. Milling at slower speeds yields finer grinding but requires considerably longer milling times. Finer grinding may also be achieved, in most cases, by using smaller grinding media and/or by wet milling.

Wet milling utilizes a liquid in which the material to be ground is insoluble. If necessary, this liquid may also contain additives, such as surfactants, to prevent particle flocculation. Wet milling is usually attempted when it is found that dry milling causes caking of the material to the balls and the chamber wall, which in turn acts to cushion both the impact and attrition action in the mill. This diminishes milling efficiency and creates problems in recovery of caked material from the mill.

The amount of grinding media and powder charge may vary in the mill but is very important factors with regard to milling efficiency and fineness of grind. The grinding media usually occupy from 30% to no greater than 50% of the mill chamber volume. The powder charge is usually gaged to fill the volume of the grinding media interstices with enough excess to just cover the top of the grinding-media bed. This is not a hard and fast rule, but should act as the upper limit, because large powder charges tend to cushion and absorb the impact energy of the grinding media.

The disadvantages of the ball mill include its difficulty to clean, long milling times, and high power requirements (considerable energy is expended in moving and lifting the grinding media for grinding). However, the mill is very well suited for milling highly abrasive materials. Typical materials of mill construction include chrome manganese alloy and porcelain, both standard and high-density grades.

C. Hammer Mill

The hammer mill, which can be of either the horizontal- or the vertical-shaft type (Fig. 17), is one of the most versatile and widely used mills in the pharmaceutical industry. Intermediate (10 to 100 mesh) to fine (100 to <325 mesh) milling can be obtained with this mill, as well as coarse to thorough dispersion of powder mixes by simply changing hammer speeds and/or screen sizes and feed rates. Evaluation of this type of mill in the pharmaceutical industry is very limited, because the information is usually of a proprietary nature. Some data are available from mill manufacturers as to types of material milled, milling conditions, and results in terms of screen analysis and throughput rates; examples are given in Tables 3 and 4. These materials are usually pure compounds and do not include various types of tablet granulations.

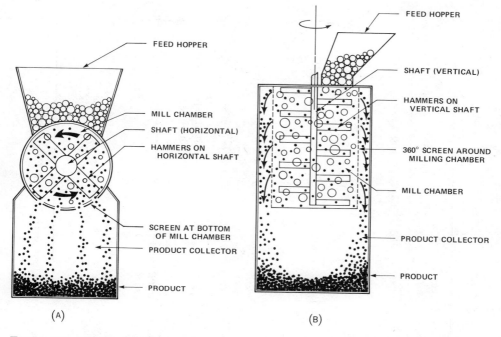

Figure 17. Schematic of two types of hammer mill. (A) Hammer mill with horizontal shaft, (B) hammer mill with vertical shaft.

    The principle of operation of the hammer mill is one of impact between rapidly moving hammers mounted on a rotor (Fig. 18) and the powder particles. The problem in design of the hammer mill is in presenting the particles to the hammers such that enough force is imparted to the particles to shatter them. This can be difficult, because the air currents created by the rotating hammers cause the powder particles to travel in the same direction as the hammers. Because of their low mass and the fluid drag forces, the particles seldom reach the velocity of the hammers, so some impact is achieved. One mill (Fig. 19)[*] is equipped with specially designed deflectors around the mill inner periphery, which alter the path of the traveling particles by deflecting them back into the path of the hammers.

    A much greater velocity differential between powder particles and hammers is achieved by deflectors, resulting in increased milling effectiveness. For the deflectors to work properly, there is apparently a critical clearance between the hammers and the deflectors: if the clearance is too great, the particles will not deflect, and if the clearance is too small, considerable heat may be developed during milling.

---

[*]Pulverizing Machinery, Mikopul Corporation, Subsidiary of United States Filter Corporation, Summit, New Jersey 07901.

Table 3

Commercial Milling Data

Material	Character	Remarks	Mill model	Hammers	Speed (rpm)	Screen	Grind	Output (lb hr^{-1})	Horse-power
Aspirin	Brittle, light	None	1SH	LFS	9,600	020HB	98.2% < 150 mesh 96.0% < 200 mesh	200	3
			1SI	Rigid, sharpened	986	1/8Rd.	53.4% < 110 mesh 22.0% < 60 mesh	2,140	Idle
Alginic acid	Fibrous, light, slightly hygroscopic	Runs hot	Bantam	FT	14,000	020Rd.	94.8% < 100 mesh	30	1/2
Ascorbic acid	Brittle, light	None	1SH	LFS-SS	8,000	035HB SS	2.4% < 100 mesh 16.2% < 200 mesh 81.4% < 325 mesh	667	3
Benzoic acid	Brittle, heavy	None	1SH	1/8 x 1 in.	8,000	3/64HB	99.7% < 30 mesh 82.5% < 100 mesh	860	–
Caffeine	Fibrous, light, soft	None	1SH	Lead-lined	3,000	1/4Rd.	99.3% < 40 mesh	425	Idle
Sugarcane	Brittle, heavy, free flowing	None	2TH	1/8 x 1 in.	1,750	020HB	88.7% < 40 mesh 51.2% < 60 mesh 35.5% < 100 mesh 19.8% < 200 mesh	2,400	3

Source: Courtesy Pulverizing Machinery Div., MikroPul Corporation, United States Filter Corporation, Summit, New Jersey 07901.

Table 4

Commercial Milling Data: Medium-Grade Sucrose

	Original	Run 1	Run 2	Run 3	Run 4
Milling variables					
Rpm		5,000	7,200	7,200	7,200
Screen hole size (in.)		0.020	0.020	0.010	0.012
Blade type		125	125	125	125
Forward		Impact	Impact	Impact	Impact
Feed size and type		S-throat	4 × 4	4 × 4	4 × 4
Feed setting no.		Gravity	3.0	3.0	1.0
Rotor amperes		-	12.0	16.0	11.0
Equipment model no.		DASO6[a]	VFS-DASO6	VFS-DASO6	VFS-DASO6
Sieve analysis (%) Mesh (U.S. Standard)					
>20	0.18	0	0	0	0
20-50	67.1	0	0	0	0
50-60	12.1	0	0	0	0
60-100	14.4	0	0	0	0
100-140	4.6	31.0	17.7	21.4	0
140-200	0.4	13.7	17.7	25.0	5.0
200-325	0.9	31.0	28.6	28.5	45.0
<325	0.09	24.1	36.8	25.0	50.0

[a] Fitzpatrick Mill model number.

Source: Courtesy Fitzpatrick Company, South Plainfield, New Jersey 07080.

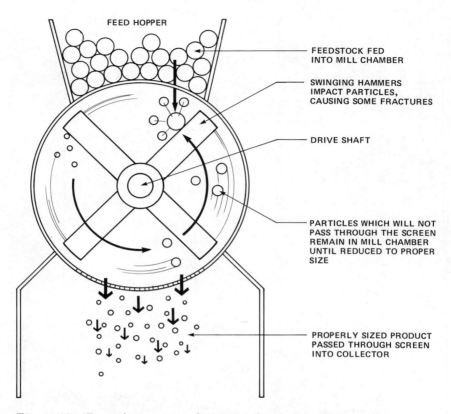

Figure 18. Particle impact and sizing in hammer mill.

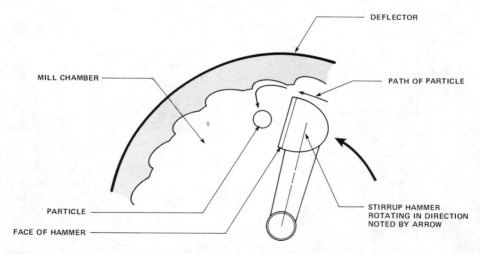

Figure 19. Hammer mill with deflector. (Courtesy Pulverizing Machinery, MikroPul Corp., Subsidiary of United States Filter Corporation, Summit, New Jersey 07901.)

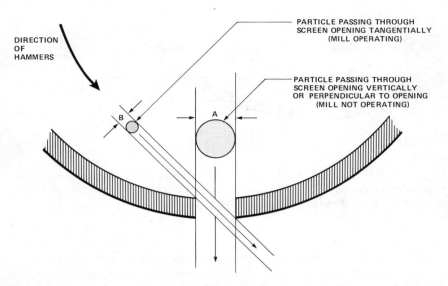

Figure 20. Effect of angle of exit through mill screen on size of exiting particle. A, diameter of screen opening; B, diameter of particle passing tangentially through screen while mill is operating. (Courtesy Fitzpatrick Company, Elmhurst, Illinois 60126.)

Another device used with the hammer mill is a screen placed over the milling chamber outlet (the bottom of the horizontal shaft mills and 360° around the vertical shaft mills). These screens serve to retain the larger particles in the milling chamber for further size reduction and also act in part as a classifier in allowing only certain-size (or smaller) particles to pass out of the milling zone into the collector. The screens do not act as sieves; one cannot expect the largest particle leaving the mill to be 20 mesh if the mill is fitted with the equivalent of a 20-mesh screen. This is due to the particle velocity and the angle at which it approaches and exits through the screen (Fig. 20).

Screen thickness is also a factor in the exiting particle size. If one assumes the same particle velocity for different screen thicknesses, Figure 21 illustrates the effect of screen thickness on particle size.

The screen is usually an integral part of the hammer mill in the pharmaceutical industry, and because of the large forces they are subjected to, they are usually not of the wire-woven type seen in hand screens and the oscillating granulator. The screen strength required for much of hammer milling is obtained by using sheet metal of various thicknesses with perforated holes or slots, as shown in Figure 22. The holes may range in size and open area (Table 5). The slots may also vary in size and pattern. Slot patterns often used are the herringbone or cross-slot configuration, also shown in Figure 22. Table 6 shows typical applications of various screen configurations.

Hammers may take several shapes, as shown in Figure 23. However, the two basic shapes are the stirrup and the bar, the bar-shaped hammers being used extensively in tablet granulating. The hammers are usually made of hardened steel, stainless steel, or a mild steel with impact surfaces made of an extremely abrasive

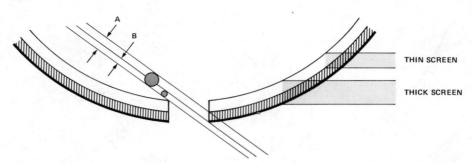

Figure 21. Effect of mill screen thickness on size of exiting particle. A, diameter of particle passing tangentially through opening in thin screen; B, diameter of particle passing tangentially through opening in thick screen.

resistant material such as haystellite (which has embedded carbaloy particles) or carbaloy. Most of the work in pharmaceuticals does not require the hardest alloy hammers; in most cases, stainless steel will suffice.

Hammers (Fig. 24) may also be free-swinging. The free-swinging hammer has the advantage or disadvantage of increasing hammer-to-screen clearance if excessive buildup occurs within the mill. This will minimize mill damage of the milled raw material fuses from heat, or it may decrease output rate if the material is extremely difficult to mill.

As mentioned previously, the hammers may be mounted on either a horizontal or a vertical shaft. Vertical-shaft mills, such as the Stokes Tornado* mill, have feed inlets at the top where powder enters the milling chamber perpendicular to the swing of the hammers. There is some tendency to segregate the powder or powder mix by size, because the smallest particles exit through the screen near the top, whereas the larger particles, which have more mass, have a tendency to fall to the bottom of the mill before complete dispersion through the screen. This is in contrast to having the powder feed tangential to the hammer swing, as found in the horizontal-shaft Micropulverizer** and Fitzpatrick† mills. Vertical-shaft mills, by virtue of the 360° surrounding screen, normally have higher throughput potential than does horizontal-shaft equipment, in which the screen is mounted at the mill chamber outlet.

There is also an air-swept hammer mill very similar to the ball mill depicted in Figure 15, where air is forced through the milling chamber, entraining and carrying the smaller particles out of the milling chamber. This air

*Sharples-Stokes, Division Pennwalt Corporation, Clark, New Jersey 07066.
**Pulverizing Machinery, Mikopul Corporation, Subsidiary of United States Filter Corporation, Summit, New Jersey 07901.
†Fitzpatrick Company, Elmhurst, Illinois 60126.

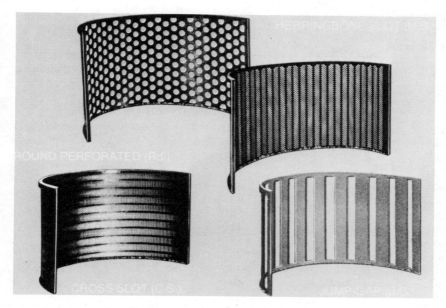

Figure 22. Different screen configurations. (Courtesy Pulverizing Machinery, Division of MikroPul, Subsidiary of United States Filter Corporation, Summit, New Jersey 07901.)

suspension of particles passes through a classifier, where the larger particles are further separated and recirculated back to the mill and the small particles are collected. This type of mill is particularly useful where a small uniform particle size is required with heat-sensitive materials (i.e., the circulating air cools the particles and the mill). This type of mill is normally used for the milling of non-heat-sensitive raw materials but is not commonly used in the preparation of tablets.

Maximum mill versatility is obtained by utilizing a hammer with a cutting blade on the trailing edge of the bar. With a simple mechanical manipulation, the cutting edge is available for use in the mill. In the case of the Fitzpatrick mill, the milling head is so designed that a 180° rotation exposes the cutting edge.

The particle size of a milled material is inversely proportional to the hammer speed, which may vary from 1000 to 20,000 ft min^{-1}, depending on hammer length and rpm. Changes in speed are accomplished by a variable-speed drive or by manually changing the hammer drive and motor pulley ratio.

The advantages of the hammer mill include:

1. Ease of setup, teardown, and cleanup
2. Minimum scale-up problems provided that the same type mill is used
3. Ease of installation
4. Wide range in size and type of feedstock that can be handled
5. Small space requirements

Table 5

Model D6 Screens

Number	Hole size (in.)	Open area (%)	Gage	Old number
		Round-hole screens[a]		
1532-0020	0.020	24	28	000
1532-0024	0.024	24	26	00
1532-0027	0.027	23	24	0
1532-0033	0.033	29	24	1
1532-0040	0.040	30	22	1A
1532-0050	0.050	33	22	1B
1531-0065	0.065	26	18	2
1531-0079	0.079	41	18	2AA
1531-0093	0.093	33	18	2A
1531-0109	0.109	45	18	2B
1531-0125	0.125	40	18	3
1531-0156	0.156	46	18	3AA
1531-0187	0.187	51	18	3A
1531-0218	0.218	45	18	3B
1531-0250	0.250	48	18	4
1531-0312	0.312	47	18	4A
1531-0375	0.375	51	18	4B
1531-0500	0.500	47	18	5
1531-0625	0.625	47	18	5A
1531-0750	0.750	51	18	6
1531-1000	1.000	58	18	7
		Square-hole screens		
1533-0200	0.200	64	18	15S
1533-0250	0.250	45	18	14S
1533-0312	0.312	51	18	516S
1533-0375	0.375	56	18	38S
1533-0437	0.437	64	18	716S
1533-0500	0.500	53	18	12S
1533-0625	0.625	59	18	58S
1533-0687	0.687	54	18	1116S
1533-0750	0.750	57	18	34S
1533-0875	0.875	68	18	78S
1533-1000	1.000	64	18	100S
1533-1125	1.125	53	18	1-18S
1533-1500	1.500	64	18	1-12S

(continued)

Table 5 (continued)

Mesh screens[b]

Number	Mesh size	Number	Mesh size
1536-0004	4	1536-0040	40
1536-0006	6	1536-0050	50
1536-0008	8	1536-0060	60
1536-0010	10	1536-0080	80
1536-0012	12	1536-0100	100
1536-0014	14	1536-0120	120
1536-0016	16	1536-0150	150
1536-0020	20	1536-0200	200
1536-0024	24	1536-0250	250
1536-0030	30	1536-0325	325

Special screens[c]

Number	Type of hole	Hole size (in.)	Open area (%)	Gage	Old number
1532-5001	Round	0.020	30	26 (18 BF)	N-000
1539-0018	Square	0.625	59	14	58S
1539-0019	Square	0.687	54	14	1116S
1539-0032	Square	0.875	68	14	78S
1539-0020	Square	1.000	64	14	100S
1539-0021	Square	1.125	53	14	118S
1539-0022	Square	1.500	64	14	112S
1539-0024	Square	1.000	64	12	100S
1539-0025	Square	1.125	53	12	1-18S
1539-0026	Square	1.500	64	12	1-12S

[a] The first six screens are mounted on 18-gage 18-hole backing frames.
[b] All mesh screens reinforced with suitable backing frames.
[c] All screens are of 18-8 stainless steel, except nickel material on screen 1532-5001.
Source: Courtesy The Fitzpatrick Company, Elmhurst, Illinois 60126.

The disadvantages include:

1. Potential clogging of screens
2. Heat buildup during milling, with possible product degradation
3. Mill and screen wear with abrasive materials

D. Cutting Mill

The use of cutting mills in tablet making is primarily for the dispersion of powder mixes, milling wet and dry granulations, and size reduction of tablet batches

Table 6

Applications of Various Mill Screen Configurations

Perforation shape	Recommended use	Comments
Round holes	Fibrous materials	Clogs more quickly; lower hole size limited because of structural strength
Herringbone slots	Amorphous and crystalline material	Slightly coarser grind than equal-diameter round perforation
Cross-slots	Amorphous and crystalline material	Same grind size as equal-size round perforation; finer slot size attainable than round perforations

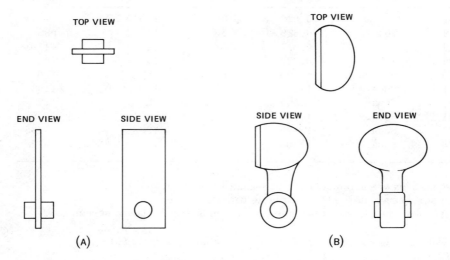

Figure 23. Two popular hammer mill hammer shapes. (A) Bar hammer, (B) stir-rup hammer.

requiring rework for one reason or another. This equipment is similar to the ham-mer mill because the cutters are usually on the trailing edge of the bar hammers. In some cases, hammers can easily be replaced with cutters, using the same shaft and milling chamber. The cutters are used with both woven and perforated-hole screens, and in some cases, as with soft, dry or wet granulations, size reduction or powder dispersion may not require a screen.

Although size reduction is primarily the result of shearing action, the same variations encountered with the hammer mill must be considered when using the

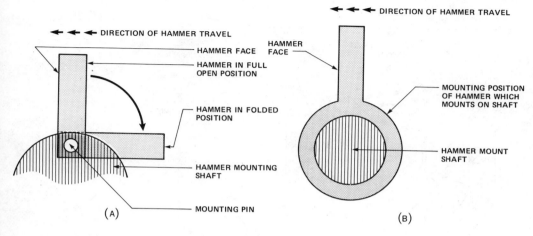

Figure 24. Swinging (A) and fixed (B) hammers.

cutting mill (i.e., size and size distribution of the feedstock, cutter speed, screen size and feed rate).

E. Oscillating Granulator

The oscillating granulator* (Fig. 25) is used in the pharmaceutical industry almost exclusively for the size reduction of wet and dry granulations, and to some extent for reducing tablets and compactions that must be recompressed. This equipment consists of an oscillating bar contacting a woven-wire screen. A hopper above the oscillator and screen provides a receptacle for the feedstock, which is forced through the screen by the oscillating motion of the bar. Size reduction is primarily by shear, with some attrition. Collection of the product may be directly onto trays in the case of wet granulations, or into drums via a sleeve from a specially fitted collector funnel that minimizes dust during the processing of a dry granulation. The oscillator speed is constant, whereas the screens, which are readily interchangeable, range in size from 4 to 20 mesh.

The outstanding characteristic of the oscillating granulator is the narrow size range and minimum amount of fines obtained during size reduction of a dry granulation, and the very uniform wet granulation size, which promotes uniform drying. The disadvantages of this equipment are the low throughput rates, wear on the screens, the possibility of product contamination by metal particles chipped away from the screen by the oscillator, and the fact that size reduction of large particles or granules (4 mesh or larger) must be done stepwise (i.e., passed through successively smaller screens until the desired granule size is obtained).

*Sharples-Stokes, Division Pennwalt Corporation, Clark, New Jersey 07066.

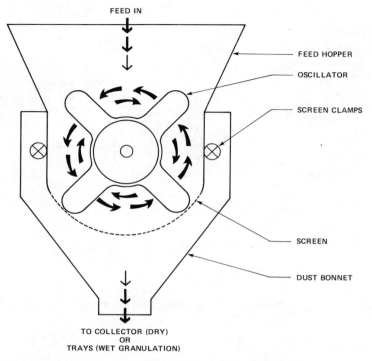

FEED IN

FEED HOPPER

OSCILLATOR

SCREEN CLAMPS

SCREEN

DUST BONNET

TO COLLECTOR (DRY)
OR
TRAYS (WET GRANULATION)

Figure 25. Schematic of oscillating granulator.

To illustrate the effect of different milling conditions, using a hammer and cutting mill and an oscillating granulator, an acetaminophen wet granulation was prepared using the following formula:

Acetaminophen	88%
Microcrystalline cellulose	10%
Polyvinylpyrrolidone (PVP)	2%
Deionized water	(q. s. to make a 7.5% PVP solution)

The wet granulation was not milled but spread on trays and dried to 1% moisture at 45°C.

Equal portions of the dry granulation were put through a Model D Fitzpatrick[*] Mill at the same feed rate under the following operating conditions:

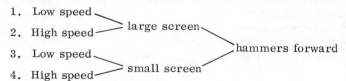

1. Low speed
2. High speed — large screen
3. Low speed
4. High speed — small screen — hammers forward

[*]Fitzpatrick Company, Elmhurst, Illinois 60126.

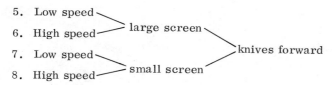

The same granulation was passed through a Stokes Oscillating Granulator* using a large screen (10 mesh woven wire) and then a small screen (14 mesh woven wire). A screen analysis was performed on each milled granulation and on the unmilled granulation using 12, 20, 30, 40, 70, and 140 U.S. Standard mesh screens. The screens were nested from the largest mesh opening (12 mesh) to the smallest, with a collector pan nested below the smallest screen (140 mesh). One hundred grams of sample was coned and quartered out of each mill sample and placed at the top of the nest of screens, each of which was preweighed. The nest of screens and the collector pan were mounted in the Rotap† screen shaker and allowed to shake for 15 min at which time the screens and collector pan were removed and individually weighed. The differences in weight were calculated and expressed as a percent of the total collected on each screen (i.e., amount collected less than 12 mesh but greater than 20 mesh) and plotted as shown in Figures 26 to 30.

In Figure 26, note that at low speed using the large screen, very little change in size distribution takes place when compared to the unmilled granulation (compare ϕ and 1). However, a change to a smaller screen reduces the granule size considerably (compare ϕ and 3). At high speed the screen size does not yield as big a change as that seen at low speed (compare 2 and 4). Mill speed changes using the large screen (compare 1 and 2) do not show as great an effect on the granule size distribution as that seen with the small screen (compare 3 and 4).

Figure 27 shows that the basic changes in granulation size distribution with screen size and mill speed are very similar to those seen with the hammer mill.

Using both large and small screens, Figure 28 illustrates that the hammer mill yields a smaller particle size than the cutting mill at high speeds. Note that except for the distribution obtained using knives forward with a small screen (No. 8), the size distributions are all very similar (nearly parallel lines) but differ in average particle size at high mill speed.

Screen size or mill type makes very little difference in granulation size distribution at low speeds, as shown in Figure 29.

Although reduced in size, Figure 30 shows that the screen sizes used did not make much difference in the size distribution of the acetaminophen granulation passed through the oscillating granulator.

Only the most general conclusions may be drawn from work of this type, because granulations with different characteristics will give differing results on the same equipment using the same milling conditions.

---

*Sharples Stokes, Division Pennwalt Corporation, Clark, New Jersey 07066.
†W. S. Tyler, Inc., Mentor, Ohio 44060.

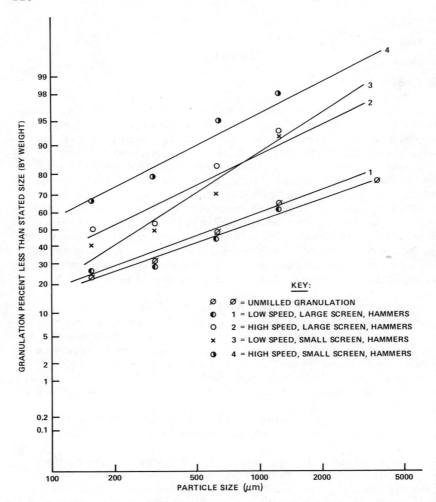

Figure 26. Effect of screen size and speed on acetaminophen granulation size distribution using a hammer mill.

F. Extruder

The extruder (Fig. 31) is considered here only because it is a means of uniformly sizing a wet granulation. The extruder is used primarily for continuous wet granulating. The dry, premixed powder and granulating solution are metered into the equipment, and the two components are mixed. The resulting mass is forced out of a series of small orifices. This yields a spaghetti-shaped mass that is easily broken up and may be dried on trays, in fluid-bed driers, in a continuous-belt drier, or in a drum-type drier.

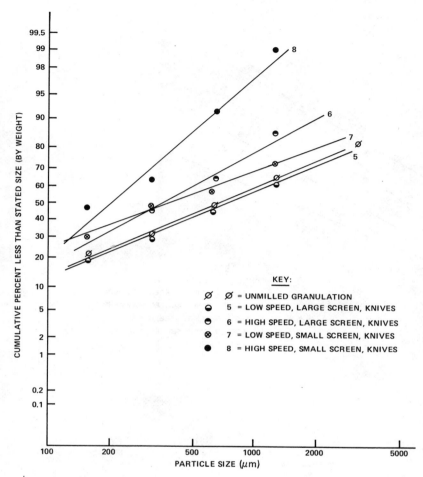

Figure 27. Effect of screen size and speed on acetaminophen granulation size distribution using a cutting mill.

G. Hand Screens

Hand screens, the forerunners of the oscillating granulator, are used in tablet making primarily for screen analysis of powder raw materials or granulations. They are also used in product development for size reduction of wet and dry granules on a small scale, and in the mixing of small amounts of powder ingredients. It should be noted that screens used in the manufacture of a granulation should not be used for screen analysis work, because forcing material through a screen alters the spacing of the woven wires. This leads to nonuniformity in size opening over the screen surface, which would lead to inaccurate screen analysis results.

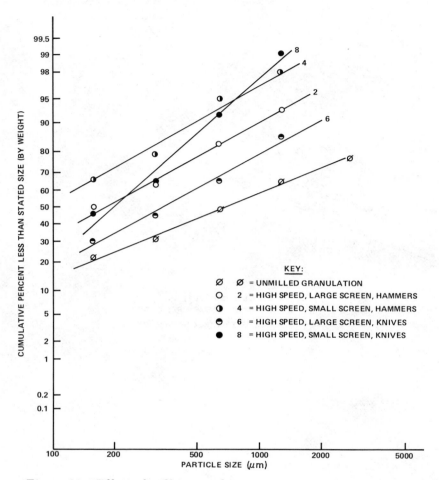

Figure 28. Effect of mill type and screen size on acetaminophen size distribution at high speed.

Hand screens are made of brass or, preferably, of stainless steel. They consist of a woven-wire cloth stretched in a circular or rectangular frame (Fig. 32), the upper portion of the frame being constructed high enough above the wire cloth to contain a dry or wet powder mass which is to be screened. Table 7 lists available mesh sizes and their corresponding openings in microns.

III. Powder Characterization

The effect of milling is evaluated by comparing the characteristics of a powder before and after milling. Even at the present level of mathematical and computer

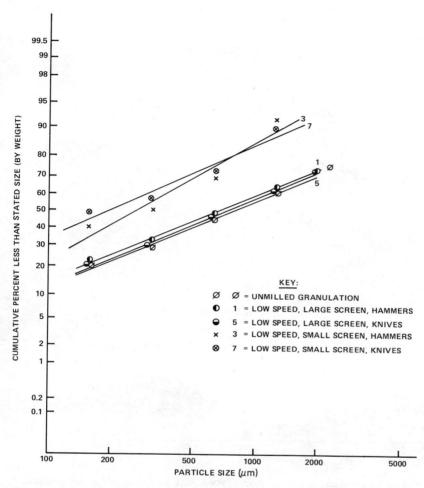

Figure 29. Effect of mill type and screen size on acetaminophen granulation size distribution at low speed.

sophistication, the basic properties of particles escape expression in a single precise mathematical term. As a result, it is necessary to treat these characterizing properties as separate and sometimes overlapping entitites. In order to discuss the characterization of powders and their constituent particles, the term "particle" is defined in the scope of this text as having:

1. Single- or multiple-ingredient composition
2. Homogeneous or heterogeneous mixture
3. Nonporous or porous structure
4. Approximate particle size range between 2000 μm (10 mesh) and 0.5 μm

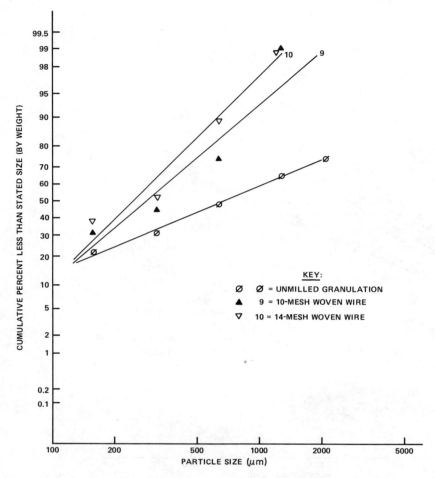

Figure 30. Effect of oscillating granulator screen size on acetaminophen granulation size distribution.

Powder composed of spherical or irregularly shaped particles of a single size or of a distribution of sizes is characterized by a number of parameters, including density, porosity, surface area, shape, and particle size and distribution.

A. Sampling

Characterizing a powdered or granular material, whether it is milled or unmilled, is heavily dependent upon the method of obtaining a sample from the bulk, since it must be representative of the entire lot or batch of material.

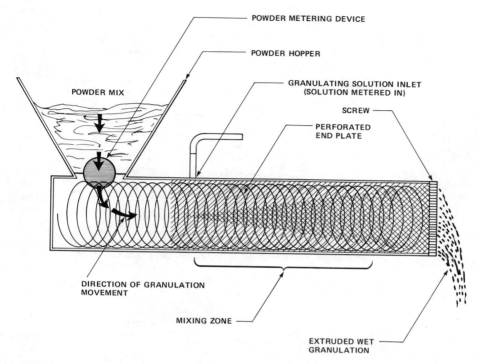

Figure 31. Schematic of extruder.

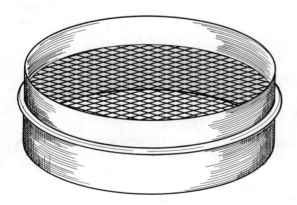

Figure 32. Hand screen.

Table 7

U.S. Standard Screen Sizes

U.S. Standard	Equivalent		Mesh openings	
	British standard	Tyler	in.	μm
325		(325)	0.0017	44
270	(300)	(270)	0.0021	53
230		(250)	0.0024	62
200		200	0.0029	74
170	170	170	0.0035	88
140	150	150	0.0041	105
120	120	115	0.0049	125
100			0.0059	149
80	85		0.0070	177
70	72		0.0083	210
60			0.0098	250
50			0.0117	297
45		42	0.0138	350
40			0.0165	420
35	30		0.0197	500
30		28	0.0232	590
25			0.0280	710
20			0.0331	840
18			0.0394	1000
16			0.0469	1190
14			0.0555	1410
12			0.0661	1680
10			0.0787	2000
8			0.0937	2380
7			0.111	2830
6			0.131	3360
5			0.157	4000
4			0.187	4760

Sampling small lots of material is fairly uncomplicated because the sample can simply be coned and quartered or riffled. Coning and quartering involve thorough premixing of the entire sample and then careful pouring of the sample into a pile, which usually forms a cone with a base angle referred to as the angle of repose of the powder. The cone is then divided into four approximately equal quarters (Fig. 33).

Two opposite quarters are combined and mixed well while the remaining two quarters are returned to the original container. This procedure is repeated at least four times, until the desired size sample is obtained. If four repeats cannot

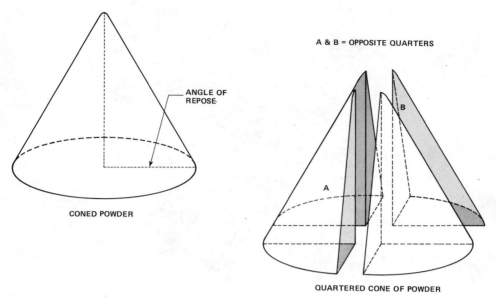

Figure 33. Coning and quartering.

be made because of a small sample size, the procedure is repeated using the material returned to the original container.

The second method is via the riffler, which is a mechanical splitting device, shown schematically in Figure 34. After each pass through the splitter, one or several portion(s) is (are) retained, depending on the number of portions developed by one pass through the riffler (this may vary from two to eight). The number of passes through the riffler will depend on the desired end sample size.

The two sampling methods described above may be satisfactory for batch sizes of powders or granules which can be manipulated on a benchtop; however, batches of hundreds or even thousands of kilograms require a different approach. Usually, unmilled, homogeneous raw material as received from the source is not blended before sampling for identification and purity. On the other hand, if physical characteristics such as bulk density and particle size distribution are a part of the initial testing or the powder is a heterogeneous mixture, representative sampling is essential.

One of the more common sampling instruments for sampling large bulks is the grain thief (Fig. 35). This instrument is made up of an inner and an outer tube, with matching openings along its length which can be closed off by rotating the inner and outer tubes to a point where the openings to the inner tube are covered.

The closed shaft is inserted vertically to the bottom of the drum and the inner tube is rotated to open the sampling chamber. The powder (theoretically) fills the thief chamber, the inner tube is rotated to close the sampling chamber, and the thief, with its sample, is withdrawn from the drum of powder. Although the

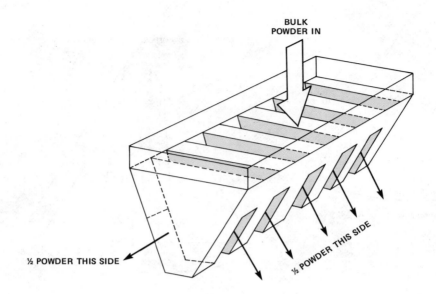

Figure 34. Schematic of powder riffler (splitter).

procedure appears to be simple, a number of problems may prevent a representative sampling:

1. The contents of the drum may have segregated on handling (small particles have sifted through the larger particles to the bottom of the drum). The contents of the lower sections of the drum may be packed material which will not flow freely, while the contents of the upper section may be the less packed, more free flowing larger particles. As the thief is opened for sampling, the larger, free-flowing particles enter from the top opening and flow down to the bottom of the thief. This prevents adequate sampling of the lower portion of the drum, thus biasing the particle size distribution.
2. The thief, when inserted into the powder, may carry a portion of the upper contents to the middle or lower sections of the drum, thus biasing the sample particle size distribution.
3. The thief may have to be moved to obtain a sample of packed powder. During movement, crystals or granules may be reduced in size, thus biasing the sample particles size distribution.
4. As the powder sample is emptied via the upper end of the thief by tipping it vertically, the smaller particles may become airborne because of the rapid powder flow and/or impact on the collecting surfaces. This dust or some fraction of the fine-particle segment of the particle size analysis is lost, and the analysis again becomes biased.

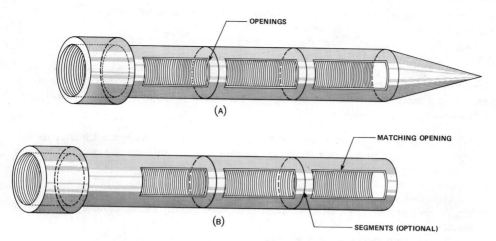

Figure 35. Grain thief. (A) Outer tube, (B) inner tube. The inner tube is inserted into the outer tube.

Several things may be done to minimize deviations that may take place during sampling with a thief:

1. To eliminate the top portion of sample from filling the lower end of the thief, use a segmented thief (i. e., each opening is a compartment separated by a divider in the inner tube). A segmented thief also minimizes dusting that occurs during pouring, because the sample must be removed by opening the sample chambers.
2. Use multiple samples from a drum which are mixed thoroughly to represent the drum contents. Coning and quartering can then be used to give the desired sample size.
3. Run duplicate particle size analyses. Usually, agreement of two or more analyses indicates satisfactory sampling. However, this does not mean that the sample may not be biased. The person taking the sample must make macro observations for obvious size separation.
4. There is no substitute for care during the sampling procedure and while handling the sample(s).

A second sampling method, which is used quite frequently but is totally unacceptable when sampling for physical characterization, is done by removing the cover from each container and taking a scoop of powder from the top of the contents. The pitfalls of this method are obvious, and the method should be avoided. For continuous processes where granulation must be sampled, timed mechanical devices are used to sample at one convenient point in the process, such as when a conveyor is carrying granulation from a drying oven or at the exit from a

continuous blender. In essence, particle size analysis data are only as representative as the sample being studied.

For sampling large bulk batches, the following methods may be used, listed in
order from the best to the worst in terms of obtaining a representative sample.
Experience dictates that one can never be certain of the container-to-container or
overall uniformity of size distribution of a powder material received from a vendor, or as a powder is collected in containers from a mill and/or handled in tran-
sit from one place to another:

1. Blend the entire batch and remove two or more samples from the blender using
   a grain thief sampler. Mix the samples thoroughly and cone and quarter to the
   desired sample size.
2. If the batch is too large to blend as one unit, select $\sqrt{n + 1}$ (where n is the
   total number of containers in the lot being tested as suggested in the Military
   Standards [20]) containers at random and blend them. Thief-sample from the
   blender as in method 1 above.
3. One may also proceed as in methods 1 and 2 above, but return the blend to the
   containers and thief-sample these containers.
4. Thief-sample all containers with no blending.
5. Select $\sqrt{n + 1}$ containers at random, and thief-sample them with no blending.

B. Density and Porosity

Density is the weight/volume ratio of a substance, expressed in g cm^{-3} or lb ft^{-3}.
For powders of pharmaceutical interest, several different densities can be manipulated to give useful information about a powder and its constituent particles.

First, the true or absolute density is the weight/volume ratio of only the solid
portion of the powder particles. True density is determined by degassing (vacuum) an accurately weighed sample of the powder in a container of known volume
and emitting a fluid that wets but does not dissolve the powder. In this way, the
void spaces around the powder particles, particularly irregularly shaped particles,
can be measured. The volume determination of the powder particles is shown
schematically in Figure 36.

The calculation is straightforward:

$$\rho_t = \frac{W}{V_c - V_{cs}}$$

where

ρ_t	= true density
W	= weight of the powder sample
V_c	= volume of container
V_{cs}	= volume of container less the volume of the powder sample
$V_c - V_{cs}$	= volume of powder particles

Since very few substances completely lack void spaces, the pharmacist usually
deals with powder particles and granules that have varying degrees of internal
porosity which cannot be easily measured and usually are not used in characterizing powder particles or granules in quality control.

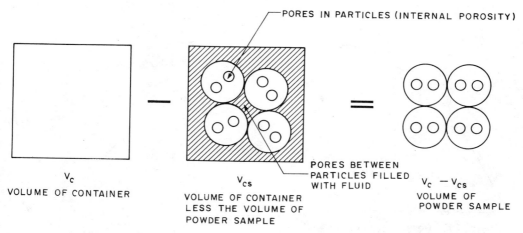

Figure 36. True density volume of a sample of known weight.

The most common method of accurately determining the volume of the solids in true density determinations is by weighing the fluid occupying the void space around the powder particles at a specific temperature and calculating its volume via the density formula

$$\text{Volume of fluid} = \frac{\text{weight of fluid}}{\text{density of fluid}}$$

We will illustrate this method using a modified ASTM density procedure [21].

A container known as a pycnometer (Fig. 37) with a known volume is accurately weighed:

Weight of pycnometer = 22.000 g

The pycnometer is filled with water at 25° C and accurately weighed (assume that the water will not solubilize the powder sample):

Weight of pycnometer + water = 42.000 g

The pycnometer is emptied and dried and a water-insoluble powder sample is added and an accurate weight is taken:

Weight of pycnometer + sample = 26.000 g

Water is added to the pycnometer containing the powder sample, and another accurate weight is taken:

Weight of pycnometer + sample + water at 25° C = 48.000 g.

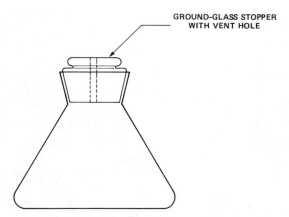

Figure 37. Powder pycnometer.

The density calculation is as follows:

Weight of water at 25°C = b - a = 42.000 g - 22.000 g = 20.000 g

Weight of sample at 25°C = c - a = 25.000 g - 22.000 g = 3.000 g

Weight of sample + water at 25°C = d - a = 47.000 g - 22.000 g = 25.000 g

Weight of water displaced by sample = g - e - f = 25.000 - 20.000 - 3.000
    = 2.000 g

$$\text{Volume of sample} = \frac{\text{weight of water displaced}}{\text{density of water at 25°C}}$$

$$= \frac{2.000 \text{ g}}{0.99707 \text{ g cm}^{-3}} = 2.006 \text{ cm}^3$$

$$\text{"True" density} = \frac{3.000 \text{ g}}{2.006 \text{ cm}^3} = 1.496 \text{ g cm}^{-3}$$

The second density term is the bulk density, or the ratio of the weight of a powder to the volume it occupies expressed in the same terms as the true density. This density term accounts not only for the volume of the solid portion of the particles (true density) and the voids within each particle (internal porosity), but also for the voids between the particles. Because of its dependence on particle packing, the bulk density should be reported at a particular packing condition. For example, the poured bulk density of a powder sample is determined by taking 50 g of the powder and gently pouring it into a 100-ml graduated cylinder and recording the volume. The packed bulk density may be determined by dropping the graduated cylinder containing the poured 50-g sample three times at 1-sec intervals through a distance of 1.90 cm [22]. The packing may be extended by tapping any number of times until the volume ceases to change. This is shown schematically in Figure 38.

$$\text{BULK DENSITY} = \frac{\text{SAMPLE WEIGHT}}{\text{SAMPLE VOLUME}} = \rho b = \frac{W}{V}$$

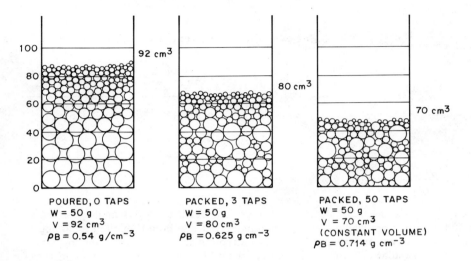

POURED, 0 TAPS
W = 50 g
V = 92 cm^3
ρB = 0.54 g/cm^{-3}

PACKED, 3 TAPS
W = 50 g
V = 80 cm^3
ρB = 0.625 g cm^{-3}

PACKED, 50 TAPS
W = 50 g
V = 70 cm^3
(CONSTANT VOLUME)
ρB = 0.714 g cm^{-3}

Figure 38. Bulk density volume.

Bulk density is very important in determining the size of containers needed for handling, shipping, and storage of raw material and granulation. It is also important in sizing hoppers and receivers for milling equipment and for sizing blending equipment in the scale-up to pilot and to commercial production.

Porosity is the measure of void spaces within a powder and can be calculated by manipulating the true and bulk densities. For example, using the densities determined above, porosities can be calculated by subtracting the reciprocal of the true density from that of the bulk density

Reciprocal $(1/\rho)$

ρ_b = bulk density = 0.498 g cm^{-3} =   2.008 cm^3 g^{-1}

ρ_t = true density = 0.722 g cm^{-3} =   1.385 cm^3 g^{-1}

Volume difference or porosity   =   0.623 cm^3 g^{-1}

The porosity may also be expressed in percent void space:

$$\% \text{ Voids} = \frac{0.623}{2.008} \times 100 = 31.0\%$$

Reciprocals $1/\rho$ (From Fig. 38)

	Poured	3 Taps	50 Taps constant volume
$\dfrac{1}{\text{Bulk density}}$	$= 1.852 \text{ cm}^3 \text{ g}^{-1}$	$1.600 \text{ cm}^3 \text{ g}^{-1}$	$1.400 \text{ cm}^3 \text{ g}^{-1}$
$\dfrac{1}{\text{True density}}$	$= 1.385 \text{ cm}^3 \text{ g}^{-1}$	$1.385 \text{ cm}^3 \text{ g}^{-1}$	$1.385 \text{ cm}^3 \text{ g}^{-1}$
Porosity $1/\rho_b - 1/\rho_t$	$0.467 \text{ cm}^3 \text{ g}^{-1}$	$0.215 \text{ cm}^3 \text{ g}^{-1}$	$0.015 \text{ cm}^3 \text{ g}^{-1}$
% Void space $\dfrac{1/\rho_b - 1/\rho_t}{1/\rho_b} \times 100 =$	25.2	13.4	1.1

The porosity of a powder indicates the type of packing a powder undergoes when subjected to vibration; when stored; when being fed into tablet machine feed hoppers or feed frames; and when being emptied from drums, tote bins, or hoppers. A powder or granulation with more void spaces will have a greater change of flowing freely than will a densely packed, low-porosity powder.

Milling may affect the density of a powder in several ways:

Bulk Density Decrease: Powder particle size has been reduced and more air is adsorbed onto the surface of each particle, yielding a high porosity (loose packing). Very small particle size powders, by virtue of their size, may not flow, even though their porosity is high because of adsorbed moisture and/or van der Waals forces, which may act to agglomerate the powder particles.

Bulk Density Increase: Powder particle size distribution has been changed such that smaller particles filter into the interstices created by the orientation of the large particles.

True Density Increase: This may occur when the internal porosity has been minimized as a result of reducing the powder particle size.

True Density--No Change: Powder particles essentially lack internal porosity and size reduction has no effect on true density.

C. Surface Area

The effectiveness and efficiency of a size reduction operation is measured by the change in a powder's particle size distribution and/or the corresponding change in its surface area. As the particle size distribution shifts to the smaller size range, the surface area increases as a result of the new surface created.

Surface area may be calculated from particle size distribution data, assuming that the particles are spherical. In this manner, calculations can be made using only one dimension, the diameter of the particle. For example, assume that a powder is composed of spheres of three different diameters, having a certain number of particles at each diameter. Given that the surface area of a sphere $= 4\pi r^2$, the number of particles at each stated size, the surface area for each size and for the total number of particles of each size is as follows:

Diameter		Surface area per particle (cm^2)	Number of particles at the stated diameter in 1 g of powder	Total surface area for all particles (cm^2)
μm	cm			
20	2×10^{-3}	1.26×10^{-5}	100	1.26×10^{-3}
40	4×10^{-3}	5.03×10^{-5}	200	10.05×10^{-3}
60	6×10^{-3}	1.13×10^{-4}	300	33.93×10^{-3}
	Total powder particles/gram of powder =		600	45.24×10^{-3}

The sum of the surface areas = the total calculated surface area for 1 g of powder, or 45.24×10^{-3} cm^2.

Problems arise when the particles are irregular in shape rather than spherical, because the calculation now becomes an estimate the accuracy of which depends on how closely the particle shape approaches that of a sphere. Unfortunately, spherical particles are the exception rather than the rule.

Surface area may be measured by a number of methods. Probably the most popular technique is the Brünauer-Emmett-Teller or BET method, which measures specific surface area by the volume of nitrogen adsorbed as a monomolecular layer on the surface of a unit mass of powder [23-26].

Referring to Figure 39, the basic steps in determining surface area by the BET method include:

1. Determining the volume of each section of the apparatus by filling it with known volume of gas at a known pressure.
2. Pretreating the sample by degassing it. More rapid degassing may be accomplished if thermal stability of the sample permits heating to above 100°C.
3. The sample in its container L of known volume (to value A) is attached to the apparatus, immersed in a liquid-nitrogen bath, and degassed (the temperature dependence of the method dictates that the system be maintained at liquid-nitrogen temperature in the Dewar flask, 0).
4. The adsorption isotherm (constant-temperature conditions) is determined by introducing clean, dry nitrogen in small increments and recording the pressure as each equilibrium point is reached. Since the volumes of both the sample and the container are known, any difference in pressure is a measure of the number of molecules adsorbed on the sample surface per the ideal-gas law:

$$\text{Number of molecules} = \frac{\text{(volume) (change in pressure) (Avogadro's number)}}{\text{(gas constant) (absolute temperature)}}$$

or

$$n = \frac{V \times \Delta P \times 6.23 \times 10^{23}}{0.082 \times T}$$

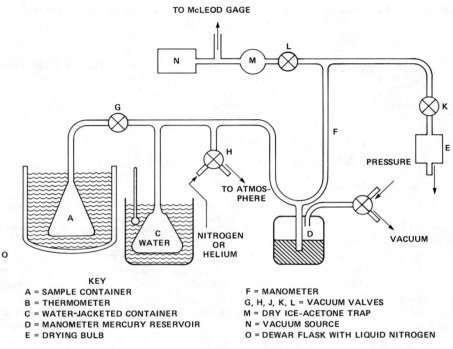

TO McLEOD GAGE

KEY

A = SAMPLE CONTAINER
B = THERMOMETER
C = WATER-JACKETED CONTAINER
D = MANOMETER MERCURY RESERVOIR
E = DRYING BULB

F = MANOMETER
G, H, J, K, L = VACUUM VALVES
M = DRY ICE-ACETONE TRAP
N = VACUUM SOURCE
O = DEWAR FLASK WITH LIQUID NITROGEN

Figure 39. Schematic of Emmet-type setup for BET surface-area determination (Adapted from Herdan, G., Small Particle Statistics, Academic Press, New York, N.Y.)

where

$$V = \text{volume, liters}$$
$$P = \text{pressure, atm}$$
$$\text{gas constant} = 0.082, \text{ liter atm mol}^{-1} \text{ deg}^{-1}$$

5. Each of these points are plotted as shown in Figure 40, and the linear portion of the line is extrapolated to the y axis, which is a measure of the number of molecules adsorbed as a monolayer on the sample surface.

The cross-sectional area of a nitrogen molecule is 16×10^{-16} cm^2. This constant, multiplied by the number of molecules in the monolayer, is a measure of the surface area of the sample and, divided by the number of grams in the sample, yields the specific surface area or surface area per gram.

For example, if the line in Figure 40 is extrapolated to point y (25×10^{20} molecules) for a 2.2-g sample, the surface area would be

$$\frac{(25 \times 10^{20}) (16 \times 10^{-16} \text{ cm}^2)}{2.2 \text{ g}}$$

or

$$1.82 \times 10^6 \text{ cm}^2 \text{ g}^{-1} \quad \text{(specific surface area)}$$

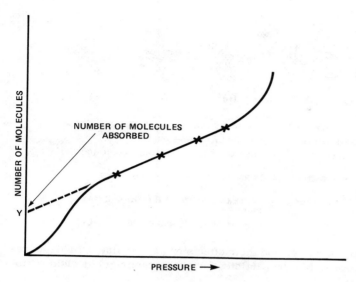

Figure 40. Example of BET absorption isotherm. (Adapted from Carstensen, J. T., Pharmaceuticals of Solids and Solid Dosage Forms, John Wiley & Sons, New York, N.Y., 1977.)

Table 8

Average Griseofulvin Blood Levels[a] in Humans as a Function of Specific Surface Area

Specific surface area (m^2 g^{-1})	Dose (g)	Fourth-hour blood levels (μg ml^{-1}) (suspension dosage form)
0.41	0.5	0.70
1.56	0.5	1.60

[a]Average of 6 to 12 subjects per group.
From: Atkinson, et al., Antibiotics of Chemotherapy 12 232 (1962).

The advantage of using surface-area measurement is the exactness with which milling effectiveness can be measured, particularly in the milling of small-particle-size raw materials. Surface-area measurement normally is not used to evaluate the milling of tablet granulations, although it can be.

Surface-area data are useful, because the surface area may be the cause of dissolution-rate differences in milled lots of raw materials and subsequently have a significant effect on the absorption rate of an active ingredient, as shown in Table 8 [27].

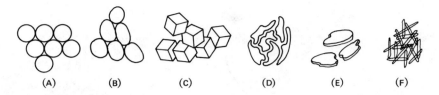

(A)   (B)   (C)   (D)   (E)   (F)

(A) SPHERICAL PARTICLES	— NORMALLY FLOWS EASILY
(B) OBLONG SHAPES WITH SMOOTH EDGES	— NORMALLY FLOWS EASILY
(C) EQUIDIMENSIONALLY SHAPED SHARP EDGES SUCH AS CUBES	— DOES NOT FLOW AS READILY AS (A) OR (B)
(D) IRREGULARLY SHAPED INTERLOCKING PARTICLES	— NORMALLY SHOWS POOR FLOW AND BRIDGES EASILY
(E) IRREGULARLY SHAPED TWO DIMENSIONAL PARTICLES SUCH AS FLAKES	— NORMALLY SHOWS FAIR FLOW AND MAY BRIDGE
(F) FIBROUS PARTICLES	— VERY POOR FLOW AND BRIDGES EASILY

Figure 41. General particle shapes and their effects on powder flow. Bridging refers to the stoppage of powder flow by particles forming a semirigid or rigid structure within the powder bulk.

The big disadvantage in evaluating milled raw materials and granulations by surface-area measurement is the care and lengthy time involved in evaluating each sample.

D.   Particle Shape and Dimension

The first step in characterizing a powder by shape and size is an examination of the units that make up the powder. In the case of granules and powder particles greater than 40-60 mesh, a macroscopic observation reveals the shape of the particle. Below 60 mesh (250 μm) it is necessary to observe particle shape through a microscope. This is done by dispersing a small amount of powder sample in a mineral oil or other liquid medium in which the particles are easily wetted and not solubilized. A drop of this slurry is placed on a slide with a coverslip. The slide is mounted on the microscope stage and the field is scanned with a magnification between 20 and 200 x, depending on the size range of the particles in the sample.

Figure 41 illustrates several general particle shapes and how they contribute to powder flow in general. The generalizations in Figure 41 pertain to powder particles greater than 200 mesh (74 μm), because surface characteristics such as static charge and adsorbed moisture usually overshadow the particle shape effect on powder flow characteristics below this size.

Particle shape also plays an important role in particle size analysis. Spherical particles are ideal not only for surface-area calculations but also for measuring particle size and size distribution. However, since irregular particle shape is the rule, the single diameter dimension that amply describes a sphere's size which

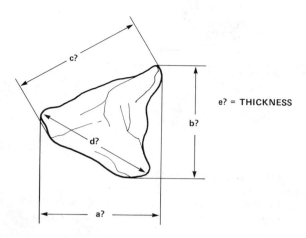

Figure 42. Particle dimension possibilities.

must be defined when sizing particles in a single plane (e.g., observation of particles through a microscope or by microprojection). For example, a number of
possible particle diameters may be used to size the particle in Figure 42.

A number of approaches have been used to solve this dilemma:

1. Volume of the Equivalent Sphere: The volume of the particle is determined by
   displacement of a liquid, and the diameter of an equivalent sphere is calculated:

$$d = \sqrt[3]{\frac{6V}{\pi}}$$

This method cannot be used per se but is the principle on which the stream
scanning, electrical resistant particle counter is based (see Sec. III.E).

2. Projected Area of an Equivalent Circle: Particles of a powder sample are
   projected down onto a white working surface or are photographed and enlarged.
   The area is measured with a planimeter and the equivalent circle diameter is
   calculated:

$$d = \sqrt{\frac{4A}{\pi}}$$

This method is time consuming when measuring hundreds of particles, but is
the principle on which stream scanning, light obstruction, electronic particle
counting equipment is based (see Section III.E).

3. Statistical Particle Diameters: For counting particles by microscopic observation, microprojection, or from photomicrographs, two statistical approaches
   to dimensioning irregularly shaped particles are used, known as Feret's and
   Martin's diameter. The use of Feret's and Martin's diameters fixes the

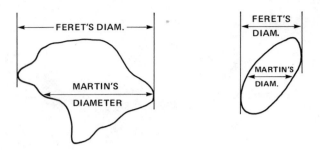

Figure 43. Statistical diameters. Martin's diameter is the mean length of the line parallel to the direction of measurement that bisects the particle and terminates at the particle boundaries. Ferret's diameter is the mean length of the line parallel to the direction of measurement that terminates at the two tangents to the outermost boundaries of the particle.

direction in which the particle is measured regardless of its orientation [25] in the microscopic field, as shown in Figure 43. The significance of measuring particle diameter by this method will be discussed later in the chapter.

E. Particle Size Analysis

From a practical point of view, particle size distribution change is more easily visualized, and is the physical measurement of choice in characterizing unmilled and milled raw materials, powder mixtures, and granulations in tablet making. Particle size analysis is the means by which the change in size distribution of powder particles is determined as a result of milling. For purposes of tablet making, it can be divided into two ranges (the exact cutoff points are arbitrary):

1. Subsieve size range: 100 μm (140 mesh) or below
2. Sieve size range: 44 μm (200 mesh) or larger

Although there is an area of overlap, each particle size range requires different methods of analysis, but both ranges use essentially the same mathematics to characterize the size distribution. The basic steps in performing a particle size analysis include:

1. Sampling the material to be analyzed (discussed earlier in the chapter)
2. Preparing the sample for analysis (see the discussion in Sec. IV)
3. Generating the data
4. Treatment and presentation of the data

F. Particle Size Statistics

In generating the data, individual particles or groups of particles from each sample are sized and counted. The sizing and counting follow a particular pattern in

Table 9

Microscopic Count Data

Class interval (μm)	Mean of the class interval (μm)	Number of particles counted in each class interval
0–5	2.5	96
5–10	7.5	105
10–15	12.5	116
15–20	17.5	129
20–25	22.5	150
25–30	27.5	212
30–35	32.5	148
35–40	37.5	127
40–45	42.5	114
45–50	47.5	101
50–55	52.5	92
55–60	57.5	88

order to put the data into an orderly, meaningful form that can be statistically analyzed for interpretive and comparative purposes. For example, it will be assumed that initial microscopic observation of a sample reveals a size range between 0.5 and 60 μm. To begin the statistics, this range is divided into convenient equal parts known as class intervals and the mean of each class interval
is determined. For convenience of calculation, the lower limit of the first class
interval is assumed to be zero. The particles are sized, counted, and tallied
under their proper class interval, as shown in Table 9.

For statistical calculation, all the particles counted in each class interval are
assumed to be equal to the mean of their respective class interval. These data
can now be put into bar graph or histogram form, as shown in Figure 44. If the
means of each class interval are connected by a smooth line, a distribution curve
results, as shown in Figure 45. This frequency curve is bell-shaped and is known
as a Gaussian curve if symmetrical. The sample represented by the curve is said
to have a Gaussian distribution. To normalize the data, the percentage of particles can be calculated in each class interval (Table 9), added cumulatively, and
plotted to give the number distribution curve seen in Figure 46.

The cumulative percent as plotted in this graph is interpreted as the percent
of the number of particles that are less than the stated size. For example, in
Table 10, 99.4% of all the particles are less than 57.5 μm, and 50% of the particles are less than 28 μm in diameter (assume the particles to be spherical).
Note that this curve is typically S-shaped. If these data are plotted on probability paper as shown in Figure 47, a straight line can usually be drawn if the distribution has a relatively narrow size range. This would be characteristic of the
milling of soft granules and more-friable raw materials. These materials are
said to have a "normal" distribution.

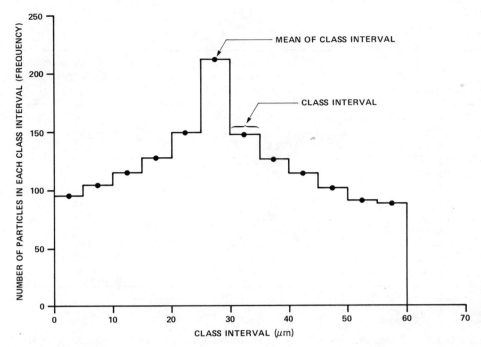

Figure 44. Histogram.

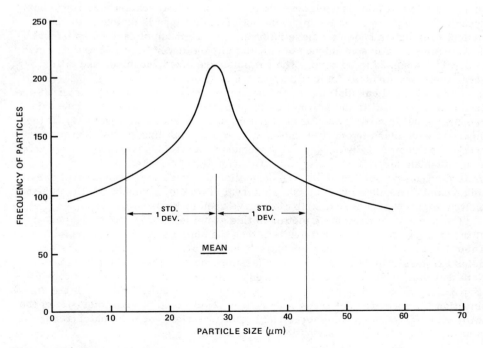

Figure 45. Frequency curve.

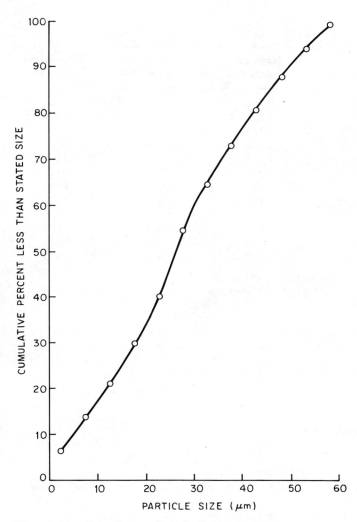

Figure 46. Cumulative distribution curve.

The 50% point on this normal probability plot approximates the arithmetic mean or average particle size of the sample (Table 11). A second very important term is used in combination with the mean to describe the scatter or dispersion around the mean. This term is the "standard deviation," which can be approximated graphically by taking the 16 and 84% points on the line, which come out to be 10.7 and 44.8 μm, respectively [25]. By subtracting the size at 50% from the size at 84% (28 - 10.7 - 17.3 μm), or subtracting the size at 16% from the size at 50%

Table 10

Calculations of Cumulative Percent

Class interval (μm)	Mean (μm)	Number of particles	Percentage of particles	Cumulative percent
0–5	2.5	96	6.5	6.5
5–10	7.5	105	7.1	13.6
10–15	12.5	116	7.8	21.4
15–20	17.5	129	8.7	30.1
20–25	22.5	150	10.1	40.2
25–30	27.5	212	14.3	54.5
30–35	32.5	148	10.0	64.5
35–40	37.5	127	8.6	73.1
40–45	42.5	114	7.7	80.8
45–50	47.5	101	6.8	87.6
50–55	52.5	92	6.2	93.8
55–60	57.5	88	5.6	99.4

Total = N = 1478

(44.8 - 28 = 16.8 μm) the standard deviation is approximated. The standard deviation is also illustrated on the frequency curve in Figure 45 to better show the range covered by this term. The standard deviation and the mean can also be determined more accurately by calculations using the following equations:

$$\overline{X}_a = \frac{\Sigma n_i X_i}{N}$$

where

$\overline{X}_a$ = arithmetic mean or average particle size

n_i = frequency or number of particles in each class interval in the series
   $n_1 + n_2 + n_3 + n_4 + \cdots + n_i$

X_i = mean of each class interval in the series $X_1 + X_2 + X_3 + X_4 + \cdots + X_i$

N = total number of particles in the distribution

Σ = summation

$$S_a = \sqrt{\frac{\Sigma n_i X_i^2 - (\Sigma n_i X_i)^2/N}{N - 1}}$$

where S_a is the arithmetic standard deviation.

The following is an example of the calculation of the mean and standard deviation of the data plotted in Figure 47 (from Table 11).

$$\overline{X}_a = \frac{43,046}{1478} = 29.1 \ \mu m$$

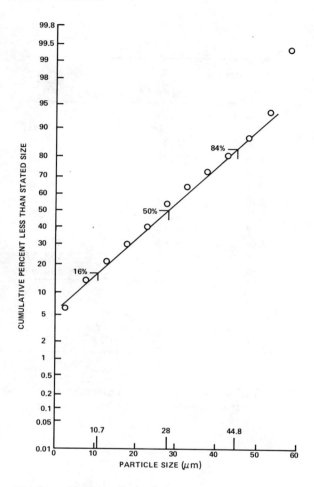

Figure 47. Normal–probability plot.

$$S_a = \sqrt{\frac{1,613,655 - (43,046)^2/1478}{1478 - 1}} = 15.6 \ \mu m$$

If the distribution has a wide range in size, the data should be plotted on log probability paper, which will usually straighten out the S curve obtained on arithmetic paper (a wide distribution range is more convenient to plot on log probability paper because of the range attainable with the log scale). This is known as a log–normal distribution and is typical of results seen from the milling of hard granules and less–friable raw materials.

Empirical data from numerous milling studies show that milled materials fit a log–normal distribution as a rule rather than a normal distribution. Therefore, the calculations that describe the log–normal distribution are important in particle

Table 11

Calculation of the Arithmetic Mean

Class interval (μm)	Mean of class interval, X_i (μm)	Frequency, n_i	$n_i X_i$	$n_i X_i^2$
0–5	2.5	96	240	600
5–10	7.5	105	788	5,910
10–15	12.5	116	1,450	18,125
15–20	17.5	129	2,258	39,515
20–25	22.5	150	3,375	75,938
25–30	27.5	212	5,830	160,325
30–35	32.5	148	4,810	156,325
35–40	37.5	127	4,762	178,575
40–45	42.5	114	4,845	205,912
45–50	47.5	101	4,798	227,905
50–55	52.5	92	4,830	253,575
55–60	57.5	88	5,060	290,950

$$\Sigma\, n_i = N = 1,478$$

$$\Sigma\, n_i X_i = 43,046$$

$$\Sigma\, n_i X_i^2 = 1,613,655$$

size analysis. The difference in the normal and log-normal size distribution means is shown in Table 12 with the data obtained from a material that was ball-milled. The equation for the geometric mean $\overline{X}_g$ is

$$\log \overline{X}_g = \frac{\Sigma\, n_i \log X_i}{N}$$

$$= \frac{10,712}{15,656} = 0.6842$$

$$\overline{X}_g = \text{antilog } 0.6842 = 4.83 \ \mu m$$

The arithmetic mean $\overline{X}_a$ for these same data is then calculated:

$$\overline{X}_a = \frac{\Sigma\, n_i X_i}{N} = \frac{80,906}{15,656} = 5.17 \ \mu m$$

The geometric mean is always smaller than the arithmetic mean. The geometric standard deviation S_g may be calculated from the plot of Table 12 data in Figure 48, using the equation

$$S_g = \frac{50\% \text{ point}}{16\% \text{ point}} = \frac{84\% \text{ point}}{50\% \text{ point}} = \frac{5.9}{3.8} = 1.55 \ \mu m$$

Table 12

Particle Size Data from Ball-Milled Material

Class interval (μm)	Mean of class interval, X_i (μm)	Log X_i	Frequency, n_i	$n_i X_i$	n_i log X_i	Percent by weight	Cumulative percent
1–3	2	0.301	1,097	2,194	330	7.00	7.00
3–5	4	0.602	7,365	29,460	4,434	47.00	54.00
5–7	6	0.778	5,014	30,084	3,901	32.00	86.00
7–9	8	0.903	1,567	12,536	1,415	10.00	96.00
9–11	10	1.000	423	4,230	423	2.70	98.70
11–13	12	1.079	141	1,692	152	0.90	99.60
13–15	14	1.146	39	546	45	0.25	99.85
15–17	16	1.204	8	128	10	0.05	99.90
17–19	18	1.255	2	36	2	0.01	99.99

$$\Sigma\, n_i = N = 15{,}656$$

$$\Sigma\, n_i X_i = 80{,}906$$

$$\Sigma\, n_i \log X_i = 10{,}712$$

Except for the ball-milling data above, the examples depicting the basic statistics have been based on the count or numbers of particles in each class interval. It is more convenient and meaningful if these data are converted to a distribution based on the particle surface area or the volume or weight of the particle.

Particle size distribution by number may be converted to a distribution by surface or by volume by assuming that all the particles are spherical and calculating the total surface or volume in each class interval. Cumulative surface or volume percentages are calculated and plotted against the mean of the corresponding class interval. The plots of these three distributions in Figure 49 show the differences between the means. It must be noted, however, that the conversion from number to surface or volume distribution is an approximation if the particles are not spherical. This estimate should be used only for comparisons of the same milled material, because it is particle-shape-dependent.

Table 13 is a tabulation of the various means or average particle sizes that can be calculated from their corresponding mathematical equations.

A comparison of the means calculated from the data in Table 10 is shown in Tables 14 and 15.

The deviations of the various particle size means are not presented in this chapter, but the reader may review them in texts by Herdan [25] and Cadle [28].

As discussed above, different average particle sizes based on number, weight, and so on, can be obtained from a single powder sample. Table 16 lists the more common methods of counting particles and the average particle size obtained from the current data.

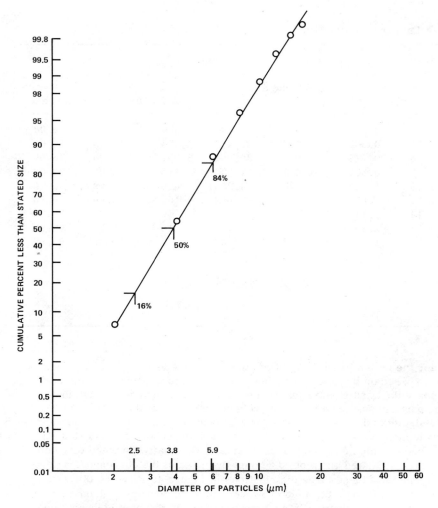

Figure 48. Log-probability plot for size of ball-milled material.

IV. Methods of Particle Size Analysis

There are many methods of determing particle size analysis. However, the discussion here is limited to the most common and practical methods (items 1 to 5, Table 16) used in tablet production and raw material processing.

A. Optical Microscope

The most common method of sizing and counting particles in the subsieve size range is by optical microscope. The advantage of this method is the relatively

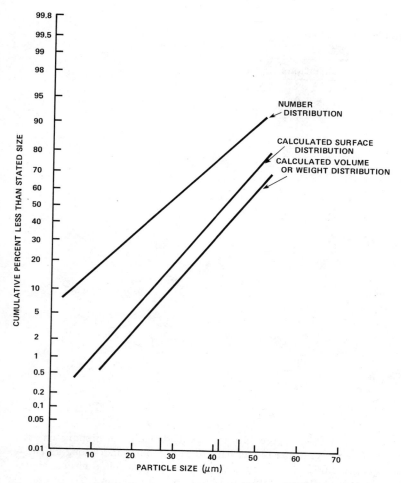

Figure 49. Three types of distribution obtained from the same number of frequency data.

low cost for equipment with fairly good accuracy. The big disadvantage is the length of time required to size a powder sample.

The optical microcsope method consists of:

1. Preparing a slurry of several mg of powder in a liquid dispersion medium in which the sample is insoluble. (Assume that the bulk powder has been sampled properly, as discussed previously.) A refractive index difference between the sample and the suspending medium should be at least 0.02 [29], since duplicate refractive indices will render the sample particles invisible if they are not opaque.

A good all-round suspending medium is light mineral oil, but oils of different refractive indices are available. It is important that a thorough dispersion of the powder particles be obtained; otherwise, size distributions of the particles and

Table 13

Equations for Calculating Various
Particle Size Means

Mean diameter	Equations
Arithmetic mean, $\overline{X}_a$ =	$\dfrac{\Sigma\, n_i X_i}{N}$
Surface mean, $\overline{X}_s$ =	$\sqrt{\dfrac{\Sigma\, n_i X_i^2}{N}}$
Volume mean, $\overline{X}_v$ =	$\sqrt[3]{\dfrac{\Sigma\, n_i X_i^3}{N}}$
Volume surface mean, $\overline{X}_{vs}$ (Sauter mean) =	$\dfrac{\Sigma\, n_i X_i^3}{\Sigma\, n_i X_i^2}$
Weight mean, $\overline{X}_w$ =	$\dfrac{\Sigma\, n_i X_i^4}{\Sigma\, n_i X_i^3}$

their flocculates will be obtained. To obtain the desired degree of dispersion, it
may be necessary to use a small ultrasonic bath to aid dispersion as long as particle size is not degreded during insonation. This should be checked microscopic-
ally. The dispersion should also contain a minimum of air bubbles. To aid the
counting of particles 3 μm and smaller, it is necessary to minimize Brownian motion of particles by using a suspending medium with a high viscosity.

   2. One of two drops of the well-mixed slurry or mull is placed on a clean microscope slide, and a coverslip is applied. The thickness of the mull between the
slide and the coverslip should be such that only one layer of motionless particles
is observed.

   3. Usually, direct lighting through the sample is used, and a magnification is
selected such that the entire range of particles can be counted under one magnification.

   4. Several random fields are selected for counting. The particle sizing may
be accomplished in several ways:

      a. A calibrated graticule is placed in one of, or the objective eyepiece(s).
          One of the more popular graticules is the Patterson-Cawood, which
          consists of a series of graded black and open circles (Fig. 50).

Table 14

Calculations for Composition of Means

Class interval (μm)	Class interval mean, X_i (μm)	Frequency, n_i	$n_i X_i$	$n_i X_i^2$	$n_i X_i^3$	$n_i X_i^4$
0–5	2.5	96	240	600	1,500	3,750
5–10	7.5	105	788	5,910	44,325	332,438
10–15	12.5	116	1,450	18,125	226,562	2,832,031
15–20	17.5	129	2,258	39,515	691,512	12,101,469
20–25	22.5	150	3,375	75,938	1,708,605	38,443,612
25–30	27.5	212	5,830	160,325	4,408,938	121,245,781
30–35	32.5	148	4,810	156,325	5,080,562	165,118,281
35–40	37.5	127	4,762	178,575	6,696,562	251,121,094
40–45	42.5	114	4,845	205,912	8,751,260	371,928,550
45–50	47.5	101	4,798	227,905	10,825,988	514,210,656
50–55	52.5	92	4,830	253,575	13,312,688	698,916,094
55–60	57.5	88	5,060	290,950	16,729,625	961,953,438

$\Sigma\ n_i = N$ 1,478

$\Sigma\ n_i X_i\ =$ 43,046

$\Sigma\ n_i X_i^2\ =$ 1,613,655

$\Sigma\ n_i X_i^3\ =$ 68,477,628

$\Sigma\ n_i X_i^4\ =$ 3,138,207,194

The field is scanned from one side to the other using a mechanical microscope stage, and particles are sized according to the nearest equivalent circle area. The sized particles are tallied under their appropriate class interval.

b. A calibrated micrometer mechanical stage may also be used for sizing the particles. The particles are sized by locating the cross hairs at the outermost or midpoint of the particle (Feret's or Martin's diameter, discussed previously). A micrometer zero reading is taken and the stage is moved to the opposite limit of the particle. A micrometer reading is taken, and the difference between the final reading and the zero reading is the particle diameter. It is stressed that the particles should be measured in only one direction of the stage movement regardless of the particle orientation, since the randomness of the powder particles in the sample will give a statistical reproducible distribution.

Again, the sized particles are tallied under their appropriate class interval.

Table 15

Calculated Mean Particle Sizes

Mean diameter		Equation		Calculation		Calculated mean (μm)
Arithmetic mean, $\overline{X}_a$	$=$	$\dfrac{\Sigma\, n_i X_i}{N}$	$=$	$\dfrac{43,046}{1,478}$	$=$	29.1
Surface mean, $\overline{X}_s$	$=$	$\sqrt{\dfrac{\Sigma\, n_i X_i^2}{N}}$	$=$	$\sqrt{\dfrac{1,613,655}{1,478}}$	$=$	33.0
Volume mean, $\overline{X}_v$	$=$	$\sqrt[3]{\dfrac{\Sigma\, n_i X_i^3}{N}}$	$=$	$\sqrt[3]{\dfrac{68,477,628}{1,478}}$	$=$	35.9
Volume surface mean, $\overline{X}_{vs}$	$=$	$\dfrac{\Sigma\, n_i X_i^3}{\Sigma\, n_i X_i^2}$	$=$	$\dfrac{684,477,628}{1,613,655}$	$=$	42.4
Weight mean, $\overline{X}_w$	$=$	$\dfrac{\Sigma\, n_i X_i^4}{\Sigma\, n_i X_i^3}$	$=$	$\dfrac{3,138,207,194}{68,477,628}$	$=$	45.8

*Data taken from Table 14.

5. The data are handled per the microscope data illustrated in Tables 9 to 11 and then are plotted. The greatest chance for error is that too few particles will be counted, making the statistics less valid. Attempts should be made to count no less than 500 and preferably 1000 particles per sample. It is also best to count two separate samples, to determine reproducibility of the sample and the counting method.

B. Sedimentation in Gas or Liquid

A weight distribution of a powder sample can be determined by using one of several available sedimentation methods. In each method the weight distribution is obtained by allowing a dispersed powder to settle in air or in a liquid in which it is not soluble, and weighing the particles in each class interval separately or cumulatively on a balance. The relationship between the particle settling time and the size of the particle is expressed in the Stokes equation

$$d = 10^4 \sqrt{\dfrac{18\eta h}{(\rho - \rho_0)gt}}$$

Table 16

Common Particle Counting Methods and Resulting Average Particle Size

Method of counting	Approximate size range covered	Resulting average particle size
1. Optical microscope	0.5–100 μm (140 mesh)	Average by number, $\overline{X}_a$ Average by surface, $\overline{X}_s{}^a$ Average by volume, $\overline{X}_v{}^a$
2. Sedimentation in gas or liquid	2–200 μm (70 mesh)	Average by weight, $\overline{X}_w$
3. Electronic sensing zone	1–300 μm (50 mesh)	Average by volume, $\overline{X}_V$ (volume of equivalent sphere)
4. Light obstruction	2–300 μm (50 mesh)	Average by volume, $\overline{X}_V$, as calculated from cross-sectional area of an equivalent sphere
5. Sieve	44 μm (325 mesh)–4700 μm (2 mesh)	Average by weight, $\overline{X}_w$
6. Air permeation	0.05–150 μm (100 mesh)	Average by surface and volume, $\overline{X}_{vs}$

[a] Per calculations shown from number distribution.

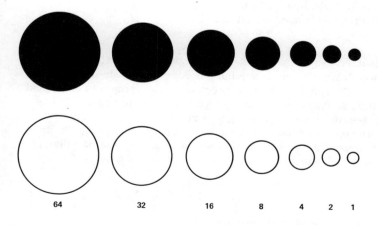

64   32   16   8   4   2   1

Figure 50. Open and closed circles in graticule.

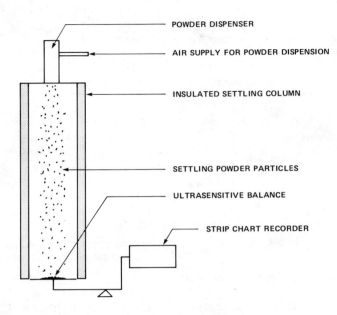

POWDER DISPENSER

AIR SUPPLY FOR POWDER DISPENSION

INSULATED SETTLING COLUMN

SETTLING POWDER PARTICLES

ULTRASENSITIVE BALANCE

STRIP CHART RECORDER

Figure 51. Schematic of air sedimentation apparatus.

where all particles are assumed to be spheres, and

d $\quad$ = particle diameter, μm
η $\quad$ = viscosity, poise
h $\quad$ = distance of fall, cm
ρ $\quad$ = absolute density of the powder particles, in g cm^{-3}
ρ_0 = density of the fluid settling medium, g cm^{-3}
g $\quad$ = gravity acceleration constant = 981 cm sec^{-2}
t $\quad$ = time, sec

Using either the Micromerograph[*] (where the powder particles settle in air), or the Cahn Sedimentation Balance[†] (where the powder particles settle in a liquid), shown schematically in Figures 51 and 52, respectively, the sample is dispersed in its respective settling medium and the powder particles settle per the Stokes equation onto an ultrasensitive balance. Weight is recorded cumulatively against time, the time being the only variable in the equation creating the change in diameter (i.e., all other components in the equation are constant, so that the diameter change is dependent on time change).

---

[*]Sharples Corporation, Philadelphia, Pennsylvania.
[†]Cahn Division, Ventron Instruments Corporation, Paramount, California 90723.

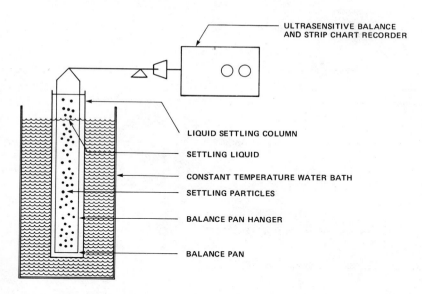

Figure 52. Schematic of liquid sedimentation apparatus.

    Each of the pieces of equipment mentioned above record these data electron-
ically, which yields a strip-chart size distribution curve. The diameter axis is
adjusted to the constants in the Stokes equation, and the data can be replotted on
normal or log-probability paper for final representation.
    Another method that is still in common use is the Andreasen Pipet. This ap-
paratus, shown in Figure 53, is also based on the Stokes equation. This apparatus
is designed for a settling liquid medium that will not dissolve the sample and can
be easily and completely evaporated by heat and/or vacuum. With this apparatus,
the settling liquid is filled to the top line and the sample weighed and predispersed
in a small amount of the settling medium. This dispersion is then added to the
top of the settling-medium column and time zero is recorded. At specified recorded time intervals that have been predetermined from the Stokes equation and
the constants used, 5-, 10-, or 20-ml samples are withdrawn into clean, pre-
tared evaporating pans. The settling medium is evaporated and each sample is
weighed. Diameters are calculated and cumulative weight percents are plotted
against them on normal or log-probability paper for presentation. An example
of an Andreasen pipet sedimentation determination is shown in Table 17, and the
plotted data are shown in Figure 54.
    Each of the sedimentation methods described is accurate and reproducible,
but each has a lower particle size limit of about 2-3 μm because of the inordinately
long settling times required with very fine powder particles. Several precautions
must also be observed when using sedimentation methods:

1. Temperature control of the settling medium is critical because of possible
    changes in density with temperature.

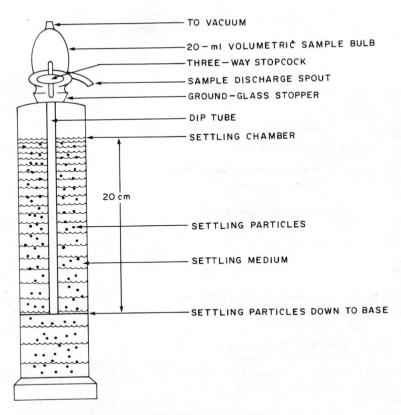

Figure 53. Schematic of Andreasen pipet.

2. Microscopic examination of the predispersed sample is essential to determine that dispersion is complete and that the particle size range is within the 2-200 μm limits.
3. Particle concentration in the settling medium. It has been shown that the higher the particle concentration, the higher the settling velocity of the powder particles. It may be necessary to try several sample concentrations until duplication of distribution is obtained at two different concentrations.

C. Stream Scanning

There are essentially two stream scanning methods in wide use today, which are based on electrical resistance and light obstruction. Both methods are electronic, count large numbers of particles (10,000 to 100,000) very rapidly, and yield highly reproducible results. Because of the large numbers of particles, the statistics yield a high level of confidence in the distribution of a sample.

Table 17

Sedimentation Data

Time of sample, t (sec)	Mean of class interval of corresponding equivalent spherical diameter (μm)	Weight of sample collected (mg)	Weight percent of sample	Cumulative weight percent
25	80	–	0	0
29	75	1	0.5	100.0
33	70	2	1.3	99.5
39	65	4	2.7	98.2
45	60	8	6.5	95.5
54	55	14	9.0	89.0
65	50	21	14.0	80.0
81	45	30	17.0	66.0
102	40	90	16.7	49.0
133	35	37	14.7	32.3
182	30	20	8.0	17.6
262	25	13	5.2	9.6
410	20	7	2.8	4.4
728	15	3	1.2	1.6
1638	10	1	0.4	0.4
6553	5	–	0	0

Total weight = 251

p = 2.2 g cm^{-3}; h = 0.005 poise; g = 981 cm sec^{-2}
p = 0.8 g cm^{-3}; h = 25 cm

A schematic of the electrical conductivity[*] method is shown in Figure 55 [30], which labels the basic parts. The counter determines the number and size of particles suspended in an electrically conductive liquid in which the sample is not soluble. This is accomplished by forcing a thoroughly dispersed suspension of particles through a small orifice on either side of which is an electrode. As each particle passes through the aperture, it changes the resistance between the electrodes because the volume of the particle displaces an equivalent volume of electrolyte.

This, in turn, produces a short-duration voltage pulse of a magnitude proportional to the volume of the particle. These pulses are sized and counted electrically. The data yield volume (or weight) distribution of equivalent spheres. Precautions that should be noted in using this equipment include the selection of

---

[*]Coulter Electronics, Inc., Hialeah, Florida 33010.

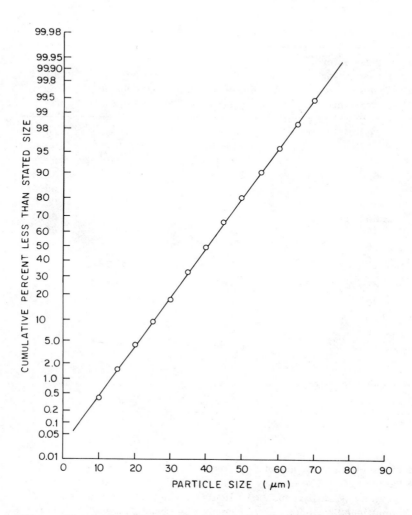

Figure 54. Andreasen pipet sedimentation distribution plot.

the proper size aperture for counting the sample size range; and adjusting the particle concentration such that only single particles pass through the aperture, thus preventing coincidence counting (i. e. , counting of two or more particles at one time). The disadvantages associated with electrical resistance counting include the cost of equipment, possible sensor blockage, the selection of an electrolyte in which the material to be counted is insoluble, and the possibility of picking up background electrical "noise, " which could lead to erroneous results.

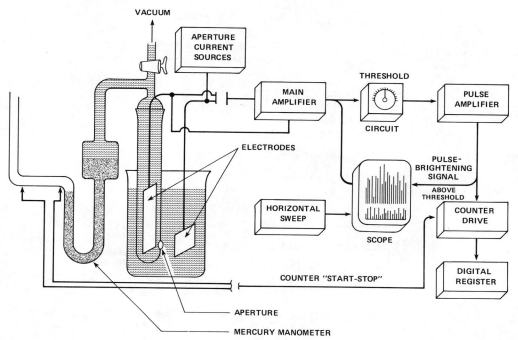

Figure 55. Schematic of the Coulter Counter. (Courtesy Coulter Electronics, Inc., Hialeah, Florida 33010.)

The light obstruction method[*] is shown schematically in Figure 56 [31]. A liquid in which the sample disperses easily and is not dissolved passes a window that is transversed by a light source. The light source is detected by a photodetector which senses loss of light transmitted through the suspending medium when a particle interrupts the light beam.

The amount of light blocked from the detector by a particle is proportional to the cross-sectional area of the particle. This creates short-duration electrical pulses which are sized and counted electrically. The data yield a distribution based on the cross-sectional area of equivalent spheres which is easily converted to a weight distribution, as shown in Section II.F.

The precautions with this equipment include keeping the sensing-zone windows clean, adhering to particle concentrations that will prevent coincident counting, selecting the proper sensor for the particle size being counted, and making certain that a thorough dispersion of particles is obtained.

The disadvantages with this method are the cost of the equipment and possible sensor blockage.

---

[*]HIAC Instrument Division, Pacific Scientific Company, Montclair, California, 91763.

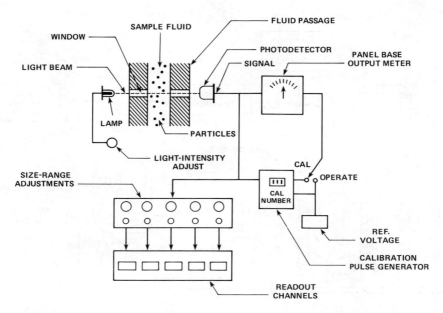

Figure 56. Schematic of HIAC particle counter. (Courtesy HIAC Instrument Division, Pacific Scientific Company, Montclair, California 91763.)

D. Sieve Analysis

This is the most widely used method of determining the size distribution of a granulation. The method is described in Section II.E for the comparison of the effect of milling conditions on an acetaminophen granulation.

The data collected from the difference in the tare weight of each screen and the total weight of the tare and the powder is entered in table form and the cumulative percentages calculated. The class intervals are restricted to the selection of sieve sizes available as shown in Table 7. For the screen analysis shown in Figures 26 to 30, screens were selected such that each smaller screen was one-half the size opening of the screen preceding it.

The mean of the class interval was obtained by taking the average of each pair of adjacent screens in the nest [e.g., 12 mesh = 1680 μm and 20 mesh = 840 μm: the mean of the class interval would calculate to be (1680 + 840)/2 = 1260 μm].

A sample calculation for the unmilled acetaminophen granulation is shown in Table 18.

There are other methods of particle size analysis to which the reader is referred if more sophisticated equipment is at hand for scanning image analysis [32], acoustical counters [33], light scattering [34], electron microscopy [35], centrifugal sedimentation [36], and laser halography [37].

Table 18

Sample Screen Analysis Data of Unmilled Acetaminophen Granulation

U.S. Standard sieve size	Sieve opening (μm)	Mean of class interval (μm)	Granulation weight on the smaller screen (cm)	Percent	Cumulative percent
>12	1680		32.7	33	98
12–20	1680–840	1260	16.7	17	65
20–40	840–420	630	17.4	17	48
40–70	420–210	315	8.9	9	31
70–140	210–105	157	21.0	21	22
< 140	105		0.9	1	
			98.6	98	

References

1. Snow, R. H., Bibliography of Size Reduction, 9 vols. National Technical Information Service, Springfield, Va., 1974.
2. Schönert, K., Fortschr. Verfahrenstech., 10(B2):204 (1970/1971).
3. Dustin, L. G., Powder Technol., 5:1 (1971/1972).
4. Herschhorn, J. S., Powder Technol., 4:1 (1970/1971).
5. Gupta, V. K., and Kapur, P. C., Powder Technol., 12:81 (1975).
6. Berg, O. T. G., and Avis, L. E., Powder Technol., 4:27 (1970/1971).
7. McCabe, W. L., and Smith, J. C., Unit Operations of Chemical Engineering, 2nd ed. McGraw-Hill, New York, 1967, p. 809.
8. Perry, R. H., ed., Chemical Engineers' Handbook, 4th ed. McGraw-Hill, New York, 1963.
9. Ramanujam, M., and Venkateswarlu, D., Powder Technol., 3:92 (1969/1970).
10. Melloy, T., Open Forum: Future Directions for Research in Powder Technology held at the International Powder and Bulk Solids Handling and Processing Conference/Exhibition 76, Chicago, 1976.
11. Prescott, L. F., Steel, R. F., and Ferrier, W. R., Clin. Pharmacol. Ther., 11:496 (1970).
12. Ullah, I., and Cadwallader, D. E., J. Pharm. Sci., 60:230 (1971).
13. Brooke, D., J. Pharm. Sci., 62:795 (1973).
14. Ikekawa, A., and Kaneniwa, N., Parts I-IX, Chem. Pharm. Bull., 15-17 (1967-1969).
15. Dobson, B., and Rothwell, E., Powder Technol., 3:213 (1969/1970).
16. Ramanujam, M., and Venkateswarlu, D., Powder Technol., 3:92 (1969/1970).
17. Snow, R. H., in: Advances in Particle Science and Technology (D. Wasan, ed.), Academic Press, New York, 1973.

18. Snow, R. H., Powder Technol., 5:351 (1971/1972).
19. Snow, R. H., Powder Technol., 10:129 (1974).
20. Ref. Military Standard
21. Standard Method of Test for Specific Gravity of Pigments, ASTM D153-54. American Society for Testing and Materials, Philadelphia, 1954 (reapproved, 1961).
22. Drug Stand., 20:222 (1952).
23. Brünauer, S., Emmett, P. H., and Teller, E., J. Am. Chem. Soc., 60:309 (1938).
24. Emmett, P. H., deWitt, Ind. Eng. Chem. Anal. Ed., 13:28 (1941).
25. Herdan, G., Small Particle Statistics. Academic Press, New York, 1960.
26. Carstensen, J. T., Pharmaceutics of Solids and Solid Dosage Forms. Wiley, New York, 1977.
27. Atkinson, R. M., Bedford, C., Child, K. J., and Tomich, E. G., Antibiot. Chemother. 12:232 (1962).
28. Cadle, R. D., Particle Size Theory and Industrial Applications. Reinhold, New York, 1965.
29. Yamati, G., and Stockham, J. D., in: Particle Size Analysis, 2nd printing. (J. D. Stockham and E. G. Fochtman, eds.). Ann Arbor Science Publishers, Ann Arbor, Mich., 1978, Chap. 3.
30. Instruction Manual, Coulter Counter Industrial Model B.
31. High Accuracy Products, Operation and Service Manual--HIAC S, Montclair, Calif.
32. Sturgess, G. L., and Braggin, D. W., Microscope, 20:275 (1972).
33. Kaiuhn, Proceedings, International Conference on Particle Technology III, Research Institute, Chicago, 1973, p. 202.
34. Stull, V. R., Proceedings, International Conference on Particle Technology III. Research Institute, Chicago, 1973, p. 52.
35. Drummond, D. C., Trans. R. Micro. Soc., Spec. Ed. (1950).
36. Bradley, D., Chem. Proc. Eng., 43:634 (1962).
37. Particle Characteristics Conference, Dept. of Chemical Engineering, Loughborough University of Technology, 1969.

4

Compression

Eugene L. Parrott

University of Iowa
Iowa City, Iowa

Compression is the process of applying pressure to a material. The process of compression as encountered in the preparation of pharmaceutical tablets may be considered to occur in the following stages:

1. <u>Transitional Repacking or Particle Rearrangement</u>: The control of the particle size distribution of a granulation determines the initial packing or bulk density as the granulation is delivered into the die cavity. During the compression cycle, most of the punch and particle movement occur at low pressure. The particles flow with respect to each other, with the finer particles entering the void between the larger particles, and the density of the granulation is increased. Spherical particles undergo less particle arrangement than do flaky particles, as the spherical particles assume a closer packing arrangement initially.

2. <u>Deformation at Points of Contact</u>: When stress or a force is applied to a material, deformation (alteration of form) occurs. If the deformation disappears entirely on release of the stress, it is an elastic deformation. A deformation that does not completely recover after release of the stress is known as a plastic deformation. The force required to initiate a plastic deformation is termed the yield value. When the particles are so tightly packed that no further filling of the void may occur, the compressional force increases, and plastic deformation at the points of contact occurs, increasing the area of contact and the formation of potential bonding areas. Both plastic and elastic deformation may occur, although one type generally predominates for a given material.

3. <u>Fragmentation</u>: Under higher pressure the deformed particles may fragment, with an increase in new, clean surfaces that are potential bonding areas. Fragmentation furthers densification, with the infiltration of the fragments into the voids.

4. <u>Bonding</u>: Absolutely clean surfaces of a solid will adhere with the bulk strength of the material, whereas contaminants or adsorbed films on a particle restrict bonding. Under pressure, the new, clean surfaces formed by deformation and/or fragmentation promote intermolecular interaction at the points of contact.

5. Deformation of the Solid Body: As the pressure is further increased, the now-bonded solid is consolidated toward a limiting density by plastic and/or elastic deformation.

6. Ejection: After the axial pressure has been removed, there is a lateral pressure from the die wall. As the tablet is ejected, it undergoes elastic recovery, with an increase in volume as it is removed from the die.

The process of compression may be depicted in terms of the relative volume (ratio of volume of the compressed mass to the volume of the mass at zero void). In the initial stage of transitional repacking, the particles are packed to an arrangement in which the particles are immobile and the number of intergranular points of contact has increased. The decrease in relative volume caused during transitional packing is represented by segment AE in Figure 1. With a further increase in pressure, temporary columns (supporting forms between bodies) may be formed, as represented by segment EF. Plastic deformation or fragmentation with bonding is represented by the segment FG as the pressure is further increased. At higher pressures bonding and densification occur more rapidly than fragmentation, and the volume is reduced as indicated by segment GH.

For the compressional process, Heckel [1] has proposed the equation

$$\ln \frac{V}{V - V_\infty} = kP + \frac{V_O}{V_O - V_\infty} \tag{1}$$

where V is the volume at pressure P, V_O the original volume of the powder including voids, k a constant related to the yield pressure of the powder, and V_∞ the volume of the solid (equal to the weight of the solid divided by the true density of the solid as determined by a suitable pycnometer). The Heckel equation has been used to distinguish between the mechanisms of tablet formation. A linear relation is obtained when the material undergoes plastic deformation without fragmentation. If fragmentation occurs during compression, a plot of the Heckel equation is not linear.

The Heckel plot permits an interpretation of the mechanism of bonding. For sodium chloride the plot is linear, indicating that sodium chloride is not fragmented but rather undergoes plastic deformation during compression. With no significant change in particle size during compression, the strength of the compressed tablet depends on the original particle size of the sodium chloride [2]. A Heckel plot for lactose, which undergoes fragmentation during compression, is nonlinear. As lactose fragments during compression, the tablet strength is essentially independent of the original particle size. This suggests that analyses of materials by use of the Heckel relationship may be indicative of the influence of the original particle size of a granulation on the tablet strength.

The materials compressed in pharmacy are nonmetallic and are generally mixtures of organic compounds. The relative significance of each stage in compression depends on the mechanical properties (plastic behavior, crushing strength) of the material, its chemical nature and surface effects (friction, adsorbed films, lubrication).

Higuchi [3] and Train [4] were probably the first pharmaceutical scientists to study the effect of compression on the physical characteristics of tablets. In a series of articles, Higuchi et al. [5-12] presented the physics of tablet compression in terms of static factors (density, disintegration time, hardness, porosity, and specific surface area) and dynamic factors (energy expenditure and

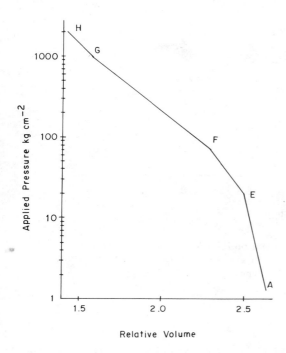

Figure 1. Stages of compression in terms of the relationship of applied pressure and relative volume. (See the text for a discussion.) (From Ref. 27.)

distribution of pressure on the die wall). With the increased concern as to the bioavailability of a medicinal compound from a tablet, the most recent interest has been in the influence of compressional pressure on dissolution.

It is desirable that a theory permit an examination of the physical and chemical properties of a material in relation to the variables of the compressional process so that a formulation and a tableting procedure, which would produce a compressed tablet with the desired properties, could be predicted. Commercial compressed tablets usually contain several ingredients (binding agent, disintegrating agent, diluent, and lubricant) in addition to the medicinal compound. Each of these ingredients has different physical properties that affect the compressional process and contribute to the structure of the tablet. The complexity of the mixtures being compressed has made it difficult to develop and apply a satisfactory theory of compression to pharmaceutical tablets.

The relationships between compressional force and apparent density and ejection force are independent of the material being compressed; thus, the compression profiles are predictable. The relationships between compressional force and hardness, friability, disintegration, and release of the medicinal compound depend on the material being compressed and are unpredictable. These properties are affected more by the formulation and nature of the medicinal compound than they are by the compressional force.

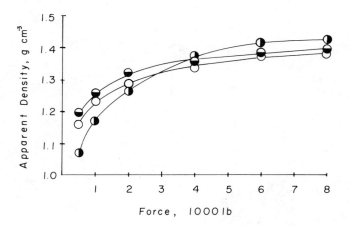

Figure 2. Effect of compressional force on the apparent density of various tablets. O, Aspirin; ◔, lactose; and ◑, lactose–aspirin. (From Ref. 8. Reproduced with permission of the copyright owner.)

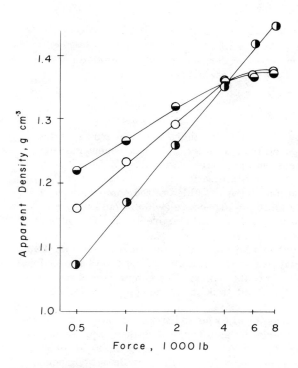

Figure 3. Linear relationship of apparent density to the logarithm of compressional force for various tablets. ◔, Aspirin; ◑, lactose; O, lactose–aspirin.
(From Ref. 8. Reproduced with permission of the copyright owner.)

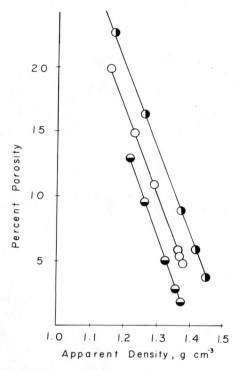

Figure 4. Plot of porosity against apparent density of various tablets. ◖, Aspirin; ◑, lactose; ○, lactose-aspirin. (From Ref. 8. Reproduced with permission of the copyright owner.)

I. Properties of Tablets Influenced by Compression

A. Density and Porosity

The apparent density of a tablet is the quotient of the weight and the geometric volume. The apparent density of a tablet is exponentially related to the compressional force (or pressure) as shown in Figure 2, until the limiting density of the material is approached [8]. As shown in Figure 3, a plot of the apparent density against the logarithm of compressional force is linear except at high forces.

As porosity and apparent density are inversely proportional the plot of porosity against the logarithm of compressional force is linear with a negative slope, as shown in Figure 4.

When equal weights of aspirin and lactose are compressed with 10% starch, the porosity of the lactose-aspirin tablet, as indicated in Figure 5, is of a magnitude between that of the individual lactose and aspirin tablets at corresponding force. Thus, in tablet formulation it can be anticipated that a change in percent composition will have a corresponding arithmetic (or averaging) effect on porosity and apparent density.

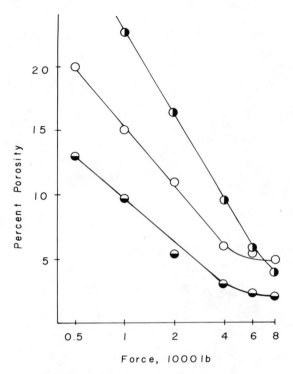

Figure 5. Effect of compressional force on the porosity of various tablets. ◖,
Aspirin; ◑, lactose; O, lactose-aspirin. (From Ref. 8. Reproduced with permission of the copyright owner.)

B. Hardness and Strength

Although hardness is not a fundamental property, its use in in-process quality
control during tablet production warrants consideration. There is a linear relationship between tablet hardness and the logarithm of compressional force, except
at high forces. As shown in Figure 6 for lactose-aspirin tablets, compressed mixtures have hardness values between those of tablets composed of the individual ingredients.

  The strength of a tablet may be expressed as a tensile strength (breaking stress
of a solid of unit cross section, in kg cm^{-2}). As shown in Figure 7, the tensile
strength of crystalline lactose is directly proportional to the compressional force.

  The fracture strength of compressed tablets varies inherently as a property of
the material, regardless of how carefully controlled the test conditions are. The
Weibull distribution may be used to express this strength variability and to characterize materials. The probability P_f that a tablet from a large batch of tablets
will exhibit a tensile strength of σ_t is expressed by the equation

$$P_f = 1 - \exp\left[-\left(\frac{1}{m}!\right)^m\left(\frac{\sigma_t}{\bar{\sigma}_t}\right)^m\right] \tag{2}$$

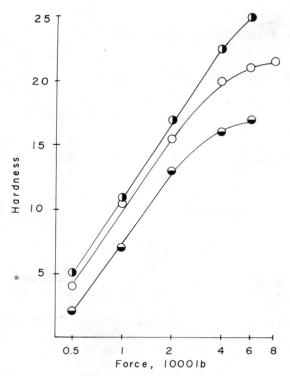

Figure 6. Effect of compressional force on the hardness of various tablets. ◖,
Aspirin; ◑, lactose; ○, lactose-aspirin. (From Ref. 8. Reproduced with permission of the copyright owner.)

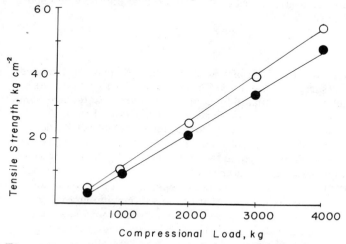

Figure 7. Tensile strength of tablets of crystalline and spray-dried lactose prepared at various compressional forces. ●, Crystalline lactose; ○, spray-dried
lactose. [From J. T. Fell and J. M. Newton, J. Pharm. Sci., 59:688 (1970).
Reproduced with permission of the copyright owner.]

Table 1

Influence of Compressional Force on Tensile Strength and Strength Variability (Weibull Modulus)

Pressure (MN·m^{-2})	Tensile strength (MN·m^{-2})	Weibull modulus
12.6	0.25	23.6
13.3	0.27	26.6
21.6	0.68	39.1
34.6	1.62	43.3
73.5	4.80	20.2
76.4	4.94	17.4
78.2	5.09	22.8

Source: Ref. 13.

where m (the Weibull modulus) is a reciprocal measure of strength variability of material, (1/m !) is a standard functional tabulated in mathematic handbooks, and $\bar{\sigma}_t$ is the mean tensile strength of the batch.

It has been suggested [13] that tablet strength could be expressed by a variety of terms, such as tensile strength and Weibull modulus, as shown in Table 1.

For material in which the granules retain their identity and the fracture of the tablet occurs at the bonding surface between these granules, the tensile strength and hardness are independent of the size of the granules. For material in which the granules are bonded as strongly as the crystal lattice and the fracture of the tablet occurs across the grain, at a given pressure a stronger tablet is formed from smaller granules than from larger granules. The Heckel plot may be used to determine the mechanism of bonding.

C. Specific Surface

Specific surface is the surface area of 1 g of material. The influence of compressional force on the specific surface area of a tablet is typified by Figure 8. As the lactose granules, which were granulated by adding 10% starch paste, are compressed into a tablet, the specific surface is increased to a maximal value (four times that of the initial granules), indicating the formation of new surfaces due to fragmentation of the granules. Further increases in compressional force produce a progressive decrease in specific surface as the particles bond. A similar relation is shown for aspirin containing 10% starch. When an equal weight of aspirin and lactose is blended with 10% starch and then compressed, a similar relationship, in which the specific surface is between that of the aspirin and lactose tablets individually, is observed [8]. As the relationship between compressional force and apparent density is independent of the material being compressed, the influence of starch on the specific surface and porosity is not significant.

For these aspirin, lactose, and aspirin-lactose tablets, the maximum specific surface area occurs at a porosity of approximately 10%, even though the forces at which the maxima occur vary with the different materials [8].

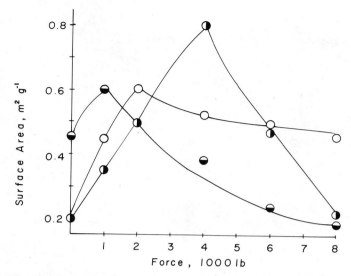

Figure 8. Effect of compressional force on the specific surface area of various tablets. ◖, aspirin; ◑, lactose; O, lactose-aspirin. (From Ref. 8. Reproduced with permission of the copyright owner.)

D. Disintegration

Usually, as the compressional force used to prepare a tablet is increased, the disintegration time is longer [14]. Frequently, there is an exponential relationship between disintegration time and compressional force, as shown for aspirin and lactose in Figure 9.

In other formulations there is a minimum value when the compressional force is plotted against the logarithm of disintegration time, as shown in Figure 9 for aspirin-lactose tablets with 10% starch. For tablets compressed under small forces, there is a large void, and the contact of starch grains in the interparticular space is discontinuous. Thus, there is a lag period before the starch grains, which are swelling due to imbibition of water, contact and exert a force on the surrounding tablet structure. For tablets compressed at a certain force, the contact of the starch grains is continuous with the tablet structure, and the swelling of the starch grains immediately exerts pressure, causing the most rapid disintegration, as demonstrated by a minimum in a plot of compressional force against the logarithm of disintegration time. For tablets compressed at forces greater than that producing the minimum disintegration time, the porosity is such that more time is required for the penetration of water into the tablet, with a resulting increase in disintegration time.

As shown in Figure 10 for sulfadiazine tablets, the concentration of a disintegrating agent influences the relationship between compressional force and disintegration time. For low starch concentrations, a small change in compressional force causes a large change in disintegration time. Thus, for formulations

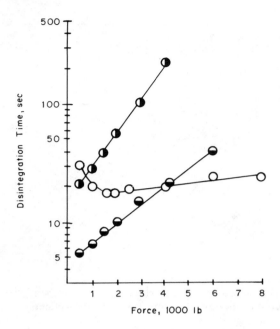

Figure 9. Effect of compressional force on the disintegration time of various tablets. ◖, Aspirin; ◗, lactose; ○, lactose-aspirin. (From Ref. 8. Reproduced with permission of the copyright owner.)

containing a small percent of starch, fluctuations in force during tablet production cause a large variance in disintegration time.

E. Dissolution

The effect of compressional force on dissolution rate may be considered from the viewpoint of nondisintegrating tablets and disintegrating tablets. Shah and Parrott [15] have shown that under sink conditions, the dissolution rate is independent of compressional forces from 270 to 11,000 kg for nondisintegrating 1.27-cm spheres of aspirin, benzoic acid, salicylic acid, an equimolar mixture of aspirin and salicylic acid, and an equimolar mixture of aspirin and caffeine. Mitchell and Savill [16] found the dissolution rate of aspirin disks to be independent of pressure over the range 2000 to 13,000 kg cm^{-2} and independent of the particle size of the granules used to prepare the disks. Kanke and Sekiguchi [17] reported that the dissolution rate of benzoic acid disks is independent of particle size and compressional force.

The effect of compressional force on the dissolution of disintegrating tablets is difficult to predict; however, for a conventional tablet it is dependent on the pressure range, the dissolution medium, and the properties of the medicinal compound and the excipients. If fragmentation of the granules occurs during compression,

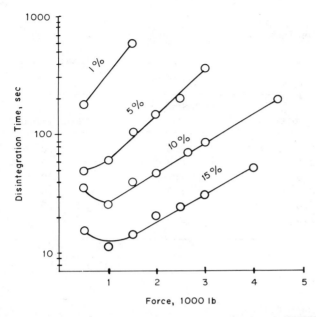

Figure 10. Effect of compressional force on the disintegration time of sulfadiazine tablets with various percentages of dried cornstarch. (From Ref. 8. Reproduced with permission of the copyright owner.)

the dissolution is faster as the compressional force is increased, and the fragmentation increases the specific surface area. If the bonding of the particles is the predominate phenomenon in compression, the increase in compressional force causes a decrease in dissolution [18].

The four general dissolution-force relations are: (1) the dissolution is more rapid as the compressional force is increased; (2) the dissolution is slowed as the compressional force is increased; (3) the dissolution is faster, to a maximum, as the compressional force is increased, and then further increases in compressional force slow dissolution; and (4) the dissolution is slowed to a minimum as the compressional force is increased, and then further increases in compressional force speed dissolution.

The complexity of tablets is demonstrated in Table 2 for sulfadimidine tablets prepared by wet granulation using three different granulation agents [19]. When starch paste was used as the granulation agent, dissolution was faster as the compressional force was increased. When methylcellulose solution was used as the granulation agent, dissolution was slowed as the compressional force was increased. When gelatin solution was used as a granulating agent, the dissolution became faster as the compressional force was increased to a maximum, and then further increases in compressional force slowed dissolution.

Table 2

Effect of Compressional Force on Dissolution of Sulfadimidine Tablets Prepared
with Various Granulating Agents

	$t_{50\%}$ (min)		
Pressure (MN·m^{-2})	Starch paste	Methylcellulose solution	Gelatin solution
200	54.0	0.5	10.0
400	42.0	0.8	4.5
600	35.0	1.1	3.0
800	10.0	1.2	4.6
1000	7.0	1.4	4.9
2000	3.3	1.8	6.5

Source: Ref. 19.

II. Measurement of Compressional Force

Instrumented tablet machines are designed on the principle that the force on a
punch is proportional to the force transmitted to other parts of the tablet machine. Early instrumented tablet machines had strain gages at some practical
position of the machine that would undergo a force proportional to the force exerted by the upper punch.

A strain gage is a coil of highly resistant wire mounted on a paper backing.
During compression the force applied causes a very small, elastic deformation
of the two punches. If a suitable strain gage is firmly bound to the punch shank
as close to the compression site as practical, it is deformed as the punch is deformed. With the deformation, the length of the resistance wire is decreased
and its diameter is increased. The resulting decrease in electrical resistance
is measured by a Wheatstone bridge used with a recording device. If a reference strain gage is placed in the opposite arm of the Wheatstone bridge, temperature fluctuation is compensated. Torsional movement of the punch may be
compensated by multiple gages mounted at the periphery of the punch.

In their early work, Higuchi et al. [6] instrumented a Stokes A-3 single-
punch tablet machine and as a function of time simultaneously recorded any two
of the three variables--upper punch force, force transmitted to the lower punch,
and displacement of the upper punch during actual operating conditions. A schematic diagram is shown in Figure 11.

The upper punch displacement is measured by a linear variable differential
transformer (A) bolted to the side of the frame. The transformer consists of
three coaxial windings on a hollow ceramic cylinder. One winding is placed at
the middle of the form and acts as the primary of the transformer. The two secondaries are placed adjacent to and on each side of the primary. The movable
core of the transformer is linked to the upper punch assembly by a threaded rod

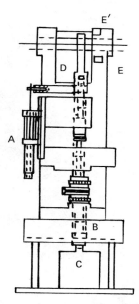

Figure 11. Diagrammatic representation of instrumented Stokes A-3 single-punch tablet machine. A, differential transformer; B, lower plunger extension; C, load cell; D, linkage to transformer core; E and E', strain gages. (From Ref. 6.)

and cross-arm (D). The primary of the differential transformer is excited by a 2500-Hz signal from an oscillator integral to strain gage amplifiers. The secondaries of the transformer are connected in series opposition, so that when the core is as much in the field on one secondary as it is in the field of the other, there is no net voltage output. Displacement of the core from this zero position produces a voltage across the connected secondaries. The magnitude of the voltage is directly proportional to the distance moved by the core. The output voltage is amplified and then actuates the recording device of the oscillograph.

The force transmitted to the lower punch is measured by a load cell (C), which is placed between the base of the machine and the platform and directly below the lower punch assembly. An expandable pin (B) is placed between the loading button of the cell and the lower plunger assembly, so that the entire plunger assembly rests on the cell. Thus, the upper punch force transmitted through the tablet to the lower punch is sensed directly by the load cell. A load cell consists of a centrally positioned steel column in a cylindrical heavy steel case. Strain gages are bonded to the column, and when stress is applied, the resulting strain in the column is shared by the strain gages. The gages are connected in a Wheatstone bridge circuit, so that any strain on the column causes a change in resistance of the gages and consequently an unbalance in the bridge. The unbalanced potential is directly proportional to the force applied to the loading button of the load cell. The Wheatstone bridge is excited by a 2500-Hz signal provided by the strain gage amplifier. The voltage output of the bridge resulting from the application of force to the load cell is amplified and actuates the recording device of the oscillograph.

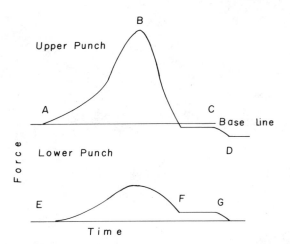

Figure 12. Diagrammatic representation of a typical record of upper and lower punch force for the compression of unlubricated granulation. (See the text.) (From Ref. 10.)

The force exerted by the upper punch is determined by two strain gages (E and E') mounted on the frame of the tablet machine. The strain gage E is mounted on the underside of the yoke supporting the drive shaft. The strain gage E' is bonded to the same yoke on the side near its upper edge. Force exerted by the upper punch has its reaction on the drive shaft and tends to straighten the yoke that holds it and consequently stretches strain gage E. Strain gage E' is compressed in a similar manner. Strain gages E and E' are arranged in opposite arms of a Wheatstone bridge so that the response to measured force is due to the sum of the two resistance changes of the two gages. The Wheatstone bridge circuit is excited by a 2500-Hz signal from an oscillator. The output signal is treated in the same manner as that described for the lower punch force arrangement.

When the tablet resists ejection from the die by the lower punch, the resulting strain in the lift rod causes the yoke to tend to bend downward, compressing the strain gage E on the underside of the yoke and stretching strain gage E' on the other side. This permits measurement of the ejection force. Details of other instrumented single-punch tablet machines have been published [16, 19, 20].

A typical force–time curve for the upper and lower punch forces is shown in Figure 12. The segment AB of the upper punch curve is transcribed as the upper punch descends and the granules are packed and compressed. As the upper punch ascents after compression, the segment BC is transcribed. The drop below the baseline is a measure of the force required to remove the upper punch from the die. As the lower punch rises and pushes the tablet from the die, the segment CD is transcribed; the recorder line drops below the zero baseline, measuring the force required to remove the tablet from the die. The segment EF of the lower punch curve is transcribed as the upper punch force is transmitted to the

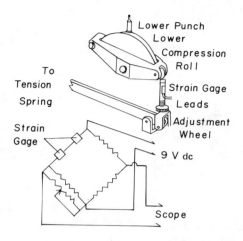

Figure 13. Diagrammatic representation of instrumentation of Stokes BB-2 rotary tablet machine for measurement of compressional force. (From Ref. 21.)

stationary lower punch. The segment FG is a measure of the force exerted by the tablet on the die wall, preventing relaxation of the lower punch assembly (the upper punch is exerting no force). This is the minimum force required to eject the tablet.

The instrumentation of rotary tablet machines has been by means of bonding strain gages to the upper and lower punch and transmitting signals from the strain gages with a radio link or by means of bonding strain gages to stationary locations near the site of compression.

In the remote instrumentation method [21] strain gages are bonded to parts (upper and lower compression release systems) remote from the punch face. A schematic representation of the instrumentation of a Stokes BB-2 rotary tablet machine is shown in Figure 13. The ejection force is measured by instrumentation of a bolt supporting a modified ejection cam, as illustrated in Figure 14. The remote instrumentation method has been criticized because (1) signals received from the remote gages may not truly represent the compressional force due to distortion of various parts of the machine transmitting the force; (2) signals received may not be limited only to the signal of a single desired event because of the fast succession of events in compression; and (3) the supporting cam during the ejection bears more than one punch at a time and may not represent the ejection force. To be assured that a remote instrumented machine is functioning properly, it should be verified by comparison with data obtained by an instrumented-punch radio system.

The remote instrumentation method can be used at normal production speed. If the pressure-release system is instrumented, each punch is monitored and can be set up in a reproducible manner. Also, for in-process control, any discrepancy during operation is detected, so that the machine may be stopped for adjustment.

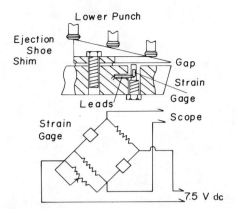

Figure 14. Diagrammatic representation of instrumentation of Stokes BB-2 rotary tablet machine for measurement of ejection force. (From Ref. 21.)

In the punch instrumentation method [22], the ratio transmitter is placed into several punch holders and one upper and lower punch is instrumented. Signals are obtained for upper and lower punch forces and for lower punch forces on ejection. Keyed punches are required to prevent rotation of the punch and the breaking of the electrical connections. Several strain gages are bonded to the shank of the punch and connected in series. The change in resistance is measured by an external Wheatstone bridge. With recent technological advances, the problem of space limitation has been surmounted, and the entire Wheatstone bridge may be bonded to the punch shank in the form of four strain gages (one for each arm of the bridge). Two are bonded parallel and two are bonded perpendicular to the major axis to compensate for temperature variation. With the proper selection of resistance gages, amplification of the signal is unnecessary.

III. Energy Expenditure

As the upper punch enters the die and begins to apply a force to the granulation, a small quantity of energy is used to rearrange the particles to a packing with less void. As the compression cycle continues, energy is expended to overcome die wall friction and to increase the specific surface as fragmentation occurs. After the tablet has been formed, energy is required to overcome die wall friction as the upper punch is withdrawn. Energy is then expended in the ejection of the tablet from the die. The energy expenditure is the sum of the energy dissipated as heat, the energy of reversible elastic strain, and the energy retained in the tablet as increased surface energy. The useful energy of compression

$$E_{compression} = E_{total} - E_{heat} - E_{elastic} \qquad (3)$$

The energy expended in the compression of granules to reduce the void and to form a tablet is the product of the force and the distance through which it acts.

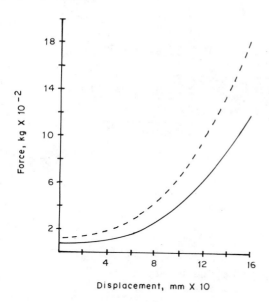

Figure 15. Diagrammatic representation of record of punch force against displacement in the compression of unlubricated and lubricated sulfathiazole granulation. -----, Upper punch force using unlubricated granulation; ——, lower punch force for lubricated or unlubricated granulation and for upper punch force for well-lubricated granulation. (From Ref. 10. Reproduced with permission of the copyright owner.)

This energy may be determined by measuring the lower punch force and the displacement of the upper punch, and then plotting the compressional force as a function of the displacement. The energy used to compress the tablet and to overcome die wall friction is equivalent to the area under the force-displacement curve (1 g cm = 2.3×10^{-5} cal).

If the granules are lubricated, the die wall friction is thus reduced and less force is required to produce a given displacement. With the use of a lubricant, less force is wasted to overcome friction, and as more of the upper punch force can then be transmitted to the lower punch, the difference between the upper and lower punch force is less than for an unlubricated granulation. Thus, the difference between the maximum value of force of the upper and lower punch can be a measure of the efficiency of a lubricant in overcoming die wall friction.

In Figure 15, the difference between the area under the curve for the compression of 0.4 g of lubricated and unlubricated sulfathiazole granules compressed at 1700 kg cm^{-2} is equal to 0.8 cal, which were required to overcome die wall friction. The 1.5 cal, as represented by the area under the curve of the lubricated granules, was used to compress the granules into a tablet. After compression of the unlubricated granules, 1.2 cal was required to withdraw the upper punch. With a lubricant, the energy to overcome die wall friction and to withdraw the upper punch was negligible. The energy required to eject the finished tablet was 5.1 cal. With a lubricant, the energy for ejection was only 0.5 cal. The energy

Table 3

Energy Expended in Compression of 0.4 g of Sulfthiazole Granulation in a Single-Punch Tablet Machine[a]

	Energy expended (cal)	
Compression	Unlubricated	Lubricated
Compression	1.5	1.5
Overcoming die wall friction	0.8	-
Upper punch withdrawal	1.2	-
Tablet ejection	5.1	0.5
Total	8.6	2.0

[a]Force of 1200 kg on lower punch using 3/8-in. flat-faced punches.
Source: Ref. 10. Reproduced with permission of the copyright owner.

expenditure for preparing the lubricated tablet and the unlubricated tablet is summarized in Table 3.

By assuming that only energy expended in the process of forming the tablet caused a temperature rise, Higuchi [10] estimated the temperature rise to be approximately 5°C. The energy expended in the process of tablet ejection, that needed to overcome die wall friction, and that used to remove the upper punch from the die were summed for a single-punch machine operating at 100 tablets per minute, and approximately 43 kcal hr^{-1} was required for unlubricated granules. For lubricated granules the value is 3 kcal hr^{-1}. A temperature rise from 4 to 30°C has been found in the compression of several formulations [23].

The temperature of compressed tablets is affected by the pressure and speed of the tablet machine. In a noninstrumented single-punch tablet machine set at minimum pressure, the compression of 0.7 g of sodium chloride caused a temperature increase of 1.5°C; when the machine was set near maximum pressure, the temperature increase was 11.1°C [24]. When the machine was operating at 26 and 140 rpm, the increase in temperature was 2.7 and 7.1°C, respectively. When the machine was operating at 26 and 140 rpm to compress 0.5 g of calcium carbonate, the increase in temperature was 16.3 and 22.2°C, respectively.

Since heating is unwanted because of wear of the punch and die and possible degradation of the tablet ingredients, lubricants are added. The chief purpose of a lubricant is to minimize friction at the die wall, although a lubricant often enhances flow of the granules by decreasing interparticular friction. A lubricant reduces the ejection force, which is directly related to the force lost to the die wall during the final phase of tablet formation. The force lost to the die wall is dependent on the area of the tablet in contact with the die wall. It is for this reason that pharmaceutical tablets are designed with a convex surface to lessen the area of tablet in contact with the die wall.

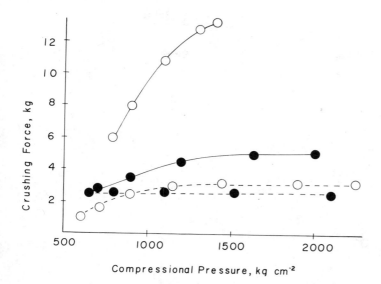

Figure 16. Effect of 2% magnesium stearate on materials that bond by plastic deformation (sodium chloride) and by fragmentation (aspirin). O, Sodium chloride; ●, aspirin; ——, unlubricated; -----, lubricated. (From Ref. 25.)

Lubrication may result from the adherence of the polar portion of the lubricant to the oxide-metal surface and the interposing of a film of low shear strength at the interface between the die wall and the tablet.

Although a lubricant is added to facilitate the operation of tableting, its presence affects the properties of the tablet. A solid lubricant is confined to the surface of the granules and is a physical barrier between the granules. If a material deforms without fragmentation during compression, a lubricant lessens bonding, with formation of soft tablets of reduced mechanical strength. As illustrated in Figure 16, 2% magnesium stearate decreases the strength of a tablet; however, in concentrations of less than 0.5%, the change in hardness is frequently not marked [25]. If a material fragments during compression, new clean surfaces for bonding are formed and the addition of a lubricant has little effect on the strength of the tablet.

The disintegration time of a tablet may be significantly prolonged by the incorporation of a lubricant, as shown in Figure 17.

Dissolution may be affected by the incorporation of a lubricant, as shown in Figure 18 [26]. Talc in concentrations from 0.1 to 5% does not alter the dissolution rates of compressed, nondisintegrating salicylic acid, aspirin, and aspirin-salicylic disks. Although it is water-soluble, polyethylene glycol 4000 does not alter the dissolution rate of these disks.

The dissolution rates of aspirin-salicylic acid disks are slowed by the incorporation of calcium stearate, glyceryl monostearate, hydrogenated caster oil, magnesium stearate, and stearic acid as a lubricant in concentrations from 0.1 to 5%.

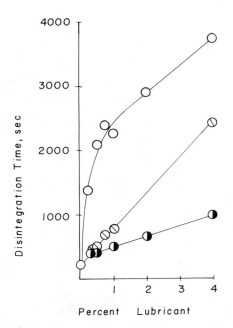

Figure 17. Disintegration time versus percent of lubricant for sodium bicarbonate granulation. O, Magnesium stearate; ⊘, stearic acid; ◑, stearyl alcohol. (From Ref. 11. Reproduced with permission of the copyright owner.)

The addition of from 0.1 to 5% cornstarch to aspirin-salicylic acid disks increases the dissolution rate, because in addition to acting as a lubricant, the starch acts as a disintegrating agent, causing flaking and increasing the effective surface.

The efficiency of a lubricant may be quantitatively expressed as the ratio R of the maximum lower punch force to the maximum upper punch force [7]. A comparison of some R values of various lubricants is shown in Table 4. In addition to the comparison of various lubricants, the R value is helpful in the determination of the concentration of a lubricant that provides an optimum lubricant effect, which for most pharmaceutical lubricants does not exceed 1%.

IV. Transmission of Force

In a single-punch tablet machine, the compressional force on the upper punch is greater than the force on the lower punch. During compression of a given weight of granules, the relationship between the upper and lower punch force is almost linear. Because of friction, the force (or pressure) distribution is not uniform in the die cavity during compression.

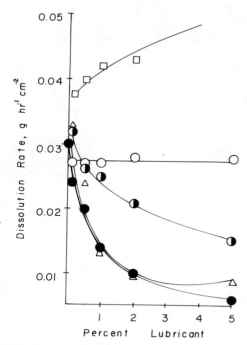

Figure 18. Effect of several lubricants in various concentrations on the dissolution rate of aspirin from a tablet composed of 0.5 M aspirin and 0.5 M salicylic acid compressed at 900 kg cm^{-2}. O, Talc; ●, magnesium stearate, ◑, glyceryl monostearate; △, calcium stearate; □, starch. (From Ref. 26. Reproduced with permission of the copyright owner.)

As a result of the nonuniform pressure distribution during compression, there are variations in density and strength within a tablet. Train [27] measured the distribution of pressure in a magnesium carbonate mass while compression was occurring, and after sectioning the extruded mass, he determined the relative densities of the sections, as illustrated in Figure 19.

The initial pressure of the upper punch produces a region (A) of high density. As the upper punch descends, its initial pressure is progressively lessened with the increasing frictional force at the face of the die wall. Consequently, less pressure is transmitted to the particles adjacent to the die wall, and the region at the bottom corners (D) is less dense than at the top corners. On the other hand, with no die wall friction and only interparticular friction, the material at the center is relatively free to move. Thus, with a greater force being transmitted, the center (C) is compressed to a greater density than region B. After compression there remains a residual die wall force (or pressure), which must be overcome to eject the tablet.

A mean value for the die wall pressure may be measured by strain gages bonded to the outer wall of the die [28]. The die wall must be thin to obtain a

Table 4

Effect of Various Substances as a Lubricant for Compression of a Sulfathiazole Granulation

Lubricant	Percent	Maximum lower punch force / Maximum upper punch force
None (control)	–	0.63
Calcium stearate	0.5	0.96
	1.0	0.98
	2.0	0.99
Sodium stearate	0.5	0.86
	1.0	0.94
	2.0	0.95
Spermaceti	0.5	0.56
	1.0	0.66
	2.0	0.68
Veegum	0.5	0.62
	1.0	0.63
	2.0	0.59
Polyethylene glucol 4000	0.5	0.76
	1.0	0.79
	2.0	0.74
Talc	0.5	0.60
	1.0	0.60
	2.0	0.63
Magnesium stearate	0.5	0.83
	1.0	0.86
	2.0	0.88

Source: Ref. 7.

measurable response. As shown in Figure 20, a part of the die wall may be ground out to increase sensitivity. One strain gage is bonded on the die wall normal to the bore of the die, and one strain gage is bonded parallel to compensate for temperature change during compression. The strain gages form a part of a Wheatstone bridge, as shown in Figure 20. Such a system does not alter the internal die bore and does not depend on the extrusion characteristics of the material being compressed.

Die wall pressure at exact points may be measured by another technique [29]. The apparatus consists of a die in which holes perpendicular to the bore of the die have been drilled and fitted with pistons, as shown in Figure 21. The die wall

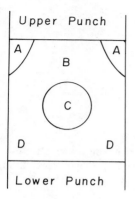

Figure 19. Variation in density within a compact. (See the text.) (From Ref. 27.)

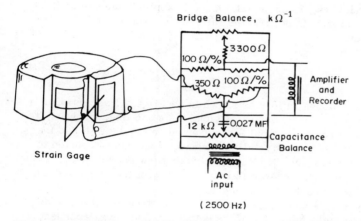

Figure 20. Diagrammatic representation of instrumentation of a single-punch tablet machine for measurement of die wall pressure. (See the text.) (From Ref. 28.)

pressure exerted on the piston is transmitted by mechanical linkage to a load cell,
which activates a recording device.

The simultaneous measurement of die wall pressure and upper punch pressure
may aid in defining the behavior of compressed materials. Axial pressure is that
force per unit area being applied in the direction in which the punch moves during
compression; its application causes a decrease in volume of the material being
compressed. The radial pressure is the force per unit area developed and transmitted at right angles from the logitudinal axis of the punch. The radial pressure
is a shearing factor causing deformation.

The compression characteristics [30] of solids under uniaxial compression
may be defined as (1) a perfectly elastic body, (2) a body with a constant yield

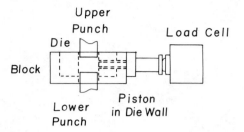

Figure 21. Diagrammatic representation of instrumentation of a single-punch tablet machine for measurement of die wall pressure. (See the text.) (From Ref. 29.)

stress in shear, and (3) a Mohr's body. The assumptions are that the die is perfectly rigid and that there is no die wall friction.

For a perfectly elastic body, when an axial force is applied, the transmitted radial force is of the same magnitude, and the ratio of the axial force σ to the radial force τ is constant:

$$\frac{\sigma}{\tau} = \nu \tag{4}$$

where ν is known as the Poisson ratio. As shown in Figure 22A, as the axial force is decreased, the radial force dissipates along the same line, and when it returns to zero there is no residual radial force exerted on the die wall and the body is free to move from the die. Crystalline phenacetin had been reported to behave similarly to an elastic body [31]. It appears that few pharmaceutical tablets are a perfectly elastic body, as force is required to eject the tablet and the ejected tablet cannot be fitted back into the die cavity.

The compression cycle of a body with a constant yield stress in shear is defined in Figure 22B. The yield value, A, of the deforming body is independent of the magnitudes of stress. The relationship between the axial and radial forces depends on the conditions of the material. When the axial force is increased to A, the body starts to deform, and thereafter

$$\sigma - \tau = 2S \tag{5}$$

where S is the yield stress in shear along AB. After point B has been reached and the axial force is decreased, the body is no longer forced to yield. The radial force decreases along BC. The slopes of BC and AO are equal. If the maximum axial force has been sufficiently large, point C will be attained, at which the radial force is greater than the axial force by an amount 2S. Yield will again occur. The difference between the radial force and the axial force ($\tau - \sigma$) will again be constant along CD. After the upper punch has been withdrawn, the tablet will exert a residual radial force of 2S on the die wall and will be restrained in the die. If the maximum axial force is not great enough, the difference ($\tau - \sigma$) will not attain a value as great as 2S. The change of slope at C, the yield point of decreased axial

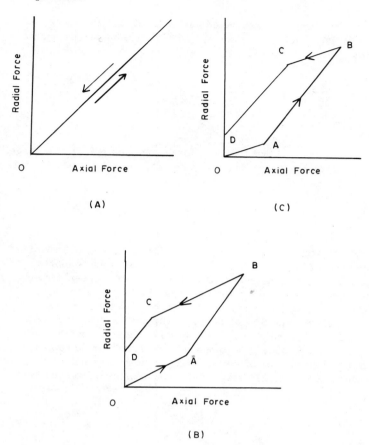

Figure 22. Theoretical compression cycles under uniaxial compression within a rigid, frictionless die. (A) Perfect elastic body, (B) body with constant yield stress in shear, (C) Mohr's body. (See the text.)

force, will not be evident from the graph of the pressure cycle. Pressure cycles for sucrose granules, sucrose crystals, and sodium chloride crystals are similar in behavior to a solid body with a constant yield stress in shear [30].

The compression cycle shown in Figure 22C defines a Mohr's body. The Mohr's body is also rigid, but after yield has occurred, the shearing stress in a plane of slip depends on the value of the normal stress σ_n acting in the same plane. The yield stress in shear is a function of the normal stress on the plane of shear. Where the body yields,

Shearing stress $= S + \mu\sigma_n$

(6)

where μ is a proportionality constant interpreted in terms of friction. The normal stress on the plane of shear equals $(\sigma + \tau)/2$, and the shearing stress equals $(\sigma - \tau)/2$. Thus, at the yield

$$\sigma - \tau = 2S + \mu(\sigma + \tau) \tag{7}$$

$$\tau = \frac{(1 - \mu)\sigma - 2S}{1 + \mu} \tag{8}$$

With decreased axial force, provided that the axial force has been sufficiently large, B', the radial force, will diminish according to the equation $\tau = \sigma$, and then when the material yields again at point C',

$$\tau = \frac{(1 + \mu)\sigma - 2S}{1 - \mu} \tag{9}$$

The slope A'B' equals $(1 - \mu)/(1 + \mu)$. The slope C'D' equals $(1 + \mu)/(1 - \mu)$.

An acetaminophen granulation prepared using acetone behaves as a Mohr's body [30]. The slope CD is 1, and the slope AB is 0.4. Acetaminophen granulated with 3% povidone behaves as a body with a constant yield stress in shear. The slopes CD and AB are 0.4. Acetaminophen on compression tends to cap and laminate; however, if granulated with 3% povidone, no capping is observed. For acetaminophen, the change from a capping tablet to a solid one is associated with the transformation from a Mohr's body type to one with a constant yield stress in shear. This suggests that the analyses of the pressure cycles of materials may be indicative of the formation of a satisfactory or unsatisfactory compressed tablet.

V. Bonding

Several mechanisms of bonding in the compression process have been conceived, but they have not been substantiated by experimentation and have not been useful in the prediction of the compressional properties of materials [32]. Three theories are the mechanical theory, the intermolecular theory, and the liquid-surface film theory.

The mechanical theory proposes that under pressure the individual particles undergo elastic, plastic, or brittle deformation and that the edges of the particles intermesh, forming a mechanical bond. If only the mechanical bond exists, the total energy of compression is equal to the sum of the energy of deformation, heat, and energy adsorbed for each constituent. Mechanical interlocking is not a major mechanism of bonding in pharmaceutical tablets.

According to the intermolecular forces theory, under compressional force the molecules (or atoms or ions) at the points of contact between newly sheared surfaces of the granules are close enough so that van der Waals forces can interact. A microcrystalline cellulose tablet has been described as a cellulose fibril in which the crystals are compressed close enough together so that hydrogen bonding between them occurs [33]. It appears that very little deformation or fusion occurs in the compression of microcrystalline cellulose. Although aspirin crystals undergo slight deformation and fragmentation at low pressure, it appears

that the hydrogen bonding has strongly bonded the tablets, because the granules retain their integrity with further increases in pressure [34].

The liquid-surface film theory attributes bonding to the presence at the particular interfaces of thin liquid films, which may be the consequence of fusion or
adsorbed moisture. For materials that may be compressed directly, the liquid-
surface film theory proposes that the liquid film is a result of fusion or solution
at the surface of the particle induced by the energy of compression. Gross melting does not occur during the compression of most tablets because the energy expended (2 cal for 0.4 g of sulfathiazole) causes only a small temperature rise (5 to
10°C), which is not sufficient to melt the material being tableted.

During the compression process, the compressional force is exerted only on
the granules in direct contact with the punches. Stress in the mass of granules
is a result of granule-to-granule contact. As irregular granules have a very
small area at the points of contact, the pressure there is very high. The effect
of this high pressure on the melting point and solubility of a material is essential
to the bonding.

The relation of pressure and melting point is expressed by the Clapeyron equation,

$$\frac{dT}{dp} = \frac{T(V_1 - V_s)}{\Delta H} \tag{10}$$

in which dT/dP is the change in melting point with pressure, T the absolute temperature, ΔH the molar latent heat of fusion, and V_1 and V_s are the molar volumes of the liquid melt and the solid, respectively.

As the latent heat of fusion is positive, the Clapeyron equation states that for
a solid, which expands on melting ($V_1 > V_s$), the melting point is raised by increasing the pressure. Most solids expand on melting. Thus, the Clapeyron
equation predicts that during compression it would be unlikely that fusion would
occur. The Clapeyron equation is derived from a thermodynamically reversible
process in which the solid is uniformly exposed to a pressure. In fact, the compression of a pharmaceutical tablet is nonreversible, and the pressure is not
uniformly exerted on each granule.

Equating the free energy of the liquid and solid phases, Skotnicky [35] derived an equation relating the heat of fusion, volumes of the liquid and solid
phases, temperature, and the pressures applied to the liquid and solid phases.
For an ideal process in which the material is exposed to a uniform pressure,
the relation reduces to the Clapeyron equation. If the pressure at the points of
contact is exerted only on the solid, and the liquid phase is subjected to a constant atmospheric pressure, the relationship simplifies to

$$\frac{dT}{dP_s} = \frac{-V_s T}{\Delta H} \tag{11}$$

where ΔH is the heat of fusion, V_s the volume of the solid, and T the temperature. As dT/dP_s is always positive regardless of the expansion or contraction
of the solid, the pressure acting locally at the points of contact lowers the melting point.

For surface fusion at the points of contact, a localized temperature at least
equal to the melting point of the material must be attained. With some mixtures

the melting point may be depressed by other ingredients and fusion will occur at a temperature lower than the melting point of the pure material. For most pharmaceutical solids, the specific heat is low and the thermal conductivity is relatively slow. The heat transfer to the surface can be estimated by dividing the compressional energy by the total time of compression. Using the derivation of Carslaw and Jaeger [36] for heat transfer, Rankell and Higuchi [37] estimated for the compression of 0.4 g of sulfathiazole that if the area of contact were 0.01 to 0.1% of the total area, the surface temperature would reach the melting point of most medicinal compounds and pharmaceutical excipients, and fusion would occur. Then upon release of the pressure, solidification of the fused material would form solid bridges between the particles.

By analogous reasoning, the pressure distribution in compression is such that the solubility is increased with increasing pressure. With an increase in solubility at the points of contact, solution usually occurs in the film of adsorbed moisture on the surface of the granule. When the pressure is released, the solubility is decreased, and the solute dissolved in the water of crystallization or in the adsorbed water crystallizes in small crystals between the particles. The strength of the bridge depends not only on the amount of material deposited, but on the rate of crystallization. At higher rates of crystallization, a finer crystal structure and a greater strength are obtained.

The poor adhesion of most water-insoluble materials and the relative ease of compression of water-soluble materials suggests that pressure-induced solubility is important in tableting. The moisture may be present as that retained from the granulating solution after drying or that adsorbed from the atmosphere. Granulations that are absolutely dry have poor compressional characteristics [38]. Water or saturated solutions of the material being compressed may form a film that acts as a lubricant, and if less force is lost to overcome friction, more force is utilized in compression and bonding, and the ejection force is reduced. In formulations using solutions of hydrophilic granulation agent, there may be an optimum moisture content. It has been reported that the optimum moisture content for the starch granulation of lactose is approximately 12% and of phenacetin is approximately 3% [39].

VI. Nature of Material

A. Chemical and Crystalline Structure

Jaffe and Foss [40] investigated the role of crystal properties on the ability of materials to form tablets. They found that compounds (ammonium halides, potassium halides, methanamine) that have cubic crystal lattice often could be compressed directly, and that substances (ferrous sulfate, magnesium sulfate, sodium phosphate) having water of crystallization could be compressed directly but did not form a tablet if the water of crystallization was removed.

The compressibility of a material may be expressed in terms of the slope of a plot of the logarithm of compressional force against porosity. In Figure 23, the slope $dP/d(\log F)$ is greater for methacetin than for phenacetin, indicating that methacetin is more compressible than phenacetin. The chemical nature of phenacetin and methacetin is very similar, yet phenacetin caps readily and is less compressible; thus, there is no correlation between their chemical structure

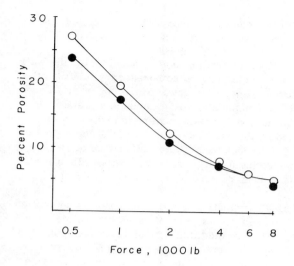

Figure 23. Effect of compressional force on the porosity of methacetin and phenacetin tablets. O, Methacetin; ●, phenacetin. (From Ref. 9.)

and compressional behavior [9]. A general similarity of compressional behavior
among formulations of the sulfa drugs and the alkali halides has been reported [5,
7, 28].

Unfortunately, no general relationship, which would allow the prediction of
compressibility of a formulation based on the chemical nature and crystalline
structure of its constituents, has been demonstrated.

B. Mechanical Properties

There is a direct proportionality between bonding and the contact area of the solid
surfaces on which intermolecular forces act. Solids, which undergo plastic deformation to a large extent, have a greater area of contact for a given pressure
and, consequently, a greater degree of bonding. The plasticity of a crystal lattice contributes to bonding regardless of the mechanism involved.

Sodium chloride is compressed by particle rearrangement and plastic deformation without significant fragmentation [41]. With sodium chloride at a
given pressure, the smaller granules form a mechanically stronger tablet than
do the larger granules [42]. When the tablet is crushed, it fractures across
the crystals, indicating that the bonding between the granules is as strong as
the bonding in the bulk of the solid. With sodium chloride, axial recovery is
completed before ejection from the die.

Lactose, dicalcium phosphate dihydrate, and sucrose [2, 35, 41] are fragmented during compression. When fragmentation is the chief mechanism in compression, tablet strength, or the ability to form a tablet, is independent of the
size of the granules. Heckel [1] used sodium chloride and lactose as examples
to distinguish between the mechanism of bonding.

When the upper punch is withdrawn and the axial force no longer applied, the tablet may crack perpendicular to the compression axis (cap) during the ejection phase.

Capping has been attributed to the effect of entrapped air. Shear at the die wall and punch may prevent the escape of air, which is then compressed within the tablet structure by the compressional force. Upon withdrawal of the upper punch and removal of the compressional force, the compressed air expands and cracks the tablet. Capping may occur by this mechanism for waxy materials and fine powders.

Mechanically capping is minimized by the use of dies in which the upper portion has been tapered several thousandths of an inch to facilitate the escape of air. In some high-speed rotary tablet machines, the use of several pressure rolls allows a gradual increase in pressure with a slower release of the air before the final compression.

In tablet production the particle size distribution of the granulation is controlled so that fine powder is not present. With the proper control of the size of the granulation and proper adjustment and operation of the tablet machine, any capping that occurs is probably not caused by entrapped air but by the formulation. It has been demonstrated that the capping of methanamine tablets under a vacuum is the same as that under atmospheric pressure [43].

The elastic property of a material is responsible for the capping or splitting of a tablet. A material that is very resistant to crushing will undergo elastic deformation under compressional force. The sudden removal of axial force, which caused the elastic deformation, results in the return of the granules to their original form, breaking any bonds that may have formed under pressure.

After the upper punch has been removed, the residual die wall pressure acts on the tablet so that it cannot recover laterally. During ejection a portion of the tablet is outside the die and free of strain, while the remainder of the tablet within the die is under strain. If the strain exceeds the shear strength of the tablet, the tablet cracks. The volume of expansion of a pharmaceutical tablet due to axial and radial recovery may be from 2 to 10%.

Phenacetin is a classical example of an elastic material that caps readily [44]. In the initial stage of compression, only a small force is transmitted to the die wall, owing to the difficulty of particle rearrangement. Force-displacement curves for the compression of phenacetin indicate that at low pressure the energy is largely expended in elastic deformation and that no further increase in tablet strength is expected with increase in pressure. After compression and the removal of axial pressure, the residual die wall pressure is small, indicating that the phenacetin tends to recover axially and contract radially. As the movement of the tablet is restricted by the residual die wall pressure and the friction with the die wall, the stress from its axial elastic recovery and the radial contraction causes splitting.

The strengths of tablets vary due to differences in their elastic recovery. The industrial pharmacist reformulates a tablet that caps by the incorporation of a stronger binding agent, so that the bond strength exceeds the elastic recovery.

References

1. Heckel, R. W., Trans. AIME, 221:671, 1001 (1961).
2. Hersey, J. A., Rees, J. E., and Cole, E. T., J. Pharm. Sci., 62:2060 (1973).

3. Higuchi, T., Arnold, R. D., Trucker, S. J., and Busse, L. W., J. Am. Pharm. Assoc., Sci. Ed., 41:93 (1952).

4. Train, D., and Hersey, J. A., Powder Metall., 6:20 (1960).

5. Higuchi, T., Rao, A. N., Busse, L. W., and Swintosky, J. V., J. Am. Pharm. Assoc., Sci. Ed., 42:194 (1953).

6. Higuchi, T., Nelson, E., and Busse, L. W., J. Am. Pharm. Assoc., Sci. Ed., 43:344 (1954).

7. Nelson, E., Naqvi, S. M., Busse, L. W., and Higuchi, T., J. Am. Pharm. Assoc., Sci. Ed., 43:596 (1954).

8. Higuchi, T., Elowe, L. N., and Busse, L. W., J. Am. Pharm. Assoc., Sci. Ed., 43:685 (1954).

9. Elowe, L. N., Higuchi, T., and Busse, L. W., J. Am. Pharm. Assoc., Sci. Ed., 43:718 (1954).

→10. Nelson, E., Busse, L. W., and Higuchi, T., J. Am. Pharm. Assoc., Sci. Ed., 44:223 (1955).

11. Strickland, W. A., Jr., Nelson, E., Busse, L. W., and Higuchi, T., J. Am. Pharm. Assoc., Sci. Ed., 45:51 (1956).

12. Strickland, W. A., Jr., Higuchi, T., and Busse, L. W., J. Am. Pharm. Assoc., Sci. Ed., 49:35 (1960).

13. Newton, J. M., and Stanley, P., J. Pharm. Pharmacol., 27:5P (1975).

14. Lowenthal, W., J. Pharm. Sci., 61:1695 (1972).

15. Shah, S. A., and Parrott, E. L., J. Pharm. Sci., 65:1784 (1976).

16. Mitchell, A.G., and Saville, D. J., J. Pharm. Pharmacol., 19:729 (1967).

17. Kanke, M., and Sekiguchi, K., Chem. Pharm. Bull., 21:871 (1973).

18. Leeson, L. J., and Carstensen, J. T., eds., Dissolution Technology. Industrial Pharmaceutical Technology Section, Academy of Pharmaceutical Sciences, Washington, D.C., p. 133.

19. van Oudtshorn, M. C. B., Potgieter, F. J., deBlaey, C. J., and Polderman, J., J. Pharm. Pharmacol., 23:583 (1971).

20. Shotton, E., and Ganderton, D. J., J. Pharm. Pharmacol., 12:87T (1960).

21. Knoechel, E. L., Sperry, C. C., Ross, H. E., and Lintner, C. J., J. Pharm. Sci., 56:109 (1967).

22. Shotton, E., Deer, J. J., and Ganderton, D. J., J. Pharm. Pharmacol., 15:106T (1963).

ΔT →23. Bogs, V., and Lenhardt, E., Pharm. Ind., 33:850 (1971).

24. Hanls, E. J., and King, L. D., J. Pharm. Sci., 57:677 (1968).

25. Shotton, E., and Lewis, C. J., J. Pharm. Pharmacol., 16:111T (1964).

26. Iranloye, T. A., and Parrott, E. L., J. Pharm. Sci., 67:535 (1978).

27. Train, D., J. Pharm. Pharmacol., 8:745 (1956).

28. Windheuser, J. J., Misra, J., Eriksen, S. P., and Higuchi, T., J. Pharm. Sci., 52:767 (1963).

29. Nelson, E., J. Am. Pharm. Assoc., Sci. Ed., 44:494 (1955).

30. Leigh, S., Carless, J. E., and Burt, B. W., J. Pharm. Sci., 56:888 (1967).

31. Shotton, E., and Obiorah, B. A., J. Pharm. Sci., 64:1213 (1975).

32. Goetzel, C. G., Treatise on Powder Metallurgy, Vol. 1. Interscience, New York, 1949, pp. 259-312.

33. Reier, G. E., and Shangraw, R. E., J. Pharm. Sci., 55:510 (1966).

34. Khan, K. A., and Rhodes, C. T., J. Pharm. Sci., 64:444 (1975).

35. Skotnicky, J., Czech. J. Phys., 3:225 (1953).
36. Carslaw, H. S., and Jaeger, J. C., Conduction of Heat in Solids, 2nd ed.
     Oxford University Press, London, 1959, p. 75.
37. Rankell, A. S., and Higuchi, T., J. Pharm. Sci., 57:574 (1968).
38. Train, D., and Lewis, C. J., Trans. Inst. Chem. Eng., 40:235 (1962).
39. Sheth, P., and Munzel, K., Pharm. Ind., 21:9 (1959).
40. Jaffe, J., and Foss, N. E., J. Am. Pharm. Assoc., Sci. Ed., 48:26
     (1959).
41. Hardman, J. S., and Lilley, B. A., Nature (Lond.), 228:353 (1970).
42. Hersey, J. A., Bayraktar, G., and Shotton, E., J. Pharm. Pharmacol.,
     19:245 (1967).
43. Long, W. M., Powder Metall., 6:73 (1960).
44. deBlaey, C. J., deRijk, W., and Polderman, J., Pharm. Ind., 33:897
     (1971).

5

Granulation and Tablet Characteristics

Dale E. Fonner

The Upjohn Company
Kalamazoo, Michigan

Neil R. Anderson and Gilbert S. Banker

Purdue University
West Lafayette, Indiana

PART ONE. CHARACTERIZATION OF GRANULATIONS

Final tablet characteristics, such as dissolution rate, disintegration time, porosity, friability, capping tendency, and hardness, are fundamental physicochemical properties of interest to the development pharmacist. Tablets are made from granular particulate solids; therefore, granulation characteristics are of interest, as they can affect all of the aforementioned performance characteristics of the final tablet, and others. The quality of tablets, once formulated, is as a general rule primarily dictated by the quality of the physicochemical properties of the granulation from which the tablets are made. There are many formulation and process variables involved in the granulation step, and all of these can affect the characteristics of granulations produced. Where possible, the effect of these variables on granulation characteristics will be covered in this section, as well as measurement methods aimed at characterizing granulations.

After a brief introduction that will deal with granule formation and structure, the following topics will be discussed in detail:

Particle size measurement and interpretation
Shape determinations
Surface area
Densities and packings
Granule strength and friability
Electrostatic properties
Flow properties
Ease of consolidation and mechanisms

The granulation characteristics that are probably of most immediate interest to development pharmacists and therefore the most universally measured are those of bulk density, some assessment of flow, particle size distribution, and some

assessment of successful compaction into tablets. These basic granulation characteristic measurements have been used to develop and monitor the manufacture
of the many successful pharmaceutical tablet products. Conceivably, then, some
of the topics that will be discussed in this section may appear purely theoretical
and of little or no practical value. However, it is not uncommon to encounter
problems in the formulation, design, or manufacture of tablets where a knowledge of granulation characteristics and their measurement, beyond the routine
methods described above, may be of value. In some cases the resolution of tableting problems may, in fact, be completely satisfactory only if the source of the
problem is first identified by in-depth studies of granulation characteristics, beyond what the basic measurements can provide in order to solve those problems.

   The product validation concept in the Current Good Manufacturing Practices
regulations for the pharmaceutical industry requires that systems and processes
involved in manufacturing a drug product be thoroughly under control to the extent that documentation can be shown that those systems and processes are doing
what they are designed to do in a reproducible fashion.

   To gain the control and to be able to monitor the critical processing variables
within a granulate system may require that more definitive or quantitative measurements be used. It is with these ideas in mind that certain topics have been
included in the following discussion.

I. Granule Formation and Structure

A discussion of granule formation must necessarily start with a consideration of
particle-particle bonding mechanisms involved in adhesion and cohesion of particles. Several forces that can act between small neighboring particles have been
identified [1, 2]. There are valency and van der Waals forces that are usually
classified as molecular forces. Although valency forces may be 50 to 100 times
the magnitude of van der Waals forces (e.g., 100 kcal mol^{-1} versus 1 kcal mol^{-1}),
they are generally discounted in the granulation process because they can act only
over very short distances (approximately 10 Å). On the other hand, van der Waals
forces can act over distances up to 1000 Å and must be considered as able to form
interparticle bonds. Most powders possess an electrostatic charge. However,
the magnitude of these forces are generally much smaller than van der Waals
forces, and they therefore contribute very little to the final strength of a granule. However, it is reasonable to assume that electrostatic forces may play a
role in initial formation of agglomerates.

   In wet granulation, an aqueous solution containing a binder is generally added
to the powder mixture. The liquid plays a key role in the granulation process.
Liquid bridges develop between particles and the tensile strength of these bonds
increases as the amount of liquid added is increased. These surface-tension
forces and capillary pressure are primarily responsible for initial granule formation and strength. Also, during granulation, particles and agglomerates are
subjected to consolidating forces by the action of machine parts or interparticle
abrasion. For example, passing the wet mass through an oscillating granulator
serves to further consolidate granules and increase particle contact points. During drying, interparticle bonds will result from fusion or recrystallization and
curing of the binding agent, with van der Waals forces playing a significant role.

Many factors can affect granule structure, with the type of granulation equipment employed and amount of water used to granulate being most important [3, 4]. The effect of the amount of granulating solution used to granulate will be discussed throughout the section as to its effect on granulation characteristics. Certainly, the structure of granules produced by spray drying are far different than those produced through an oscillating granulator, and in general, granulation equipment influences granule structure [5, 6]. Granules produced by spray drying are approximately spherical in shape, possess a narrow size distribution, and are often hollow [7]. Therefore, spray-dried granulations are usually free-flowing, possess a low bulk density, and dissolve rapidly. Kanig [8] has shown that the flow and compressional qualities of mannitol can be greatly improved by granulating this material by a spray congealing process. Fonner et al. [9] have shown that granules produced in a V-blender are more spherical and less dense than those produced in an oscillating granulator. The effect of these and other variables on granule structure and characteristics is discussed in this section.

II. Particle Size Measurement and Interpretation

The principal intent of particle size measurement is to establish the true frequency distribution of particle size. Although the concept is simple, there are basic problems in defining both size and distribution. If powders or granulations contained only spherical particles, there would be no difficulty in defining particle size, because the size of a sphere is uniquely determined by its diameter. But particles are rarely spherical in shape, and more often than not are quite irregular in shape. Experimental methods vary greatly, and the observed particle size distribution is dependent upon the methodology and technique employed. In addition, powders and granulations pose some unique sampling problems. The amount of material subjected to a particle size analysis usually represents only a very small part of the particulate material in question. Therefore, it is essential that the sample(s) selected be unbiased and representative of the total material. In spite of these problems, it is possible to establish valid frequency distributions of particle size. The observed distribution then serves as the basis for establishing descriptive characteristics or constants, such as median diameter (by weight or number), percent by weight greater than a stated size, or standard deviation. Several good reference sources are available on particle size measurement and interpretation [10-14]. This discussion begins by covering the various methods of data presentation.

A. Methods of Data Presentation

1. Tabular Presentation

The most general method of data presentation, and perhaps the most widely used, is tabular form. Most often the table lists particle size versus one of the many ways of expressing its distribution. Table 1 illustrates the most common way of presenting data in tabular form. The distributions are presented both as frequencies and as cumulative frequencies.

Table 1

Size Distribution Data for a Hypothetical Tablet Granulation

Size (μm)	Percent frequency distribution by weight	Cumulative % by weight less than stated size
0-100	5.0	5.0
100-200	17.0	22.0
200-300	18.0	40.0
300-400	25.0	55.0
400-500	11.0	66.0
500-600	8.0	74.0
600-700	6.0	80.0
700-800	4.0	84.0
800-900	3.0	87.0
900-1000	2.0	89.0
≥1000	11.0	
	100.0	

Note that the frequency data in Table 1 are presented by weight rather than by number. The size distribution can be defined in terms of the weight or number of particles within a given size range. For pharmaceutical granulations, size distributions are normally described by weight. For example, it is far simpler to weigh the amount of granulation retained on a sieve as opposed to counting individual particles. For the granulation represented in Table 1, 5% by weight of the particles are from 0 to 100 μm, 17% by weight are in the range 100 to 200 μm, and so forth. From the cumulative percent distribution, 22% of the particles by weight are less than 200 μm in size, 40% by weight are less than 300 μm in size, and so forth. It should be pointed out that the weight distribution data of Table 1 are hypothetical, since standard sieves do not exist that produce the even 100 μm size fractions shown in the table.

2. Graphical Presentation

Although the most precise and explicit way of presenting size distribution data is by tabular form, there are several compelling reasons for presenting size distribution data graphically. Graphs are more concise than are long tables, and in some cases, numerical measurements or constants can be obtained which further describe the distribution of particle sizes. Also, skewness of the distribution and location of the mean particle size can readily be approximated. Further, graphical presentation offers a clear and concise way to compare size distribution data from two or more samples. Histograms, size frequency curves, and cumulative frequency plots represent the most common ways of graphically illustrating size distribution data. Any elementary book on statistical analysis [15] will provide the reader with additional background information concerning these types of graphical analyses.

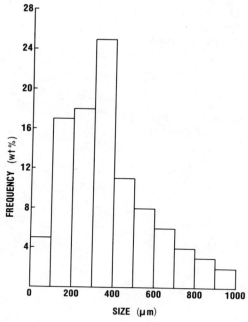

Figure 1. Histogram plot for the size frequency data given in Table 1.

Frequency Histograms

The simplest graphical form is a histogram plot in which frequency of occurrence is plotted as a function of the size range. A histogram plot of the data represented in Table 1 is shown in Figure 1. Note that the height of each rectangle corresponds to the frequency percent for the size range indicated. For example, the height of the rectangle in the range 0 to 100 μm is 5% on the frequency scale, indicating that 5% by weight of the particles are in the size range 0 to 100 μm.

Size Frequency Curves

A size frequency curve can be drawn from the histogram; this is shown in Figure 2. A size frequency curve is nothing more than a smoothed-out histogram and is obtained by drawing a continuous line through the midpoints of the top of the rectangles. In other words, it can be seen that the tops of the rectangles form a smooth curve. Some words of caution are in order concerning size frequency curves. These curves are valid only if a large number of points are utilized. Considerable error is introduced when trying to draw a size frequency curve from a small number of points. Also, the shape of the size frequency curve can become quite irregular if uneven size ranges are used. Therefore, it is preferable to draw size frequency curves employing many points and equal size intervals. Often, it is not practical to obtain size intervals in a regular progression. This is especially true when using sieving as a method of particle size analysis. In these instances, the cumulative percent plot is valuable and is discussed next.

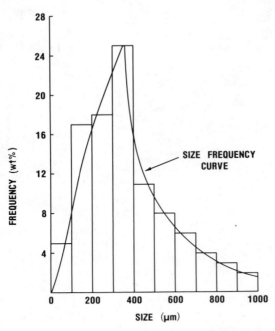

Figure 2. Illustration of the size frequency curve for the data given in Table 1.

Cumulative Frequency Curves

Cumulative frequency curves are arrived at by plotting the percent of particles less than (or greater than) a given particle size versus particle size. A cumulative frequency plot of the data contained in Table 1 is shown in Figure 3. If the summation is carried out from the top downward, as in Table 1, the result is the percent of particles smaller than the upper limit of the successive size intervals.

The cumulative frequency data in Table 1 could just as easily have been summed from the bottom upward, yielding the percentage of particles greater than the lower limit of the successive size intervals. A cumulative frequency plot of percent greater than stated size could then be drawn. The choice of whether to use percent less than, or greater than, a stated size is largely arbitrary but may be based on whether the researcher is most interested in directly identifying the fraction of particles that are "oversize" or "undersize" vis-a-vis, a particular cutoff point. It should also be clear that these graphical methods are just as applicable for size frequency data generated on a number basis.

From a mathematical standpoint, integration of the size frequency curve (Fig. 2) will give the cumulative frequency curve (Fig. 3). In a like manner, differentiation of the cumulative frequency curve will yield a smooth size frequency curve. The latter point is of practical value, as the cumulative frequency curve can be drawn from data with unequal size intervals. As was mentioned before, drawing a size frequency distribution curve from frequency data in uneven size intervals will often yield a very irregular curve. This can be overcome by

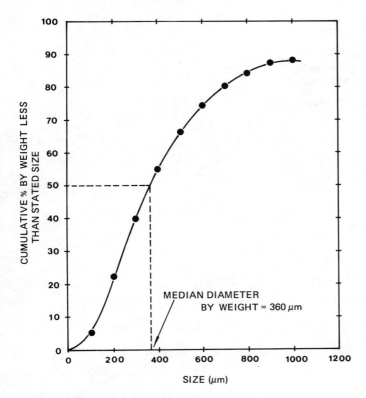

Figure 3. Cumulative frequency plot for the data contained in Table 1.

first plotting the cumulative frequency curve and then deriving the size frequency
curve from a differentiation of this plot over equal size intervals.

One useful constant or descriptive characteristic that can be obtained from
the cumulative frequency curve is the median diameter by weight (or number).
On a weight basis, the median diameter is that particle size value above and below which half the total weight of particles is found. In Figure 3, it can be seen
that the median diameter by weight is equal to approximately 360 μm.

B. Distribution Functions

1. Log-Normal Law

Perhaps the most important statistical law in nature is the log-normal distribution law [10, 11, 16, 17]. With this law it is the logarithm of the variant
that is distributed normally rather than the variant itself. Note that the size frequency curve in Figure 2 is skewed and has a long "tail" of large particles. This
skewness is characteristic of many, if not most, particulate systems. Thus, the
normal distribution law is not applicable to most particulate systems. Figure 4

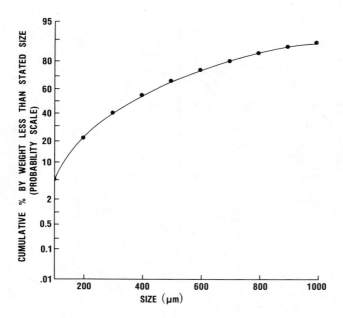

Figure 4. Cumulative frequency plot using probability paper for the data contained in Table 1.

contains a cumulative frequency plot on probability paper for the data contained in Table 1. Had the data followed a normal distribution, the points would have resulted in a straight line. However, when the cumulative percent data contained in Table 1 are plotted against the log of particle size (Fig. 5), a straight line results. The graph paper used in Figure 5 is termed log-probability paper and can be used to determine if particle size distribution data follows a log-normal distribution. The straight-line relationship shown in Figure 5 indicates that these particle size data follow the log-normal law.

To reiterate, most particulate systems will approximate the log-normal distribution rather than the normal distribution. When making a log-probability plot, it is not uncommon to find that experimental data are scattered, with the apparent degree of scattering being greater at the extremities (the very small and very large particles). When determining the best straight line, greater weight should be given to points lying closest to the 50% cumulative point [18]. Because of the distortion created by the probability axis at the extremities, some authors recommend that when fitting the best straight line, only experimental points within the 20 to 80% range be used.

Further, to minimize human error in determining the best straight line, it is suggested that regression analysis be employed if there is much "scatter" to the experimental points. Again, if the particle size distribution follows a log-normal distribution, it will always be represented by a straight line on log-probability paper.

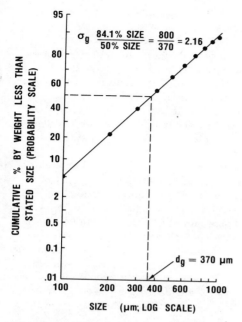

Figure 5. Cumulative frequency plot using log-probability paper for the data contained in Table 1.

Two useful constants can be derived from Figure 5, and these are the geometric mean diameter d_g and the geometric standard deviation σ_g. The value of d_g is equal to the median or 50% diameter. Mathematically,

$$d_g = \text{antilog} = \left(\frac{\sum\limits_{i=1}^{n} n_i \log d_i}{\sum\limits_{i=1}^{n} n_i} \right) = 50\% \text{ size} \tag{1}$$

where d_i are diameters and are equal to the midpoints of the particle size intervals employed, and n_i are the number or weight of particles having these respective diameters. d_g is usually determined graphically, and from the plot in Figure 5, d_g is found to be approximately 370 μm. The geometric standard deviation σ_g can be found by dividing the diameter at the 84.1% size by the 50% diameter, d_g. Mathematically,

$$\sigma_g = \text{antilog} = \sqrt{\frac{\sum\limits_{i=1}^{n} n_i (\log d_i - \log d_g)^2}{\sum\limits_{i=1}^{n} n_i}} = \frac{84.1\% \text{ size}}{50.0\% \text{ size}} = \frac{50.0\% \text{ size}}{15.9\% \text{ size}} \tag{2}$$

In the case of both d_g and σ_g, it is usually easiest to obtain these values from a graphical plot on log-probability paper as opposed to employing their mathematical counterparts [Eqs. (1) and (2)]. The derivation of the fact that σ_g = 84.1% size/50.0% size = 50.0% size/15.9% size follows from integration of the probability curve describing the log-normal distribution. The derivation will not be presented here and the interested reader is referred to the literature [19]. Again, σ_g is usually determined graphically, and from Figure 5, σ_g is found to be 2.16. Notice that σ_g is unitless and the minimum value that it can assume is 1.0 (when all particles are of the same diameter). σ_g and d_g describe completely the distribution of particle sizes and are, therefore, useful when comparing size distribution data from several samples.

Equations (1) and (2) are applicable for size frequency data derived on a number or weight basis. That is, n_i can represent either the number or weight of particles having a diameter d_i. For purposes of clarity in future discussions, d_g will be used to represent this parameter derived on a weight basis and d_g' will be used to represent this parameter derived on a number basis. It can be shown that if the particle size distribution gives a straight line on a weight basis when plotted on log probability paper, the size distribution by number will be a parallel straight line on the same coordinates [19, 20]. Thus, for a particular sample of particles, the geometric standard deviation by weight equals the geometric standard deviation by number. Therefore, only the term σ_g will be used in future discussions. It is also possible to convert the geometric mean diameter by weight to a number basis as follows [12]:

$$\log d_g' = \log d_g - 6.908 \log^2 \sigma_g \tag{3}$$

Diameters on a number basis will generally be considerably smaller than those on a weight basis. For example, if one substitutes d_g = 370 μm and σ_g = 2.16 (obtained from Fig. 5) in Equation (3), d_g' = 62.4 μm. In a like manner, Fonner et al. [21] found that for a granulation prepared by the hand screen method (No. 12 mesh), d_g and σ_g on a weight basis were 900 μm and 4.12, respectively. From Equation (3) the geometric mean diameter by number for this sample was equal to 2.19 μm. On a weight basis d_g = 900 μm, and on a number basis, d_g' = 2.19 μm. Thus, it can be seen that the contribution by smaller particles on a number basis is enormous.

2. Normal Law

If the data follow a normal distribution, one should get a straight line from cumulative plots made on probability paper. The arithmetic mean d_a and standard deviation σ can be obtained from such a plot as follows:

$$d_a = \frac{\sum\limits_{i=1}^{n} n_i d_i}{\sum\limits_{i=1}^{n} n_i} = 50\% \text{ size} \tag{4}$$

$$\sigma = \sqrt{\frac{\sum\limits_{i=1}^{n} n_i (d_i - d_a)^2}{\sum\limits_{i=1}^{n} n_i}} = 84.1\% \text{ size} - 50\% \text{ size} \tag{5}$$

If the particle size data follow a normal distribution, d_a and σ completely describe the distribution of particle sizes and are valuable for comparison purposes. As with the log-normal distribution, d_a and σ can be determined from a graphical plot on probability paper, as opposed to using cumbersome equations [Eqs. (4) and (5)]. Should particle size data not fit either the normal or log-normal distribution law, there are other distributions, such as modified log-normal distributions and empirical equations, that may be considered [10]. However, it may be well to just present the data as shown in Table 1 or Figures 1 to 3 should data not follow a normal or log-normal distribution.

C. Average Particle Size

The average particle size or mean diameter for a population of particles can be defined in many ways. We have already been exposed to two of these, the geometric mean diameter and the arithmetic mean diameter. Numerous other ways exist for calculating mean diameters, and Edmundson defines a total of 11 different ways in which a mean diameter can be computed [13]. Of these, perhaps the most important is the mean volume surface diameter d_{vs}, which is defined as follows:

$$d_{vs} = \frac{\sum\limits_{i=1}^{n} n_i d_i^3}{\sum\limits_{i=1}^{n} n_i d_i^2} \tag{6}$$

The mean volume surface diameter is often of value and interest because it is inversely proportional to the specific surface area of the sample. Therefore, if the physical or chemical properties of the particulate sample are dependent upon surface area, the mean volume surface diameter should be used to describe the mean particle size. It should be noted that d_g and d_a are of value for comparative purposes only and are not relatable or proportional to any physical properties of the particles in question. However, this is often not a serious drawback, as most studies involving pharmaceutical granulations are of a comparative nature. In other words, we are usually interested in the effect of various processing variables (e.g., granulating equipment, granulation solution, processing time, etc.) on the size distribution of granules produced. On the other hand, the surface area of the granules produced may affect dissolution rate, ease of compaction, flowability,

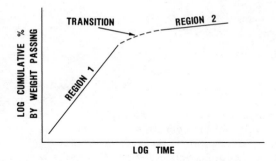

Figure 6. Typical plot of the cumulative percent by weight of material passing a sieve as a function of time.

and so on. If such characteristics are related to granule surface area and of importance to the investigator, then d_{vs} should be used to define the average particle size of the sample. Although Equation (6) can be used to compute d_{vs}, if the particle size distribution obeys the log-normal law, d_{vs} can be obtained from a knowledge of d_g [22]:

$$\log d_{vs} = \log d_g - 1.151 \log^2 \sigma_g \qquad (7)$$

For the data shown in Figure 5 ($d_g = 370$ μm and $\sigma_g = 2.16$), d_{vs} is found to be equal to 275 μm through the use of Equation (7). Thus, for the size frequency data contained in Table 1, we have now computed the mean particle diameter by three methods, with the following results:

d_g = geometric mean diameter by weight = 370 μm
d_g^1 = geometric mean diameter by number = 62.4 μm
d_{vs} = mean volume surface diameter by weight = 275 μm

Each of the above is a valid way of computing and expressing the average particle size for a sample. Of these diameters, d_{vs} has the most practical significance in that it is related to specific surface area. Opankunle et al. [23] have illustrated the use of d_{vs} as applied to drying-rate studies on lactose and sulfathiazole granulations.

D. Methods of Particle Size Determination

Sieving represents by far the simplest and most widely used method for the determination of particle size for pharmaceutical granulations and powders. For this reason, sieving will be considered in detail.

1. Sieving

Factors involved in sieving of pharmaceutical powders have been investigated [21] and an extensive study of the physical laws that govern the sieving of particles has been published by Whitby [24]. It was shown by Whitby that the sieving curve can be divided into two distinctly different regions, with a transition range in between. The sieving curve can be obtained by plotting the cumulative percent by weight passing the sieve versus time. Plots may be made on log-log paper or on log-probability paper. A typical example of the former case is given in Figure 6. Whitby found that the rate at which material passes a sieve in region 1 is a constant and closely follows the following relationship:

$$\% \text{ Passing} = at^b \tag{8}$$

where t is the sieving time, b is a constant, and a is a sieving-rate constant. Region 2 was found to follow the log-normal law. In this region all of the particles much smaller than the mesh size have already passed the sieve; consequently, particles now passing the sieve are of a constant mesh size. Exact equations for determining the amount of material passing through a sieve are given in Whitby's paper.

For all practical purposes, the sieve is considered to be at equilibrium at the time when region 2 begins, since the slight positive slope of the line is due mostly to attrition of larger-than-mesh-size particles. To minimize experimental error, it is important when determining a sieving time for a stack of sieves that one be in region 2.

Sieves are made with woven-wire cloth and have square openings. Two standard series are utilized in the United States, the Tyler Standard Scale and the United States Sieve Series. The relationship between mesh number and aperture dimension are given in Table 2 for both of these standard sieves.

Sieves are normally used for coarse particles. However, depending upon the material, they traditionally have been employed down to a particle size of about 37 μm (400 mesh). Recent developments in screen fabrication technology and the employment of an oscillating air column for particle movement through sieves allows one to go as low as 5 μm in sieving separations. These developments greatly extend the utility and versatility of the sieving method for particle size analysis.

Sieves are calibrated by manufacturers according to National Bureau of Standards specifications. Sieves, especially shop-worn sieves, should be checked periodically for proper calibration. Care should be exercised in the use and particularly in the cleaning of sieves that are employed for particle size fractionation. Brushes should be avoided in cleaning sieves, because brushing may cause disorientation of the screen wires. Soluble components should be dissolved or gently washed out of the screen surface. Insoluble materials may best be removed by running a gentle stream of water against the back side of the screen and/or by driving a compressed airstream against the reverse side of the screen surface.

Stainless or corrosion-resistant steel is recommended as a material of construction for screens. Carefully sized fractions of glass beads are available from the National Bureau of Standards for calibration purposes.

In sieve analysis, an accurately weighed sample is placed on the top sieve of a nest or stack of sieves. Each sieve has a smaller size opening in the wire cloth than the one immediately above it. The sample is then shaken through the various sieves and thereby separated into a series of fractions on the individual sieves. The amount of material retained on each sieve is then weighed. This figure can then be divided by the initial sample weight to arrive at the percent frequency for

Table 2

Relationship Between Sieve Mesh and Aperture for Tyler Standard Scale and
United States Sieve Series

United States		Tyler	
Mesh number	Aperture (mm)	Mesh number	Aperture (mm)
3 1/2	5.66	3 1/2	5.613
4	4.76	4	4.699
5	4.00	5	3.962
6	3.36	6	3.372
7	2.83	7	2.794
8	2.38	8	2.362
10	2.00	9	1.981
12	1.68	10	1.651
14	1.41	12	1.397
16	1.19	14	1.168
18	1.00	16	0.991
20	0.840	20	0.833
25	0.710	24	0.701
30	0.590	28	0.589
35	0.500	32	0.495
40	0.420	35	0.417
45	0.350	42	0.351
50	0.297	48	0.295
60	0.250	60	0.246
70	0.210	65	0.208
80	0.177	80	0.175
100	0.149	100	0.147
120	0.125	115	0.124
140	0.105	150	0.104
170	0.088	170	0.088
200	0.074	200	0.074
230	0.062	250	0.061
270	0.053	270	0.053
325	0.044	325	0.043
400	0.037	400	0.038

the described size range. For example, consider a nest of sieves as shown in the
first column of Table 3. Assume a 200 g sample of a granulation is then shaken
through these sieves, with the results being as shown in Table 3.

The first column in Table 3 indicates the mesh number of the sieve and the
order in which they were stacked from top to bottom. The second column gives
the aperture opening for each sieve in microns. The third column gives the
weight retained on each sieve in grams. Note that the total of the individual
sample weights on each sieve equals 200 g, the size of the sample taken for analysis. The fourth column gives the theoretical respective size ranges for the

Table 3

Tabular Presentation of Particle Size Data for Sieving Analysis Problem

Mesh number	Aperture (μm)	Weight retained on sieve (g)	Size range (μm)	Percent frequency distribution	Cumulative % (less than)
16	991	20	> 991	10.0	——
28	589	30	589–991	15.0	90.0
42	351	38.0	351–589	19.0	75.0
60	246	28.0	246–351	14.0	56.0
100	147	44.0	147–246	22.0	42.0
200	74	24.0	74–147	12.0	20.0
270	53	9.0	53–74	4.5	8.0
Pan	—	7.0	< 53	3.5	3.5
		200		100	

particles on each sieve in the stack. The fifth column gives the percent frequency distribution which is computed by dividing individual sample weights on each sieve by the initial sample weight of 200 g. The last column then gives the cumulative percent by weight less than stated size. This is arrived at by summing, from the bottom up, the results in the percent frequency distribution column (the fifth column). The data contained in Table 3 can then be presented graphically by any one of the methods previously described. Note, however, that the range of and midpoint between the various size ranges in Table 3 are not equal, as is typical for such sieve data.

There are numerous factors that can affect the screening operation. An awareness of these factors is important in minimizing the magnitude of sieving errors and assuring reproducibility. The more notable factors influencing the performance of the sieving operation are given below.

Sieve load and sieving time
Screen movement, particle orientation, and particle shape
Aperture size and variations
Sampling of material

From an examination of the sieving curve (Fig. 6), it is clear that different sieving times will give different results. The effect of sieving time on d_g for a lactose granulation has been studied [21]. As expected, as sieving time increases, d_g decreases. A straight line with a negative slope was obtained when log d_g was plotted against time. There is no absolute end point, but rather an arbitrary time is chosen. It has been shown that the sieving rate decreases as the initial sieve load increases [21, 24, 25]. Therefore, at constant sieving times, different size loads of the same material will give different particle size distributions. Thus, sieving analysis methods should be established to accommodate the material under test, and thereafter closely standardized for subsequent analyses.

The type and intensity of screen movement can affect the resultant size distribution. Common screen motions are circular, resonant, or linear, and the mode chosen will affect the results [26-28]. The orientation that particles present to sieve apertures are quite random. There is only a certain probability that a particle oriented in a certain fashion will pass an aperture and a certain probability that it will reach the aperture in that orientation [9].

Studies have shown that as the particle size approaches aperture size, the rate of material passing the sieve decreases rapidly [21, 24, 29]. Furthermore, the aperture sizes in a sieve are not absolutely uniform, but form a normal distribution about a mean value. During the sieving process, the more irregular the particle, the longer the time interval before peak blinding occurs [29]. Finally, if a number of samples of the same weight are withdrawn from the same material and these are sieved on the same equipment at the same speed setting for the same length of time, the sieving results will differ because of random variations in the composition of the samples. The homogeneity of the sample is determined by the extent of mixing. From a statistical sense, even if mixing is complete, small samples from the mixture will present a different size distribution than will larger samples. In general, the smaller the sample, the more biased the resultant size distribution. Therefore, from a statistical sampling standpoint, one should use large samples. At the same time, the researcher is often interested in differences in particle size distribution in various regions of a powder or granulation blend, and will run several analyses rather than one composite analysis, to determine this information. As the initial sieve load is increased, in attempting to run more representative samples, the researcher must remember that the sieving efficiency decreases, and attrition affects may be accentuated.

It has been stated that the optimal sieving load is one that results in a powder depth of one to two particle diameters. Therefore, obtaining a representative sample must be balanced against sieving efficiency. For further details on the factors affecting sieving, the reader is referred to Jansen and Glastonbury [30].

2. Other Methods for Determining Particle Size Distributions

There are many other methods for determining the particle size distribution of powders. Some of the more common methods are as follows:

1. Microscopy
2. Sedimentation
3. Light scattering
4. Adsorption methods [Brünauer-Emmett-Teller (BET) apparatus]
5. Electrolytic resistivity (Coulter counter)
6. Permeametry

When dealing with agglomerated powders, sieving is the preferred method for determining particle size distribution. However, when dealing with fine powders, such as a direct-compression powder system, one or more of the foregoing methods may be of value in particle size determinations. The chief limitation of sieving is that of particle size. When the size distribution of the powder in question is in the range 0 to 100 μm, one of the foregoing methods may be better suited than sieving. The reader is referred to the literature [10, 13, 31, 32] for an in-depth review of the various methodologies available for determining particle size.

E. Effects of Granule Size and Factors Affecting Granule Size

A survey of the literature indicates that granule size can affect the average tab-let weight [33, 34], tablet weight variation [33, 34], disintegration time [35], granule friability [34], granulation flowability [34], and the drying rate kinetics of wet granulations [23, 36]. The exact effect of granule size and size distribu-tion on processing requirements, bulk granulation characteristics, and final tablet characteristics is dependent upon formulation ingredients and their concentration as well as the type of granulating equipment and processing conditions employed. Therefore, it is up to the formulator to determine for each formulation and manu-facturing process the effects of granule size and size distribution and whether they are important or not. The literature is often conflicting as to the affects of gran-ule size, and therefore few general conclusions can be drawn.

There are many factors that can affect the size and size distribution of gran-ulations. The factor having perhaps the largest effect on mean granule size is the mesh size of the screen used to wet granulate. Other formulation and proc-essing factors that can effect granule size are illustrated in a series of papers by Chalmers and Elworthy [37-39]. In general, it can be concluded that mean granule size increases as the volume of granulating solution is increased and wet mixing time is increased. These authors further found that the type and amount of binder used, the particle size of formulation ingredients, and the method of granulation can affect mean granule size.

In working with granulations prepared in a fluid-bed dryer, Davies and Gloor [40-42] found that the following tended to increase granule size: (1) increase in the formula weight of binder, (2) increase in the amount of solution used to granu-late, (3) increase in the addition rate of granulating solution, (4) decrease in the air inlet temperature during the granulation cycle, (5) decrease in the air pres-sure to the nozzle, and (6) decrease in the nozzle height above the distribution grid. In general, it can be concluded that granule size and size distribution are the net result of many formulation and processing variables. If mean granule size is found to be important (e.g., suppose that granule size directly affects granulation flowability and tablet weight variation), then an appreciation and understanding of the factors discussed above that can affect mean granule size are important.

Chalmers and Elworthy [37-39] noted the effects of various formulation and processing variables on granule size of oxytetracycline tablet granulations proc-essed on an oscillating granulator. They found that when changing from water to 1.25% polyvinylpyrrolidone (PVP) as the granulating solution, average granule size decreased (360 μm versus 210 μm). As the volume of granulating solution was increased, granule size increased dramatically. In all cases, inclusion of the excipients alginic acid and/or microcrystalline cellulose reduced mean gran-ule size for granulations produced both by slugging and wet granulation techniques. These authors further found that as the wet mixing time was increased, mean granule size increased. The particle size of the oxytetracycline had a dramatic effect on granule size. For example, for material wet massed for a total of 15 min, the mean granule size for granulations produced from oxytetracycline having a particle size of 15 and 1.9 μm was 235 and 535 μm, respectively.

Davies and Gloor [40-42] have noted effects of various formulation and processing variables on granule size for granulations prepared in a fluid-bed dryer. They found that the following tended to increase granule size: (1) increasing the formula weight of binder, (2) increasing the amount of solution used to granulate, (3) increasing the addition rate of granulating solution, (4) decreasing the air inlet temperature during the granulation cycle, (5) decreasing the air pressure to the nozzle, and (6) decreasing the nozzle height above the distribution grid.

III. Shape Determinations

Particle behavior is a function of particle size, shape, density, and surface. These interact in a complex manner to give the total particle behavior pattern. Effects of particle shape are probably not as well appreciated as other particle characteristics. However, particle shape is important and can influence such important properties as bulk volume, particle packing arrangements, flowability, coatability, and ease of compaction [43, 9, 44].

A. Volume Shape Factor Related to Relative Sphericity

The volume of a particle is proportional to the cube of a characteristic dimension. A spherical particle is uniquely determined by its diameter and the volume is determined by

$$V = \alpha_V d^3 = \frac{\pi}{6} d^3 \tag{9}$$

where d is the diameter of the sphere and α_V a proportionality constant and in the case of a sphere equals $\pi/6$ (0.52). The proportionality constant α_V is known as the volume shape factor. Thus, for a sphere, α_V and d are easy to come by. For irregularly shaped particles, one computes α_V [by rearrangement of Eq. (9)] employing the following equation [45, 14]:

$$\alpha_V = \frac{V}{d_p^{\,3}} \tag{10}$$

where d_p is the equivalent projected diameter, defined as the diameter of a sphere having the same projected area as the particle when placed in its most stable position on a horizontal plane and viewed from above. Average particle volume is generally determined by counting out a specific number of particles and weighing them. Thus,

$$V = \frac{M_n}{\rho_g n} \tag{11}$$

where V is the average particle volume, n the number of particles weighed, M_n the mass of n particles, and ρ_g the density of the particles. The particle density ρ_g is normally computed using the pycnometer method.

Table 4

Volume Shape Factors (α_V) and Bulk Densities (ρ_b) for 20- to 30-mesh Particles Prepared by Various Granulation Methods

	Colton upright	Oscillating granulator	Hand screen	Fitzpatrick comminutor	Liquid-solid V-shaped blender
α_V	0.15	0.18	0.16	0.22	0.25
ρ_b	0.37	0.39	0.40	0.43	0.51

Source: data from Ref. 9.

The equivalent projected diameter is normally arrived at by photographing or tracing the outline of particles that have been magnified and then determining the diameter of a sphere that has the same projected area. The area of the magnified images can be obtained using a planimeter [9] or by cutting out projected images from photographs and weighing them [43]. In either case, computed areas from enlarged images must be reduced to true areas by dividing by p^2, where p is the power of magnification. Thus, it can be shown that

$$\frac{A}{p^2} = \frac{\pi d_p^2}{4} \tag{12}$$

or

$$d_p = \sqrt{\frac{4A}{\pi p^2}} \tag{13}$$

where A is the average area of the magnified images.

When computing average particle volume V and average equivalent projected diameter d_p, at least 100 or more particles should probably be used. As mentioned, $\alpha_V = \pi/6 \simeq 0.52$ for a sphere, and as the particle becomes more irregular, the value of α_V changes. Some values of α_V for lactose granulations in the 20- to 30-mesh range that were prepared by different methods of granulating are shown in Table 4. These authors also found that as the volume shape factor increased, bulk density increased (Table 4 and Fig. 7). This is as would be expected, because more spherical or more regular shaped particles produce the closest packing arrangements and hence the greater bulk density.

One can readily check the accuracy of experimentally determined α_V values through use of the following equation [12]:

$$N = \frac{1}{\alpha_V \rho_g d_p^3} \tag{14}$$

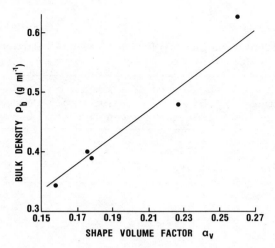

Figure 7. Relationship between bulk density and shape volume factor of 20- to 30-mesh particles prepared by five different granulation methods. (From Ref. 9. Reproduced with permission of the copyright owner.)

where N is the number of particles per gram and ρ the particle density. One can compute N and compare it with values obtained through an actual counting and weighing procedure. The more accurate α_v, ρ_g, and d_p are, the closer the computed value of N will be to actual values.

In summary, the volume shape factor is a measure of particle shape. It has been used to describe shape differences in pharmaceutical granulations [Eq. (9)].

B. Surface Shape Factor

The surface area of a particle is proportional to the square of a characteristic dimension. For a spherical particle,

$$S = \alpha_s d^2 = \pi d^2 \tag{15}$$

where S is the surface area of the particle, d the diameter, and α_s a proportionality constant. The proportionality constant α_s is termed the surface shape factor and in the case of a sphere, $\alpha_s = \pi \simeq 3.14$. For irregularly shaped particles, one computes α_s [by rearrangement of Eq. (15)] in the following manner [45, 14]:

$$\alpha_s = \frac{S}{d_p^2} \tag{16}$$

where d_p is again the average equivalent projected diameter. The determination of d_p has been discussed (p. 203). The average surface area per particle must,

Table 5

Surface Shape Factors for Various Mesh Sizes of Natural Uncrushed Sand

Mesh size	Sample number	Surface shape factor
44–60	1	3.03
	2	2.68
30–36	1	3.28
	2	2.89
18–20	1	3.54
	2	3.39

Source: data from Ref. 43.

therefore, be determined by gas adsorption, air permeability, and so on. Methods for estimating surface area are discussed later in this chapter. Since the method of determining surface area can have a pronounced effect upon the results (e.g., gas adsorption may give surface area values 10 to 100 times greater than results obtained by air permeability), the method of determining S must be stated when presenting or comparing values of α_S. Some values of α_S for various mesh sizes of sand are presented in Table 5.

The volume shape factor α_V and the surface shape factor α_S may be combined as a ratio α_S/α_V. This is called the shape coefficient and is discussed next.

C. Shape Coefficient

The shape coefficient α_{VS} is defined as follows [46]:

$$\alpha_{VS} = \frac{\alpha_S}{\alpha_V} \tag{17}$$

For a perfect sphere,

$$\alpha_{VS} = \frac{\pi}{\pi/6} = 6.0 \tag{18}$$

As particle shape becomes more irregular, the value of α_{VS} increases. For example, the α_{VS} for a cube can be calculated.

Using Equation (13) without the magnification term, the projected diameter of a cube with sides of length a is

$$d_p = \sqrt{\frac{4A}{\pi}} = \sqrt{\frac{4a^2}{\pi}} = \frac{2a}{\sqrt{\pi}} \tag{19}$$

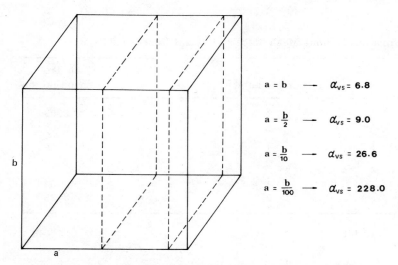

Figure 8. Shape coefficients for sections of a cube. (From Ref. 47.)

The volume of the cube $V = a^3$ and the surface area of the cube $S = 6a^2$. From Equation (10),

$$\alpha_v = \frac{V}{\sqrt{d_p^3}} = \frac{a^3}{8a^3/\pi\sqrt{\pi}} = \frac{\pi\sqrt{\pi}}{8} \tag{20}$$

$$= 0.696$$

From Equation (16),

$$\alpha_s = \frac{S}{d_p^2} = \frac{6a^2}{4a^2/\pi} = \frac{6\pi}{4} \tag{21}$$

$$= 4.71$$

Substituting into Equation (17), we obtain

$$\alpha_{vs} = \frac{\alpha_s}{\alpha_v} = \frac{4.71}{0.696} \tag{22}$$

$$= 6.8$$

The effect on the α_{vs} when various sections of a cube of width b are taken is shown in Figure 8. Ridgway and Shotton [48] found that as the shape coefficient of sand particles increased, the mean weight of die fill on a tablet machine decreased

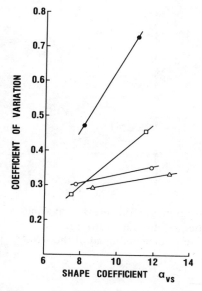

Figure 9. Effect of shape coefficient on the coefficient of variation of the die fill for different sizes of sand. $\bullet$, d_p = 805 μm; $\square$, d_p = 461 μm; $\triangle$, d_p = 302 μm; o, crushed sand having d_p = 213 μm. (From Ref. 48.)

and the coefficient of variation of die fill increased. The latter effect is shown in Figure 9. Ridgway and Rupp [43] found that as the shape coefficient decreased, bulk density decreased and angle of repose increased. The effect of the shape coefficient on bulk density is shown in Figure 10.

D. Other Measures of Shape

There are many other measurements of particle shape available and readers are referred to Pahl et al. [49] and Davies [50] for an extensive review of this literature.

IV. Surface Area

It is a fairly common practice to determine the surface area of finely milled drug powders. This is especially true with drugs that enjoy only limited water solubility. In these cases, particle size or available surface area of the drug can have a significant effect upon dissolution rate. It is not a common practice to determine the surface area of granulations. Generally, if one is interested in the effects of granulation surface area upon measurable properties of the final dosage form, the particle size of the granulation is employed. Thus, it is normally assumed that there is an inverse relationship between particle size and surface area. Furthermore, technology available for determining the surface area of coarse powders is

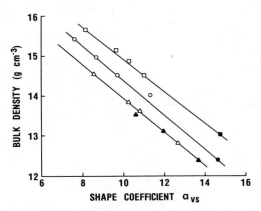

Figure 10. Bulk density as a function of shape coefficient for three sizes of sand. □, Mean projected diameter 805 μm; o, mean projected diameter 461 μm; Δ, mean projected diameter 302 μm. ■, ●, and ▲ refer to crushed sand of the same mean diameters. (From Ref. 43.)

not as advanced as it is for fine powders. Thus, available methods for determining surface areas of a solid are better suited for fine powders. For these reasons, only the fundamentals will be covered here, and the reader will be referred to reference texts for more in-depth information.

The term that is used to describe the surface area for a bed of powder or granules is the specific surface S_W, which is the surface area per unit weight. Thus,

$$S_W = \frac{\text{total surface area of particles}}{\text{total weight of particles}} \tag{23}$$

S_W is usually expressed in $cm^2 \ g^{-1}$ or $m^2 \ g^{-1}$. The S_W measurement of a powder can be used for quality control purposes, and many pharmaceutical companies specify acceptable S_W values for the tablet lubricant magnesium stearate. For example, the tablet lubricant, magnesium stearate, may be purchased having a specific surface as high as 25 $m^2 \ g^{-1}$.

A. Experimental Determination of Surface Area

The two most common methods for determining surface area of solid particles are gas adsorption and air permeability. In the first method (gas adsorption), the amount of gas that is adsorbed onto the powder to form a monolayer is a function of the surface area of the powder sample. In the latter, the fact that the rate at which air permeates a bed of powder depends upon the surface area of the powder sample is the basis of the measurement. For further details on gas adsorption, the reader is referred to Martin et al. [51], Fries [52], Shaw [53], and Adamson [54]. For more details on permeametry, the reader is referred to Edmundson [13], Herdan [11], Martin et al. [51], Irani and Callis [10], Rigden [55], and Carman [56, 57].

V. Densities and Packings

Particles may be dense, smooth, and spherical in one case, and rough, spongy, and irregular in another. It is clear that particles in these two cases are quite dissimilar and that their packings will not be similar. Measurements are available that help describe these characteristics and are discussed in this section. Thus, this section covers such topics as granule density, granule porosity, bulk density, and bed porosity. These measurements assist in describing individual particles or granules as well as how they behave en masse. Granule density, porosity, and hardness are often interrelated properties. In addition, granule density may influence compressibility, tablet porosity, dissolution, and other properties. Dense, hard granules may require higher compressible loads to produce a cohesive compact, let alone acceptable-appearing tablets free of visible granule boundaries. The higher compression load, in turn, has the potential of increasing the disintegration time. Even if the tablets disintegrate readily, the harder, denser granules may dissolve less readily. At the same time, harder, more dense granules will generally be less friable.

A. Granule Density

Since particles or granules can have open or closed pores, and surface cracks or fissures, great care must be used when expressing particulate density. The nomenclature of Heywood [14] will be used here as an introduction, and three different types of particle densities are defined:

True Density: The mass of a particle(s) divided by the volume of the particle(s), excluding open and closed pores.

Apparent Particle Density: The mass of a particle(s) divided by the volume of the particle(s), excluding open pores but including closed pores.

Effective Particle Density: The mass of a particle(s) divided by the volume of the particle(s), including open and closed pores.

When one speaks of granule density ρ_g, one is generally referring to apparent particle density or effective particle density. Two methods are basically used to determine granule density. Both methods involve the use of a pycnometer. In one case, the intrusion fluid is mercury and in the other case, a solvent of low surface tension (e.g., benzene) in which the granules are not soluble.

The mercury displacement method is described by Strickland et al. [58] and gives a value of ρ_g that approximates the effective particle density. This method is based on the fact that in a sample of granules, intraparticular pores are sufficiently smaller than between particle pores, which permits differential determination of granular volume without including open pores between particles. Mercury will not enter pores which are smaller than that indicated by the following approximate relationship:

$$D = \frac{1892}{p} \tag{24}$$

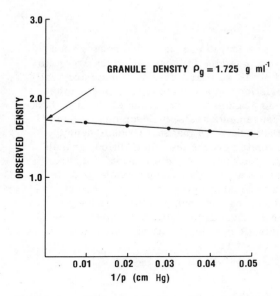

Figure 11. Mercury displacement method for determining granule density. (Data from Ref. 58.)

where p is the pressure of mercury applied in dyn cm^{-2} and D equals the minimum pore diameter in centimeters that mercury will enter at pressure p. In practice, one plots observed density against $1/p$. Extrapolation of the linear portion of this curve to the density axis yields the granule density ρ_g. This method of determining granule density includes both open and closed pores. The method is illustrated in Figure 11.

Other authors have used the pycnometer method, employing an organic solvent in which the granules are not soluble [40-42, 9]. Details of this method are outlined by Weissberger [59]. In this method of determining granule density, most open pores are excluded from the density determination and granule density approximates the apparent particle density described earlier by Heywood. When employing this method, the following equation applies:

$$\rho_g = \frac{G}{C - B/F} \tag{25}$$

where G is the weight of granules in grams, C the capacity of the pycnometer in milliliters, B the weight of the intrusion fluid in grams, and F the specific gravity of the intrusion fluid.

Davies and Gloor [40-42] have studied the effects of various formulation and processing variables in lactose granulations produced in a fluid-bed dryer. For processing variables, their results may be summarized as follows; (1) as the addition rate of water was increased, granule density increased; (2) as inlet air temperature was increased, granule density tended to increase slightly; and (3) as nozzle height above the grid was increased, granule density tended to decrease. For formulation variables, these authors found that as the formula weight of binder was increased, the granule density tended to increase. The latter effect was observed for the binders povidone, NF; hydroxypropylcellulose; Gelatin, USP; and Acacia, USP.

Strickland et al. [58] determined ρ_g for a number of different tablet granulations. Their studies included granulations that were prepared by starch paste as well as one that was prepared by slugging. Fonner et al. [9] determined the granule density for a lactose granulation that was produced from several different types of granulation equipment. In general, they found that granules produced from an oscillating granulator were the most dense ($\rho_g = 1.54$) and those produced from a Fitz mill and liquid-solid V-shaped blender were the least dense ($\rho_g = 1.42$ to 1.45). Armstrong and March [60] compared granule density of granulations prepared from various diluents that were wet-screened through an oscillating granulator and dried in a fluid-bed dryer. Chalmers and Elworthy [37-39] studied the effects of various formulation and processing variables on granule density of oxytetracycline formulations. Granules produced by slugging were significantly more dense than granules produced by the wet granulation technique. They also found that increasing the wet mixing time increased granule density for granulations produced by the wet granulation technique.

B. Granule Porosity

Granule porosity (intragranular porosity) is computed from a knowledge of ρ_g and the true particle density ρ:

$$\epsilon_g = 1 - \frac{\rho_g}{\rho} \times 100 \qquad (26)$$

where ϵ_g is the granule porosity in percent. The method of determining ϵ_g should be specified, so that one knows whether ϵ_g includes or excludes open pores in the granules.

Some studies involving granule porosity have been reported in the literature [6, 61]. These authors found that ϵ_g decreased as the amount of water used to granulate lactose powder was increased. This effect is shown in Figure 12. These authors also found that lengthening the massing time also decreased ϵ_g, but the effect was not as dramatic as that produced by varying the amount of water used to granulate. These authors also studied effects of initial lactose particle size and amount of water used to granulate on macropore size (10-80 μm) distribution in lactose granules. In general, the distribution of pores is related to the initial particle size of the lactose. Those granulations made with coarser grades of lactose had a greater percentage of large pores. Also, increasing the amount of water used to granulate lactose causes densification by rapidly eliminating larger pores, thus reducing mean pore diameter and increasing granule strength. The same authors [5], working with a calcium phosphate granulation, found that granule porosity increased as the amount of water used to granulate was increased. This unusual result was felt to be due to the fact that calcium phosphate is not readily consolidated by capillary forces during wet massing because the irregular particles cannot easily rearrange to form a closely packed system. In fact,

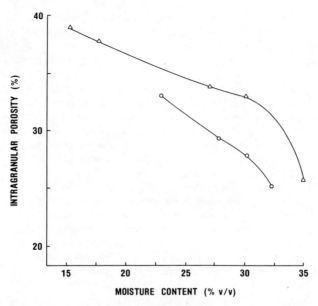

Figure 12. Effect of amount of water used to granulate on the porosity of 12- to 16-mesh lactose granules. o, Pan-granulated; Δ, massed and screened. (From Ref. 6.)

pendular or capillary liquid bonds tend to maintain a rigid, open structure. These authors further found that as massing was increased, granule porosity decreased for the three types of massing equipment evaluated. Strickland et al. [58] determined ϵ_g for a number of pharmaceutical granulations. For those cases where granulations were prepared with starch paste, $\epsilon_g \simeq 30\%$. For a slugged aspirin granulation, they found that $\epsilon_g \simeq 3\%$. Chalmers and Elworthy [38, 39] found that granules produced by slugging had much lower granule porosity values than did those produced by wet granulation. For oxytetracycline granulated with water, $\epsilon_g = 38.9\%$; for granules produced by slugging, $\epsilon_g = 17.8\%$. In the former case, the mean pore size was 0.97 μm, and in the latter, 0.10 μm. They also found that as wet mixing time was increased, granule porosity and mean pore size decreased.

The studies of these investigators show that granule density and/or porosity could be used as the characteristic(s) with which to evaluate granulation techniques, formula changes, equipment changes, and the like. Granule density and/or porosity could even be used as the measurable characteristic by which to control a granulation process.

C. Characteristics of Packings

When considering an ideal system consisting of monosized spheres, porosity or void space can range from 26% (rhombohedral packing) (i.e., ◌◌) to 48% (cubical packing) (i.e., ◌◌), depending upon the arrangement of spheres in the packing [62].

In heterogeneous systems, packing arrangements can become quite complicated. For example, smaller particles can fill interstices between large particles, thus reducing void space. On the other hand, this reduction in void space may be nullified by the fact that fine particles tend to form arches or bridges and chain formations that result in an increase in void space. For example, a very fine powder such as carbon black may have a voidage as high as 96 to 98% [63]. In the case of large particles, where cohesion effects are negligible, voidage is decreased when the particles extend over a wide range of sizes.

The arrangement of particles when poured or dropped into a container cannot be predetermined. However, it is possible to describe certain characteristics of packings once formed. Thus, such terms as bulk density and bed porosity are measures used to describe a packing of particles or granules. To date, it has not been possible to relate these measures of packings to other superficial features of the particles themselves. Particles in a container may be in a state of open packing, or the bed of particles may have been "tapped" to facilitate rearrangement and a closer packing. To attain good reproducibility, bulk density and bed porosity should be reported on the tapped product.

D. Bulk Density and Bed Porosity

The equation for determining bulk density ρ_b is

$$\rho_b = \frac{M}{V_b} \tag{27}$$

where M is the mass of the particles and V_b the total volume of packing. Another measure often used is bulk volume, which is the reciprocal of bulk density. The volume of the packing should be determined in an apparatus similar to that described by Neumann [64]. This device consists of a graduated cylinder mounted on a mechanical tapping device consisting of a specially cut cam that is rotated. An accurately weighed sample of powder or granulation is carefully added to the cylinder with the aid of a funnel. Typically, the initial volume is noted and the sample is then tapped until no further reduction in volume is noted. The volume at this tightest packing is then used in Equation (27) to compute bulk density ρ_b. Considerable variation exists in the literature as to the length of tapping or number of taps used [9, 34, 65, 66]. However, the important point is that the number of taps required to achieve the tightest packing will be dependent upon the material or granulation under study. Therefore, a sufficient number of taps should be employed to assure reproducibility for the material in question. The tapping should not produce particle attrition or a change in the particle size distribution of the material under test.

An important measure that can be obtained from bulk density determinations is the percent compressibility C, which is defined as follows [67]:

$$C = \frac{\rho_b - \rho_u}{\rho_b} \times 100 \tag{28}$$

where ρ_u is the untapped bulk density (often called loose or aerated bulk density). In theory, the more compressible a bed of particulates is, the less flowable the powder or granulation will be. Conversely, the less compressible a material is, the more flowable it will be. Carr [67] defines a material having a C value of less than 20 to 21% as being a free-flowing material.

Often, it is of interest to know bed porosity or percentage of void space in a packing. Bed porosity ϵ_b, in percent, is determined by the equation

$$\epsilon_b = 1 - \frac{\rho_b}{\rho_g} \times 100 \tag{20}$$

Bed porosity is often referred to as percent voids, void porosity, void space, interspace porosity, or extragranular porosity. As with granule density and porosity, the bulk density and porosity may be used as granulation-characterizing measurements for quality control specifications, and during product development, equipment evaluations, or raw material evaluations, for existing products, process changes, and in developing new products. Fonner et al. [9] compared the bulk density of 20-30 mesh lactose granulations prepared by five different granulation methods (Table 4). Over this narrow size range, bulk density was found to be largely dependent upon particle shape (see Fig. 7). As the particles became more spherical in shape, bulk density increased. Ridgway and Rupp [43], working with sand particles, found this same dependency of bulk density upon particle shape (see Fig. 10). Harwood and Pilpel [68] investigated the effect of granule size and shape on the bulk density of griseofulvin granulations. As granule size increased, bulk density was found to decrease. The smaller granules were able to form a closer, more intimate packing than were larger granules. Granule shape had a very great impact on bulk density. As noted previously, the bulk density for irregularly shaped granules is generally lower than the bulk density for the more spherical particles.

Davies and Gloor [40-42] investigated the effects of various formulation and processing variables on bulk density and bed porosity of granulations produced in a fluid-bed dryer, as noted, in part, earlier. The effects of water addition rate and inlet air temperature are summarized in Table 6. With Gelatin, USP, as a binder, they [42] also found that as the amount of water used to granulate was increased, bulk density increased and bed porosity decreased. Chalmers and Elworthy [38] noted that the addition of microcrystalline cellulose and/or alginic acid decreased bulk density and increased bed porosity for oxytetracycline granulated with water. The bulk density values of granules produced by slugging was again noted to be greater than bulk density values for granulations produced by the wet granulation technique.

Hunter and Ganderton [61] found that as the amount of water used to granulate lactose powder was increased, bed porosity went through a maximum value, as shown in Figure 13. This region of poor packing was found at the lower end of the "useful granulation range" and is the result of overall shape effects resulting from irregular or "fluffy" granules. The authors also found that at a given moisture content, the finer grades of lactose formed granules with more regular surfaces, promoting closer packing and a reduction in bed or extragranular porosity. In a similar study [6], these authors determined bed porosity for calcium phosphate and lactose granulations that were prepared by a rotating pan and oscillating

Table 6

Effect of Processing Variables on the Bulk Density and Porosity of Granulations
Produced in a Fluid–Bed Dryer

Processing variable	Level	Bulk density (g ml^{-1})	Porosity (%)
Addition rate (g H$_2$O/min)	85	0.41	72.4
	100	0.44	70.5
	115	0.46	69.1
	130	0.46	69.1
	145	0.48	67.9
Inlet air temperature (°C)	25°	0.54	63.8
	40°	0.50	66.6
	50°	0.44	70.7
	55°	0.41	72.6

Source: data from Ref. 40.

granulator. With both lactose and calcium phosphate, those granulations that were prepared in a rotating pan had the lowest bed porosity. The granulated lactose material that had an almost spherical shape and a dense packing had a bed porosity of 36 to 42%. On the other hand, granules from the oscillator were irregular in shape and had a bed porosity of about 50%. Their results for lactose granulations are shown in Table 7.

Eaves and Jones [69] describe the effects of increasing moisture content on the packing properties of various particulate materials. These authors found that the inherent cohesiveness of the bulk solid plays an important role in determining the effect of moisture on packing properties and tensile strength of moist beds. Their experiments covered the effect of consolidation of moist beds, which is of relevance to the granulation process. These authors concluded that agglomerate size is usually dependent upon tensile strength of the moist granule. For example, granules will disintegrate before or during drying if tensile forces are weak. In addition, final granule density is largely dependent upon the density of the moist granular bed, although some density changes may be expected during drying. At a fixed moisture content, increasing the consolidation stress produces a decrease in specific volume and an increase in tensile strength. Therefore, granulation methods that employ a consolidation step (e.g., an oscillating granulator) can be expected to produce denser granules than those that do not (e.g., rotating pan method).

Recent work in the area of particle packings is aimed at establishing a quantitative geometric description of packing [70, 71]. These authors describe radiological techniques needed to obtain a geometric description of a packing involving particles of any shape and a large range of sizes.

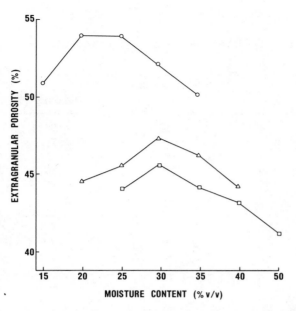

Figure 13. Effect of amount of water used to granulate on extragranular porosity
of 12- to 16-mesh granules. □, Mean particle diameter $d_m = 26$ μm; Δ, $d_m = 70$
μm; o, $d_m = 140$ μm. (From Ref. 61.)

VI. Granule Strength and Friability

A granule is an aggregation of component particles that is held together by the
presence of bonds of finite strength [1]. The strength of a wet granule is due
mainly to the surface tension of liquid and capillary forces. These forces are
responsible for initial agglomeration of the wet powder. Upon drying, the dried
granule will have strong bonds resulting from fusion or recrystallization of particles and curing of the adhesive or binder. Under these conditions, van der Waals
forces are of sufficient strength to produce a strong, dry granule. Measurements
of granule strength are, therefore, aimed at estimating the relative magnitude of
attractive forces seeking to hold the granule together. The resultant strength of
a granule is, of course, dependent upon the base material, the kind and amount of
granulating agent used, the granulating equipment used, and so on. Factors affecting granule strength will be discussed in this section. Granule strength and
friability are important, as they affect changes in particle size distribution of
granulations and consequently compressibility into cohesive tablets. Less appreciated is the fact that granule friability can also affect unit dose precision in
some tablet systems. This is especially true for hydrophobic drugs which are
poorly wetted by the granulating agent and are not firmly bound into the granulation. When such granulations undergo friability breakdown, the drug may preferentially separate from the granules, and as particle size separation occurs,
the tablets containing a higher level of fines also contain a higher concentration
of drug. In addition, the measurement of granule hardness and friability can be

Table 7

Effect of Granulating Method on the Extragranular Porosity of 12- to 16-Mesh
Lactose Granules

Granulating method	Amount of H$_2$O used to granulate (% v/v)	Extragranular porosity
Pan	23.0	39.0
	28.3	39.5
	30.6	41.0
	32.1	42.0
Oscillator	15.3	48.5
	18.4	49.5
	27.5	50.5
	30.6	50.0
	33.7	50.0

Source: data from Ref. 6.

used as a characterizing tool, together with granule size, density, and porosity, in an effort to quantitatively characterize a granulation to the extent that processing parameters can be set and controlled so that highly reproducible granulations can be manufactured. The more that is known about a process, the better that process can be controlled or problems solved and eliminated from the process. The ability to produce reproducible tablets, batch to batch and lot to lot, is directly related to the ability to produce reproducible granulations.

When determining a relative measure of granule strength, three distinct types of measurements can be made. The one that is perhaps most commonly used is that of compression strength. In this test, a granule is placed between anvils and the force required to break the granule is measured. An example of this type of apparatus is shown in Figure 14. A lab jack is used to raise the granule until it is in contact with an upper flat plate that is mounted to the bottom of a balance pan. Lead shot is then added until the granule breaks; the amount of lead shot added is termed the breaking load and taken as a measure of granule strength. A more sophisticated variation of the compression strength test was employed by Gold et al. [72] and Ganderton and Hunter [6]. In the latter case, the authors used a miniature press in which the lower platen was driven upward at a constant rate. A sensitive load cell was employed with the electrical output being fed to a recording galvanometer to give a continuous record of the signal.

Other common methods of studying granule strength are those that relate to friability measurements [9, 40, 34, 73]. Most of these methods are a variation of the American Society for Testing and Materials (ASTM) tumbler test for the friability of coal (ASTM Designation, D441-45 1945). These methods provide a means of measuring the propensity of granules to break into smaller pieces when subjected to disruptive forces. The method typically involves taking granules

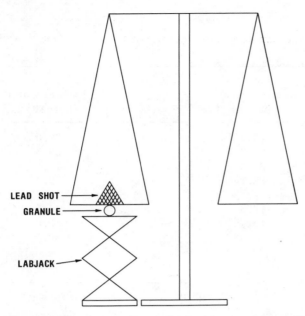

LEAD SHOT

GRANULE

LABJACK

Figure 14. Granule strength-testing apparatus. (From Ref. 68. Reproduced with permission of the copyright owner.)

that are known to be greater than a particular mesh size, say m^*. The granules are then placed in a container that is then tumbled or shaken for a predetermined period. The material is then shaken on a screen of mesh size m^*. The percentage of material passing is then taken as a measure of granule friability or strength.

A third type of measurement involves determining the indentation hardness of a granule [48, 74]. The equipment consists of a pneumatic microindentation apparatus that employs a spherical sapphire as the indenter. The diameter of the impression is determined, and from this the Brinell hardness number can be determined. This methodology for determining granule strength has limited application. One must be able to accurately determine the diameter of the impression; and to do this, regularly shaped granules having a smooth surface must be used. Most granulations do not fall into this category.

In a batch of granules, it would appear that the larger granules possess more strength than the smaller ones [68, 72, 34], as illustrated in Figure 15. It would appear that smaller granules are more poorly formed and thus less robust than are their larger counterparts.

Numerous reports exist in the literature to show that increasing amounts of binder produce granules of greater strength [68, 60, 76, 41, 75, 5]. Figure 16 illustrates this effect with dibasic calcium phosphate granules and various binding agents.

In lactose and sucrose granulations using water as the granulating fluid, granule strength was found to increase as the amount of water used to granulate was

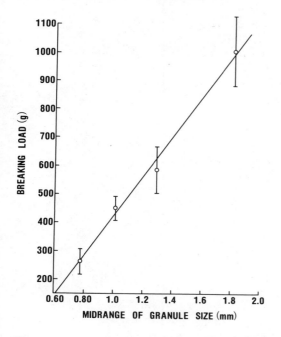

Figure 15. Plot showing relationship of strength of aspirin granules to granule size. (From Ref. 72. Reproduced with permission of the copyright owner.)

increased [75]. This same dependency of granule strength upon the amount of water used was reported for lactose granulations that had been produced on three different pieces of mixing-massing equipment [5]. However, with calcium phosphate granulations, granule strength went through a maximum as the amount of water used to granulate was increased.

Hunter and Ganderton [61] conducted a revealing study on the effect of the amount of water used to granulate and initial particle size on granule strength of lactose granulations. Their results are illustrated in Figure 17. Four different particle size grades of lactose were used. As shown in Figure 17, granule strength was found to be inversely related to the initial mean particle size of the lactose, with the increase being dramatic for the finest grade of lactose used. Granules produced from grade A lactose were much stronger, owing to the large number of bonds formed per unit volume. Essentially, the number of bonds formed with the fine grades of lactose is a function of particle size. Thus, with the finer grades of lactose, more bonds were formed during granulation and granule strength was therefore greater for these granules than for those produced from the coarse grades of lactose. As has been noted previously, as the amount of water used to granulate was increased, granule porosity decreased and granule strength increased. As the amount of water used to granulate is increased, the number of points at which liquid bonds form increases, resulting in less porous and greater strength granules upon drying.

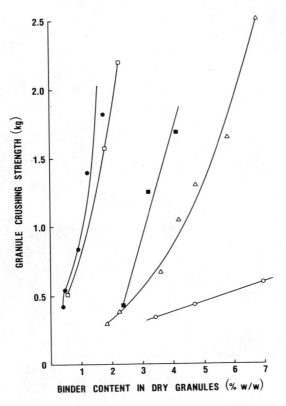

Figure 16. Crushing strength of dibasic calcium phosphate granules prepared with various binding agents. ●, Gelatin; □, potato starch mucilage; ■, acacia; △, povidone; o, polyethylene glycol 4000. (From Ref. 60. Reproduced with permission of the copyright owner.)

At a constant binder concentration in the final formula, dilution of the binder solution increases granule strength or reduces granule friability [77, 42]. This was found true for a lactose granulation prepared in a fluid-bed dryer using gelatin as a binder, as well as a lactose granulation using starch paste and produced on conventional granulating equipment.

The effect of processing variables on granule strength has been reported on by numerous authors. Processing variables of the fluid-bed technique were found to have a large impact on granule strength [40]. These included water addition rate, inlet air temperature, air pressure to the binary nozzle, and nozzle height. Fonner et al. [9] compared the granule strength of lactose granulations prepared from five different pieces of granulating equipment. Of the five pieces of equipment studied, granules produced from the oscillating granulator were the strongest and those produced in a liquid-solid V-shaped blender were the weakest. Working with a granulation of calcium phosphate, Ganderton and Hunter [6] found that

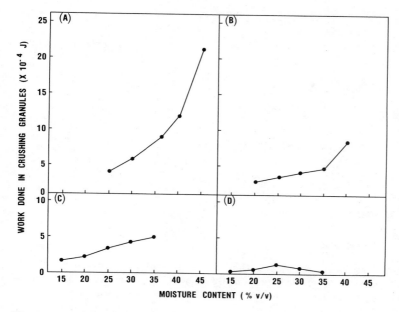

Figure 17. Effect of the amount of water used to granulate on the mean work done (joules) in crushing 14- to 16-mesh granules prepared from four grades of lactose. Grade A, d_m = 26 μm; grade B, d_m = 70 μm; grade C, d_m = 140 μm; grade D, d_m = 340 μm. (From Ref. 61.)

granules that were massed and screened were stronger than those produced in a rotating pan. When lactose was used in place of calcium phosphate, these authors found that the strength of granules from massing and screening was about equal to those produced by the rotating pan method. Chalmers and Elworthy [39] investigated the effect of wet mixing time on granule strength for oxytetracycline granulations. In general, as wet mixing time increased, granule strength increased.

Ridgway and Rubinstein [74] studied solute migration during granule drying. They worked with a magnesium carbonate granulation that utilized PVP as the binder. Material was massed and screened and then rotated in a coating pan to produce spherical granules. Selected granules were then dried in a special drying tunnel. The effect of moisture content on granule friability is shown in Figure 18. The attrition rate k is plotted against drying time and granule moisture content. Initially, the wet particles are held together by liquid-surface-tension forces and the granules are quite resistant to attrition. As drying proceeds, the granules become more friable and reach a maximum at the point when the granule surface is just dry. After this point, the interior of the granule starts to dry and granule strength increases. Working with dried granules, the authors determined granule strength as a function of depth from the granule surface. They found that Brinell hardness decreased linearly as measurements were taken from the outer surface toward the center of the granule. Finally, a point is reached where no

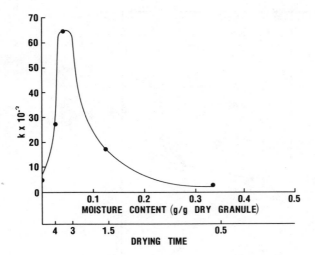

Figure 18. Effect of moisture content on the granule friability. k is the gradient
of the straight line representing the attrition time against the logarithm of the percentage weight intact, for granules shaken in the multiple-attrition-cell apparatus.
(From Ref. 74.)

further decrease in granule hardness occurs. This point provides a measure of
crust thickness residing on the outer surface of the granule. During the initial
stages of drying, PVP migrates to the granule surface and upon evaporation is
deposited, forming a crust of finite thickness.

VIII. Electrostatic Properties

Only the contact and separation of solids is necessary to induce electrostatic
charges. Static electrification is perhaps best known for its potential fire and
explosion hazards, and the importance of proper "grounding" of pharmaceutical
processing equipment cannot be overemphasized. Electrostatic forces are also
well known for the detrimental effect they may have on the mixing process. The
mixing action often results in generation of static surface charges, as evidenced
by a tendency for powders to clump following a period of agitation. Thus, the
generation of electrostatic charges during solids blending is one of the principal
factors responsible for the phenomenon of unblending. In a general sense, such
unit operations as mixing, milling, sizing, and tablet compression do induce
static electrification. All these operations lead to the overall charge development on granules and finished tablets, which can cause difficulties in the efficient
operation of processing equipment [78].
    Electrostatic forces probably do not play a significant role in the flow behavior
of granules produced by the wet granulation method or slugging. The magnitude of
these forces are negligible when compared to the weight of individual granules [79].

Further, electrostatic forces contribute very little to the overall strength of a granule; however, it is not unreasonable to assume that these forces play a part in the initial formation of aggregates [1]. Also, electrostatic forces may influence the behavior of direct compaction granulations [80].

Early work on the electrification of particles dealt with atmospheric dust [81]. In the early 1900s, it was assumed that electrification of particles was produced by friction or contact with dissimilar substances. In 1927, it was demonstrated [82] that charges could be produced by friction and contact between particles themselves, even though similar in composition. Later, Kunkel [83] demonstrated that a powder may be essentially neutral, yet practically all particles may be charged. Finally, in 1959, it was established that friction was not a prerequisite—that only contact and separation were necessary to charge particles electrostatically [84]. There is evidence to indicate that the mechanism of contact charging involves the transfer of electrons from one solid to another [85, 86]. For an in-depth review of electrostatic forces, the interested reader is referred to Krupp [87] and Hiestand [88]. Only a few reports appear in the pharmaceutical literature that deal with electrostatic forces, and these are reviewed below.

Gold and Palermo [80] utilized a commercially available ionostat to measure hopper flow electrostatics of acetaminophen formulations. Fine crystalline and crystalline acetaminophen exhibited higher induced static charges than did acetaminophen granulations prepared from ethylcellulose, starch paste, or syrup. Tablet excipients were found to have an effect on hopper flow static charge of fine crystalline acetaminophen. Lubricants such as talc and magnesium stearate at a 2% concentration level were found to dramatically reduce static charge. The addition of 0.5% water was also found to dramatically reduce hopper flow static charge. In a follow-up article, the authors [89] evaluated antistatic properties of tablet lubricants. Ten tablet lubricants at 1% concentrations were investigated for their ability to reduce static charge of anhydrous citric acid. Magnesium stearate, polyethylene glycol (PEG) 4000, sodium lauryl sulfate, and talc significantly lowered static charge. Liquid petrolatum, fumed silicon dioxide, stearic acid, and hydrogenated vegetable oil were found to have no antistatic properties. The antistatic properties of the lubricant were not altered by the material to which they were added. The lubricants found to be effective in reducing static charge of citric acid were equally as effective when added to acetaminophen and ascorbic acid. In a subsequent article [90], the effect of flow rate on hopper flow static charge of selected organic acids was studied. A summary of their data is shown in Table 8. As expected, increasing hopper flow rate results in a significant increase in induced static charge. Of the materials tested, tartaric acid resulted in the largest hopper flow static charge.

Lachman and Lin [91] describe the design and operating principles of an apparatus capable of measuring the inherent static charge on materials as well as the relative static electrification tendencies of materials. The basic equipment consists of an electrostatic tester, an X-Y recorder, and a humidifying chamber. The electrostatic tester is composed of three parts: a dual-polarity high-voltage power supply unit, a modified Faraday cage, and an electrostatic voltage-sensing pistol. The sample to be evaluated is placed in the Faraday cage, and voltage accumulation or decay can be read on the ammeter of the voltage sensing pistol or displayed on the X-Y recorder. The authors report on the relative static electrification tendencies of sodium chloride, stearic acid, sulfisomidine, and

Table 8

Flow Rates and Static Charges of Selected Organic Acids as Obtained with Different Hopper Orifices

| | Orifice diameter | | | |
| | 8.0 mm | | 15.0 mm | |
	Flow rate (g sec^{-1})	Static charge (V cm^{-1})	Flow rate (g sec^{-1})	Static charge (V cm^{-1})
Aspirin	4.77	239	37.77	600
Ascorbic acid	4.41	472	36.11	744
Citric acid, anhydrous	3.77	533	44.22	1039
Tartaric acid	5.99	1306	49.37	2289

Source: Ref. 90. Reproduced with permission of the copyright owner.

iodochlorhydroxyquin. The equilibrium potential as a percent of applied potential is shown in Table 9. The equilibrium potential of sodium chloride is much greater than that for other materials tested, which is in agreement with the concept that charge flows faster in a good conductor (e.g., sodium chloride). In the steady state, only sulfisomidine exhibited an inherent electrostatic charge (+240 V). No measurable inherent static charge was detectable for the other materials tested. The authors further obtained charge accumulation and decay data and these were plotted according to first-order kinetics. Results for stearic acid are shown in Figure 19. As noted in the figure, there are two slopes, the first being steeper than the second. The authors feel that the initial slope is due to inherent tendencies of the material to be polarized by the applied potential; and the second slope represents the saturation of the surface of the material with the applied potential, as well as a loss of charge from the material due to radiation and conduction to the surrounding air. The rate constants derived from the plots for stearic acid (Fig. 19) are shown in Table 10. Thus, it is possible to rate static electrification tendencies of materials through use of this equipment and treatment of data in accordance with first-order kinetic principles. It should, therefore, be possible to acquire fundamental knowledge that will permit a scientific approach toward alleviating static charge problems in pharmaceutical systems.

In summary, electrostatic charges may play a role in initial granule formation that may be beneficial or harmful, depending upon the extent of attractive and repulsive charges. In pharmaceutical processing systems, static charges can cause detrimental effects ranging from unblending in mixing operations to fire and explosion hazards. Several methods have been suggested to minimize the effects of electrostatic charges [78, 88]. These include modification of the crystalline habit, use of antistatic agents, and humidity control. Static

Table 9

Equilibrium Potential (%) on Powders at Applied Potential of 6000 V

Materials	Polarity of applied potential	
	+	−
Sodium chloride	85.0	90.0
Stearic acid	55.0	45.0
Sulfisomidine	60.0	48.0
Iodochlorhydroxyquin	50.2	50.3

Source: Ref. 91. Reproduced with permission of the copyright owner.

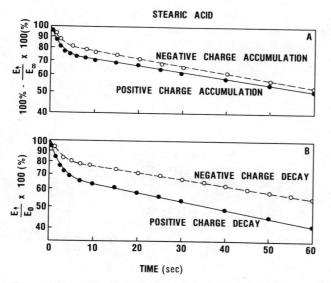

Figure 19. First-order plot of charge accumulation and decay data for stearic acid at a positive(———) and negative (-----) applied potential of 6000 V. (From Ref. 91. Reproduced with permission from the copyright owner.)

charge problems are most apparent with nonconductive materials that accumulate charges. The problem can usually be overcome by increasing the surface conductivity of powders or granules. Thus, addition of glidants, surfactants, other antistatic agents, and increased humidity are capable of dissipating accumulated static charges in nonconductors. All of the above produce a conductive path that will allow the charge to drain off or otherwise be neutralized. This can also be accomplished by making the air around the surface conductive by breaking up the

Table 10

Accumulation and Decay of Negative and Positive Electrification for Stearic Acid
at Applied Potential of 6000 V

Charge	Accumulation rate (sec^{-1})		Decay rate (sec^{-1})	
	k_1	k_2	k_1	k_2
+	8.92×10^{-2}	5.90×10^{-3}	1.06×10^{-1}	8.35×10^{-3}
−	7.90×10^{-2}	6.37×10^{-3}	5.36×10^{-2}	6.96×10^{-3}

Source: data from Ref. 91.

air into positively and negatively charged particles. This is the principle upon
which nuclear static elimination devices are based. Typically, a radioisotope
such as polonium 210 (a pure α-particle emitter) is used to ionize the air. As
the α particles streak through the air, they interact with electrons in the air,
causing them to float as free electrons, leaving the rest of the molecule positively charged.

VIII. Flow Properties

Solid particles attract one another, and forces acting between particles when they
are in contact are predominantely surface forces. There are many types of
forces that can act between solid particles. Pilpel [79] identifies five types:
(1) frictional forces, (2) surface-tension forces, (3) mechanical forces caused
by interlocking of particles of irregular shape, (4) electrostatic forces, and (5)
cohesive or van der Waals forces. All of these forces can affect the flow properties of a solid. With fine powders (≤ 150 μm), the magnitude of frictional and
van der Waals forces usually predominate [79]. However, surface-tension
forces between particles can be significant where capillary condensation can
occur [88]. Thus, small liquid bridges can be formed between particles if
moisture content is high or particles are exposed to high humidities ($\gtrsim 60\%$ relative humidity). Surface-tension forces resulting from absorbed films of gases
are generally quite small and not significant in comparison to other forces acting between particles. Although electrostatic forces of a magnitude greater than
van der Waals forces are theoretically possible, the usual presence of even
minute quantities of water are sufficient to minimize the effect of electrostatic
forces. For larger particles ($\gtrsim 150$ μm), such as granules produced by a wet
granulation technique, frictional forces normally predominate over van der Waals
forces. Thus, when evaluating interparticle forces of granules, agglomerates,
or other large particles, cohesive or van der Waals forces are often assumed to
be insignificant or equal to zero. The gravitational effect of large particles will
normally overwhelm any effects due to van der Waals forces. Also, as particles
increase in size, mechanical or physical properties of particles and their packings

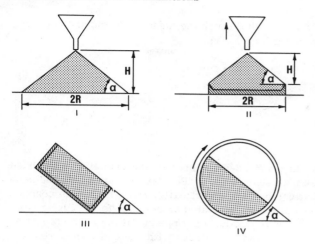

Figure 20. Four principal methods of measuring the angle of repose. I, Fixed-funnel and free-standing cone, II, fixed-bed cone; III, tilting box; IV, revolving cylinder. (From Ref. 94.)

become important. The packing density of the mass of particles and bed expansion required to develop a shear plane are important considerations with larger particles.

Many methods are available to measure extent of interparticle forces. Such measures are then commonly employed as an index of flow. Some of the more common methods that will be discussed are: (1) repose angle, (2) shear strength determinations, and (3) hopper flow-rate measurements. There are many fundamental properties of solid particles that influence their flow properties. Such properties as particle size, particle size distribution, particle shape, surface texture or roughness, residual surface energy, and surface area affect the type and extent of particle-particle interactions. Studies involving the effect of some of these properties on flow of solids are summarized in this section.

A. Repose Angle

Many different types of angular properties have been employed to assess flowability [93, 67, 92]. For example, the following angular properties have been identified: (1) angle of repose, (2) angle of slide or friction, (3) angle of rupture, (4) angle of spatula, and (5) angle of internal friction. Of these, angle of repose and angle of internal friction are perhaps the most relevant to predict particle flow. The angle of internal friction will be discussed under shear strength measurements.

The more common ways of determining angle of repose are illustrated in Figure 20. In the fixed-funnel and free-standing cone method, a funnel is secured with its tip a given height H above graph paper placed on a flat horizontal surface.

Powder or granulation is carefully poured through the funnel until the apex of the conical pile just touches the tip of the funnel; thus,

$$\tan \alpha = \frac{H}{R} \tag{30}$$

or

$$\alpha = \arctan \frac{H}{R} \tag{31}$$

where α is the angle of repose. In the fixed-cone method, the diameter of the base is fixed by using a circular dish with sharp edges. Powder is poured onto the center of the dish from a funnel that can be raised vertically until a maximum cone height H is obtained. The repose angle is calculated as before. In the tilting box method, a rectangular box is filled with powder and tipped until the contents begin to slide. In the revolving cylinder method, a cylinder with one end transparent is made to revolve horizontally when half filled with powder. The maximum angle that the plane of powder makes with the horizontal on rotation is taken as the angle of repose. Angles determined by the first three methods (Fig. 20) are often referred to as the static angle of repose, and the angle arrived at in Method IV is commonly called the kinetic angle of repose. Usually, the kinetic angle of repose is smaller than the static angle of repose. Other methods of determining the repose angle are given by Pathirana and Gupta [95] and Pilpel [79]. For a discussion of the forces involved in the formation of a conical pile of particles, including cohesion and friction, see Refs. 88, 96, and 97.

The angle of repose is best suited for particles ≥150 μm [98]. In this size range, cohesive effects will be minimal and the coefficient of friction will be largely dependent upon the normal component of the weight of the test specimen. Values for angles of repose ≤30° generally indicate a free-flowing material, and angles ≥40° suggest a poorly flowing material [79]. The value of the angle of repose for a given material is dependent upon particulate surface properties that will also affect flowability [66]. However, as mentioned previously, the flow of coarse particles will also be related to packing densities and mechanical arrangements of particles. For this reason, a good auxiliary test to run in conjunction with repose angle is the compressibility test. The measurement of this value was discussed previously and is given in Equation (28). From the angle of repose and compressibility values, a reasonable indication of a material's inherent flow properties should be possible. Carr [57] employs these two measurements together with the angle of internal friction to arrive at a flow index value for a particular material. The important point is that one can be misled if a judgment on flowability is based entirely on angle-of-repose measurements.

Several factors and granule characteristics have been studied for their effect on the angle of repose. Among them are particle size, use of glidants, moisture effects, and particle shape. Numerous authors have investigated the effect of particle size on the angle of repose. In a general sense, the repose angle normally increases as particle size is reduced, and this effect is usually quite dramatic in the small particle size range [99-102]. This effect is shown in Figure 21 for magnesia particles. It has also occasionally been observed that a plot of repose angle versus particle size goes through a minimum value [103, 99,

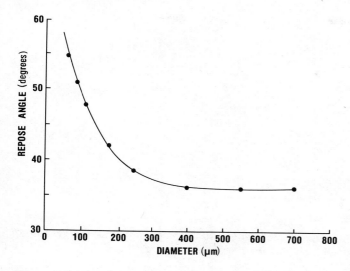

Figure 21. Angles of repose for different sieve cuts of magnesia. (From Ref. 79.)

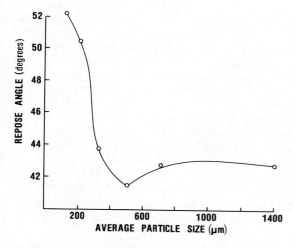

Figure 22. Repose angle as a function of sulfathiazole granule average particle size. (From Ref. 100. Reproduced with permission of the copyright holder.)

100, 101]. Figure 22 illustrates this effect for a sulfathiazole granulation that was fractionated into various sieve cuts. The repose angle goes through a minimum at about 500 μm.

Another area that has been heavily investigated deals with the effect of glidants and "fines" on angle of repose. Craik [104] and Craik and Miller [105] studied the effect of magnesium oxide fines on the angle of repose of starch and found that with this system the repose angle went through a minimum at about a 1%

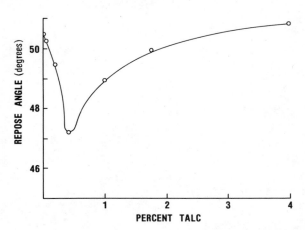

Figure 23. Effect of talc on repose angle of 60- to 80-mesh sulfathiazole granules. (From Ref. 100. Reproduced with permission of the copyright holder.)

concentration of magnesium oxide. Nelson [100] found that as the percentage of fines (100 mesh) was increased, the repose angle increased, as would be expected from the discussion above. Pilpel [79] found that for mixtures of two sieve cuts of magnesia particles, the angle of repose was inversely proportional to the size of the fine particles but was directly proportional to their weight fraction.

The effect of glidants on the repose angle of various materials has been reported in detail. In general, the angle of repose goes through a minimum and then increases as glidant concentration increases, as illustrated by the effect of small concentrations of talc on the repose angle of 60- to 80-mesh sulfathiazole granules in Figure 23. In addition to talc, investigators have tested the effects of colloidal silica on the angle of repose of lactose [106], magnesium oxide, titanium dioxide, zinc oxide, cornstarch, and magnesium carbonate [107]. Gold et al. [108] report on the effect of small concentrations of talc, magnesium sterate, silicon dioxide, and starch on the repose angle of aspirin, calcium sulfate granules, and spray-dried lactose particles. Other reports of interest are those of Nash et al. [109], Awada et al. [110], Dawes [111], Carstensen and Chan [112], and Carr [67].

When materials that take up moisture from the atmosphere are exposed to high humidities, the material generally becomes more cohesive, cake in their containers, and exhibit very poor flow characteristics. It would appear from such observations that moisture and humidity affect the angle of repose. Figure 24 illustrates the effect on starch mixtures that 24 hr of exposure to various relative humidities has on the observed angle of repose. As noted in Figure 24, as the storage humidity is increased, repose angle increases. This effect of moisture on repose angle has been noted by others [97, 113, 107, 66].

It is generally recognized that particle shape has an effect upon the angle of repose, and this has been illustrated by Ridgway and Rupp [43]. They found that as the shape coefficient of sand particles increased (particles becoming more irregular), repose angle increased. The effect of various pieces of granulating

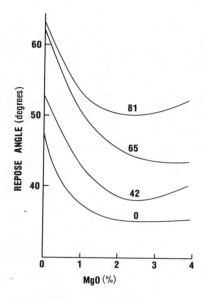

Figure 24. Angle of repose of starch and mixtures with light magnesium oxide after 24 hr of exposure to atmospheres of 0, 42, 65, and 81% relative humidity at 30° C. (From Ref. 105.)

equipment on the repose angle of 20–30 mesh lactose granulations has been reported [9]. Comparisons of hopper-flow-rate values of various materials with their respective repose angle measurements have been published [99, 106, 99]. In dealing with angle of repose of particles, it should be remembered that in general, "the angle of repose is <u>not</u> an inherent property of a solid, but a result of the interplay of properties, equipment-design parameters, and the history of the material" [114]. As mentioned previously, repose-angle measurements are applicable to relatively free flowing powders greater than 150-μm-diameter particle size; with cohesive powders, however, repose angles become inaccurate [66]. In efforts to assess the flow characteristics of cohesive powders, powder failure testing equipment (i.e., shear cells for shear strength measurements) has been used.

B. Shear Strength Measurements

A simplified schematic diagram of a shear cell apparatus is illustrated in Figure 25. Reference articles by Jenike [115–118] and others [119, 98] describe in detail this type of biaxial translatory shear tester, often called the Jenike shear cell. The Jenike shear cell is the one in most common use, but other types of shear cells have been used [109, 120, 121]. To use the shear cell (Fig. 25), the bulk solid specimen is compacted to a specific state of consolidation inside the powder chamber. A normal load P, which is less than the original consolidating load, is then applied to the cover. The powder bed is sheared by a

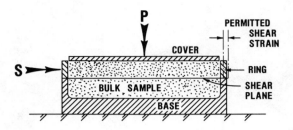

Figure 25. Schematic cross section of a shear cell ready for shear-strength measurement.

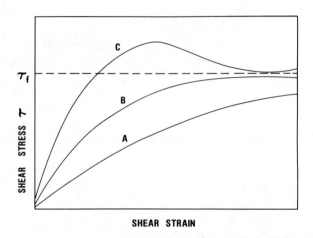

Figure 26. Typical stress/strain curves for powders; τ_f, shear stress at failure. [With permission from Pilpel, N., in: Advances in Pharmaceutical Sciences, Vol. 3 (H. S. Bean, A. H. Beckett, and J. E. Carless, Eds.), Academic Press, New York, 1971. Copyright by Academic Press Inc. (London) Ltd.]

translatory movement of the top half of the cell over the base at a constant shear strain rate. Shear force S is continuously measured by a transducer and results are plotted in the form of a stress/strain curve, shown in Figure 26. The degree of original consolidation is critical. If the consolidating force is too great, a curve such as C will result; and if the powder specimen is under compacted, a curve such as A will result. If the correct amount of consolidating force is applied, a curve such as B will result. Note that curve B reaches a limiting value that is termed the shear stress at failure, τ_f. The shear stress at failure is then obtained for a number of different reduced loads. Results are then plotted to give a so-called yield locus, and this is illustrated in Figure 27. This is generally referred to as a Mohr's shear diagram. The reader should refer to Hiestand et al. [121] for a discussion of the basic concepts involved with shear cell measurements

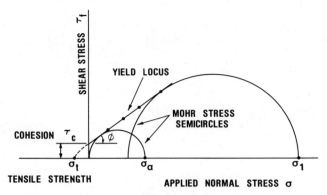

Figure 27. Typical Mohr's shear diagram.

and shear diagrams. Since the shear stress data obtained may be limited, a linear regression line may be drawn as an estimate of the yield locus.

From the yield locus, two useful measures describing particle-particle interaction influencing flow characteristics can be obtained: the cohesion value of the powder τ_c, and the angle of internal friction ϕ. The cohesion value of the powder is defined as the value of the shear stress at zero applied load and is obtained by extrapolating the yield locus curve back to the τ_f axis. The angle that the yield locus curve makes with the τ_f axis gives a rough approximation of the angle of internal friction for the powder. The angle of internal friction is a measure of the difficulty of maintaining a constant volume flow [122]. By employing tensile strength measurements, the tensile strength, σ_t, of the powder can be determined. Hiestand and Peot [123] discuss methodology for accurately determining σ_t.

Another parameter of interest in predicting flow properties of a material is a quantity known as the material's flow factor, FF [116, 118, 106]. To arrive at this quantity, shear cell testing is done, the yield locus is plotted, and two Mohr's stress circles are drawn with their centers on the σ axis, tangently to the yield locus (see Fig. 27). The smaller semicircle is constructed to pass through the origin and defines the unconfined yield stress σ_α. The larger semicircle is drawn to pass through the end point of the yield locus and defines the major normal stress σ_1. A graph is then made by plotting σ_α versus σ_1 obtained from several yield loci. The FF is then defined as the reciprocal slope of the graph. The graph is often rectilinear, but if not, then FF is defined as the reciprocal slope of the tangent to the graph at the origin of the axes [98].

York [106] has used the FF measurements from shear cell testing for assessing the effect of glidants on the flowability of cohesive pharmaceutical powders. As an example, the effect of magnesium stearate concentration on the flowability of lactose and calcium phosphate is shown in Figure 28. The optimum glidant level for lactose is 1.75% and for calcium phosphate is 2.2%.

Other investigators have made use of shear cell testing in assessing the flowability of cohesive powders that have not been covered in this section. The reader is referred to the literature for a more in-depth study [120, 124-126].

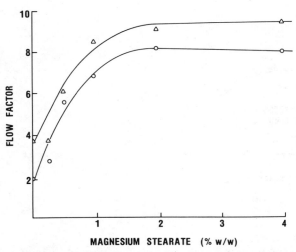

Figure 28. Graphs of changes in the flow factor of host powder-magnesium stearate mixtures at different concentrations of magnesium stearate. o, Lactose-magnesium stearate mixtures; Δ, calcium hydrogen phosphate-magnesium stearate mixtures. (From Ref. 106. Reproduced with permission of the copyright holder.)

C. Hopper Flow Rates

Hopper flow rates have been employed by numerous authors as a method of assessing flowability. In addition, in some production operations, tablet weight variation may be influenced by hopper flow rates, especially if material flow to the feed frame of the tablet press is not consistent. Most of the instrumentation employed is a variation of that described by Gold et al. [90, 106, 127, 128] and basically involves a recording balance. Instrumentation is generally quite simple and results are easy to interpret, making the method attractive from a practical standpoint. These authors compared hopper-flow-rate data with repose angle for glidant studies, investigated factors affecting the flow rate of lactose granules, and presented methods for determining uniformity of flow. The degree of correlation between hopper flow rate and repose angle was judged to be low. Talc was found to be a poor glidant for the materials studied, as it decreased flow rates at all concentrations tested. For the glidants magnesium stearate, fumed silicon dioxide, and cornstarch, optimum concentrations were 1% or lower, with flow rates decreasing at higher concentrations. When studying lactose granules, these authors found that the percent fines, the amount and type of granulating agent, particle size distribution, and the type of glidant all had a measurable effect on flow rate. In their last article, the authors describe instrumentation necessary for qualitative and quantitative evaluation of flow uniformity through a hopper orifice, and examples are presented to illustrate the utility of the instrumentation.

Davies and Gloor [40-42], in a series of publications, have described the effect of various formulation and process variables on hopper flow rates of granulations produced in a fluid-bed dryer. Increasing the addition rate of water and

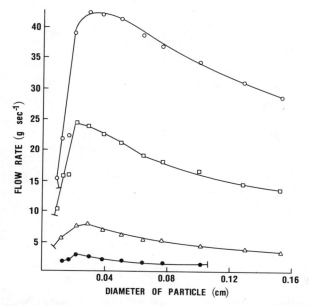

Figure 29. Flow rate of various sizes of lactose granulation through circular orifices with diameters. o, 1.905; □, 1.428; △, 0.9250; ●, 0.6530 cm; B, blocked.
(From Ref. 99. Reproduced with permission of the copyright holder.)

decreasing the inlet air temperature were found to increase hopper flow rates. The
authors conclude that the reason for this enhanced flow is because these conditions
result in better wetting of the solids and more robust granules. Increasing the formula weight (% w/w) of binder was found to decrease hopper flow rates for the three
binders tested. For example, with gelatin as a binder, the flow rate for granules
containing 2% w/w gelatin was 168.8 g min[-1]; whereas at 4.25% w/w gelatin, the
flow rate was 93.5 g min[-1]. The authors conclude that the decreased hopper flow
rates are a result of the increase in average particle size that occurs as formula
weight of binder was increased. At a constant formula weight of binder, increasing the amount of water used to granulate resulted in granules that gave a higher
hopper flow rate. Marks and Sciarra [34] and Harwood and Pilpel [68] also
found that hopper flow rate was inversely proportional to average granule size.
Others [103, 99] have reported that a plot of flow rate versus particle size goes
through a maximum. This is illustrated in Figure 29 for lactose granules.

Jones [129] presents an excellent review of the effect of glidant addition on the
flow rate of bulk particulate solids. He concludes that many glidants can improve
the flowability of bulk solids and that several mechanisms of action may be involved.
Glidants may act by one or more of the following mechanisms: reduction of interparticulate friction, change in surface rugosity, separation of coarse particles,
reduction of liquid or solid bridging, and minimization of static charge. Many
glidants are lubricants and often possess a coefficient of friction less than that of
the bulk solid to which they are added. Such lubricants may also act by reducing
surface rugosity, which will minimize mechanical interlocking of the particles
and thereby reduce rolling friction. The glidant may also function by providing

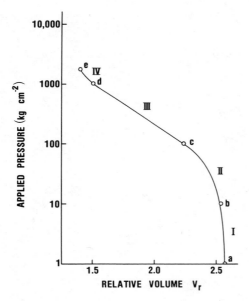

Figure 30. Relation between applied pressure and relative volume of a compact. (Data from Ref. 131.)

a physical separation of coarse particles in the bulk solid. Aggregates of glidant particles may adhere to the surface of coarse particles and thereby provide this physical separation. This is thought to reduce the action of capillary adhesion forces and also prevents formation of solid bridges between particles.

IX. Ease of Consolidation and Mechanisms

The process of consolidation and compact formation is complex owing to numerous internal events that are acting simultaneously [130]. These events include (1) particle rearrangement (consolidation), (2) particle fracture, and (3) plastic deformation. Particle rearrangement occurs mostly at low compression pressures and plastic deformation occurs at high pressures. All these events lead to a greater area of true interparticle contact, with high compression pressure, resulting in extensive areas of true particle contact. At these true areas of contact, van der Waals forces act to provide strong bonds that maintain the integrity of the compact.

A simplistic view of the consolidation process can be achieved by considering the effect of pressure on the relative volume of a compact V_r, as shown in Figure 30. It was concluded that the consolidation process proceeded in stages. During stage I (point a to b in Fig. 30), the decrease in V_r arises through interparticulate slippage of powder, leading to a closer packing. This rearrangement of particles continues until they become immobile relative to each other. Stage II (b to c) is characterized by the formation of temporary struts, columns, and vaults arising through interparticular contact points. These temporary structures in effect support the compressive load. In stage III (c to d), the increasing

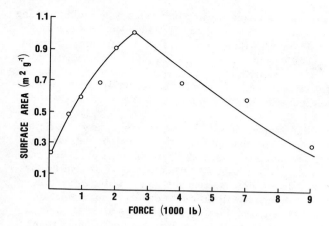

Figure 31. Effect of compressional force on the specific surface area of sulfadiazine tablets. (Data from Ref. 132.)

compressive load brings about a failure of the aforementioned temporary structures by fracture or plastic flow. The true area of particle contact begins to increase, and bonding occurs at these points. The generation of fresh surfaces has
been illustrated by Higuchi [132] using nitrogen absorption methods to measure
specific surface areas of sulfadiazine tablets. From Figure 31 it can be seen that
the surface area of the compact goes through a maximal value as the compressive
force is increased. The authors attribute this phenomenon to particle fragmentation at the lower compressive loads, with subsequent rebonding at higher compressive loads. In stage IV (d to e) of the compression cycle, rebonding is probably
occurring more rapidly than is fragmentation. Plastic flow may also occur in
this region.

Rubinstein [133] has studied granule consolidation during compaction by measuring the deformation of small cylindrical aggregates of dibasic calcium phosphate containing 10% by weight of radiographic barium sulfate. Spherical granules were lightly compressed (15 MN m^{-2}) with 3.2-mm-diameter flat-faced
punches into small cylindrical aggregates. These aggregates were placed di-
ametrically in the middle of a bed of sucrose granules and compacts were prepared at various pressure settings. X-rays were taken of the compacts, and
from the radiographs, diameter and thickness measurements of dibasic calcium
phosphate aggregates were determined using a traveling microscope. Also, these
aggregates could be recovered from the compact by dissolving out the sucrose with
water. The authors interpretation of their experimental data is as follows:

Up to 200 MN m^{-2}, there is an increase in aggregate diameter accompanied by
a corresponding reduction in thickness. The result is that there is only a relatively small reduction in aggregate volume. This phase may be attributable
to interparticulate slippage, which leads to a closer packed arrangement. The
increase in diameter is the result of granules being squeezed outward by the
descending upper punch. At about 200 MN m^{-2}, the aggregate diameter no

longer increases because solid bridges are formed between the particles making
up the granules and the die walls, preventing any further squeezing out of the
granules. From 200 to 420 MN m^{-2}, failure of the granular material occurs by
plastic deformation and a consolidation occurs by a reduction in aggregate thickness only. Finally, from 420 to 800 MN m^{-2}, a structure is formed that can support the applied load without further consolidation. This structure behaves elas-
tically, since the aggregates increase in size when removed from the compacts.

Hiestand et al. [130, 134] state that during compaction, particles undergo sufficient
plastic deformation to produce die wall pressures greater than can be relieved by
elastic recovery when the punch pressure is removed. This die wall pressure causes
enough internal stress in some materials to cause a crack to propagate and initiate
fracture of the compact in the die. If the excess stresses do not initiate fracture
upon decompression in the die, the compact will laminate or "cap" upon ejection
from the die. As the compact is ejected, the die wall pressure is allowed to go to
zero. The emerging compact will expand while the confined portion cannot, thus
concentrating shear stresses at the edge of the die and initiating fracture.
    Compacted materials that do not fracture have the ability to relieve the shear
stresses developed during decompression and/or ejection by plastic deformation.
This stress relaxation is time-dependent, and therefore the occurrence of compact fracture is also time-dependent. Intact compacts of acetaminophen, meth-
enamine, and erythromycin were made when the decompression was extended for
several hours. If rapidly decompressed, the compacts fracture. Stress relaxation could be the explanation for some practical tableting problems. Tablet lami-
nation or capping problems are often eliminated by precompression, slowing the
tableting rate and reducing the final compression pressure. In each adjustment,
the stress relaxation time is increased or the amount of stress needing to be relieved is reduced, allowing an intact compact to be formed.
    In many cases, deep concave punches produce tablets that cap. In this case,
the curved part of the tablet expands radially whereas the body of the tablet cannot, which establishes a shear stress that initiates the fracture. Flat punches
avoid this additional shear stress.

X. Summary: Characterization of Granulation Section

As noted in the introduction of this section on the characterization of granulations,
the various physical and physicochemical properties of granulations affect many
quality features of tablets, such as compressibility, unit dose accuracy, porosity,
hardness, friability, capping tendency, disintegration, and dissolution rate. Unfortunately, a single granulation property can influence many different tablet properties, improving some tablet properties while degrading others, as the granulation property is systematically changed in a given direction. In addition, adding
to the complexity of property relationships is the fact that many different granulation properties, alone and as interaction effects, often influence a single tablet
property. Nevertheless, optimization procedures [135] have been employed to
optimize tablet properties, such as dissolution rate [136]. As granulation properties are more clearly defined and the exact relationships of these properties to
tablet quality features are established, optimization of the properties of tablets
will become more realistic and feasible.

PART TWO. <u>EVALUATION OF TABLETS</u>

Pharmaceutical tablets are evaluated for their chemical, physical, and biological (bioavailability and drug performance) properties. These properties, in consort, describe the total quality of any given tablet formulation, according to its particular method of manufacture, in its package/container, under fixed storage or a range of storage conditions (including possible and reasonable environmental exposures under conditions of use). In the case of physical or chemical properties, a series of characteristics are required to fully identify the particular property. All three property classes—chemical, physical, and biological—have or may have a significant stability profile. In addition, the stability profiles may be interrelated; that is, chemical breakdown of or interactions between tablet components may alter physical tablet properties to greatly change the biological properties (notably the bioavailability) of a tablet system. Until recent decades, only the chemical stability of solid dosage forms was recognized as an important stability consideration. Pharmaceutical scientists now understand that various physical properties of tablets can undergo change under environmental or stress conditions, and that physical property stability, through its effect on bioavailability in particular, can be of more significance and concern in some tablet systems than chemical stability. In evaluating a particular formulation or establishing an expiration date for a product, the stability of all three classes of properties must be considered today.

Taking a very simplistic view, the development of a tablet dosage form can be viewed as five phases:

1. Concept phase
2. Feasibility phase
3. Development phase
4. Finalization phase
5. Production/Release phase

In the concept phase, the tablet project is initiated and the conceptual specifications for the new tablet are set.

The formulator becomes actively involved in the feasibility phase, attempting to make a prototype of the new tablet within the specifications of the conceptual design.

In the development phase, the tablet formula is perfected into a safe, efficacious, and reliable dosage form. Once designed, the finalization phase allows other operational units the opportunity to comment on the production suitability of the tablet in their operations, particularly the areas of packaging and shipping. Finally, production begins and quality assurance/quality control releases the new tablet for consumer use.

As the development of a tablet moves through each phase, the formulator becomes concerned about an increasing number of specific aspects of the tablet formula and evaluates the tablet for those properties. Therefore, as the project progresses, the total cumulative number of tablet evaluations performed increases. This scheme is graphically illustrated in Figure 32 and is used as a general outline for the following discussion of tablet evaluations.

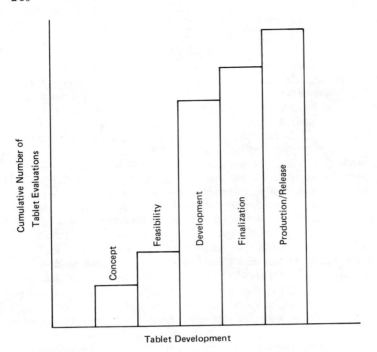

Figure 32. Tablet evaluations in the tablet development process.

XI. Concept Phase

When the concept of a new tablet is developed, approved, and the project initiated, a minimum number of measurable tablet properties are involved. These properties are generally size and shape, color, and the unique identification markings to be placed on the tablets.

A. Size and Shape

The physical dimensions of the tablet, together with the density of the materials in the tablet formulation, will determine the weight of the tablet. The size and shape of the tablet can also influence the choice of tablet machine to use, the particle size of the granulation that can be used, production lot sizes that can be made, the type of tablet processing that can be used, packaging operations, and the cost to produce the tablet. The shape of the tablet alone can influence the choice of tablet machine used. Because of the nonuniform forces involved within a tablet during compression, the more convex the tablet surface, the more likely it is to cause capping problems, forcing the use of a slower tablet machine or one with precompression capabilities [130].

Control of the size and shape of the tablet is essential to consumer acceptance, lot-to-lot uniformity, tablet-to-tablet uniformity, and trouble-free manufacturing.

Only with tooling that is uniform within specifications can tablets be uniform [137]. In 1971, the Academy of Pharmaceutical Sciences published its IPT Standard Specifications of Tableting Tools [138]. In this publication the IPT approved dimensional and tolerance specifications for tableting tools and made recommendations for the inspection and control of tools. With standardized tooling, the length and width dimensions (or diameter) and the shape become constant values for the tablet, leaving the thickness of the tablet as the only variable.

B. Tablet Thickness

Tablet thickness should be controlled within 5% or less of a standard value. Any variation in tablet thickness within a particular lot of tablets or between manufacturer's lots should not be apparent to the unaided eye to maintain product acceptance by the consumer. In addition, it is important to control thickness to facilitate packaging. Difficulties may be encountered in the use of unit dose and other types of packaging equipment if the volume of the material being packaged is not consistent. A secondary packaging problem with tablets of variable thickness relates to consistent fill of the same product container with a given number of dosage units.

At a constant compressive load, tablet thickness varies with changes in die fill and tablet weight, whereas with a constant die fill, thickness varies with variations in compressive load. Three sets of factors influence tablet thickness and tablet thickness control. These are (1) the physical properties of the raw materials, including crystal form and true and bulk density; (2) control of upper and lower punch lengths, which should be appropriately standardized; and (3) the granulation properties, including bulk density, particle size, and particle size distribution. Tablet thickness cannot be independently controlled, because it is related to tablet weight, which must also be closely adjusted and controlled, to compaction force, possibly to tablet friability, to tablet porosity, to drug release, and to bioavailability. Since we do not have the latitude to independently adjust tablet thickness, and as tablet thickness is often thought to be a specification of secondary importance to bioavailability, it is obvious that appropriate control of raw materials, machine operation, and granulation properties is fundamental to the satisfactory control of the thickness specification in practice.

The crown thickness of individual tablets may be measured with a micrometer, which permits very accurate measurements and provides information on the variation between tablets. Other techniques employed in production control involve placing 5 or 10 tablets in a holding tray, where their total crown thickness may be measured with a sliding caliper scale. This method is a much more rapid way to provide an overall estimate of tablet thickness in production operations, but it does not readily provide information on variability between tablets. However, if the punch and die tooling have been satisfactorily standardized and the tablet machine is functioning properly, the latter method is very satisfactory for production work.

Tablet crown thickness is also determined for the purpose of determining the density of tablet compacts. The volume of a tablet, standard flat face, may be computed from the formula for the volume of a cylinder ($V = \pi r^2 h$, where r is the radius of the tablet surface and h the tablet thickness). In some cases the consolidation characteristics of materials or various tablet formulas are of interest and may be evaluated by measuring the density of the tablet compacts under standard pressures and pressure loading conditions. Density equals mass per unit volume, where mass is determined by weighing the individual tablets and volume is determined as described previously. Formula or processing modifications of a particular drug product that produce a greater tablet density under given compression-loading conditions generally reflect improved consolidation of the formula and may be expected to yield a more cohesive tablet compact. The resultant tablets may be expected to have improved mechanical strength and resistance to attrition. They may also have less rapid disintegration times and dissolution rates, depending on the relationship of porosity for a particular compact to disintegration/dissolution.

C. Hardness

A tablet requires a certain amount of strength, or hardness, to withstand mechanical shocks of handling in its manufacture, packaging, and shipping. In addition, tablets should be able to withstand reasonable abuse when in the hands of the consumer (i.e., bouncing about in a purse or pocket in a partially filled prescription bottle). Adequate tablet hardness and resistance to powdering and friability are necessary requisites for consumer acceptance. More recently, the relationship to and importance of hardness as it may influence tablet disintegration and, perhaps more significantly, drug dissolution release rate have become apparent. It may be especially important to carefully monitor tablet hardness for drug products that possess real or potential bioavailability problems or are sensitive to altered dissolution-release profiles as a function of the compressive force employed.

Historically, the strength of a tablet was determined by breaking a tablet between the second and third fingers with the thumb acting as a fulcrum. If there was a "sharp" snap, the tablet was deemed to have acceptable strength [139]. More recently, however, tablet hardness has been defined as the force required to break a tablet in a diametrial compression test. To perform this test, a tablet is placed between two anvils, pressure is applied to the anvils, and the crushing strength that just causes the tablet to break is recorded. Hardness is thus sometimes termed "tablet crushing strength." Several devices operating in this manner have, and continue to be used, to test tablet hardness: the Monsanto tester [140], the Strong-Cobb tester [141], the Pfizer tester [142], the Erweka tester [143], and the Heberlein tester [144].

One of the earliest testers to be developed to evaluate tablet hardness was the Monsanto hardness tester, which was developed approximately 50 years ago. This device consisted of a barrel containing a compressible spring held between two plungers. The lower plunger was placed in contact with the tablet and a zero reading was taken. The upper plunger was then forced against a spring by turning a threaded bolt until the tablet fractured. As the spring was compressed, a pointer rode along a gauge in the barrel to indicate pressure. The pressure of fracture was recorded and the zero pressure deducted from it. The zero pressure was the gauge reading at the point at which the lower plunger barely contacted the tablet when it was initially placed in the instrument. To overcome the manual nature of this first tester and 1 min or longer time required to make an individual test, the Strong-Cobb tester was developed about 20 years later.

In the original device a plunger was activated by pumping a lever arm that forced an anvil against a stationary platform, by hydraulic pressure. The force required to fracture the tablet was read from a hydraulic gauge. In later modifications of this instrument, the force could be applied by a pressure-operated air pump rather than manually. The dial was calibrated to 30 kg in.$^{-2}$.

About another decade later, the Pfizer tester was developed and made available to the industry. This tester operates on the same mechanical principle as a pair of pliers. As the plier's handles are squeezed, the tablet is compressed between a holding anvil and a piston connected to a direct-force-reading gauge. The dial indicator remains at the reading where the tablet breaks. It is returned to zero by depressing a reset button. This tester was fairly extensively adopted over the previous testers based on its simplicity, low cost, and the rapidity with which it could be used.

Two testers have been developed to eliminate operator variation. In the Erweka tester, the tablet is placed on the lower anvil and the anvil is then adjusted so that the tablet just touches the upper test anvil. A suspended weight, motor driven, and moving along a rail, slowly and uniformly transmits pressure to the tablet. A pointer moving along a scale provides the breaking-strength value in kilograms. In the Heberlein tester, a moving anvil driven by an electric motor presses the tablet at a constant load rate against a stationary anvil. A pointer moving along a scale indicator provides the breaking-strength value. The instrument reads in both kilograms and in Strong-Cobb units. This instrument is currently the most widely employed, and has the advantage of being both fast and very reproducible.

Because of the lack of precision with the commonly used hardness testers, investigators doing work in the fields of compaction physics or tablet-breaking theory have used other means to determine the strength of compacts: for example, direct measurement instrumentation such as the Instron Tester [144] axial tensile strength tester [145], work of failure measurements [146], traversely compressed square compacts [123], impact testing [147], and conductivity measurements [148].

Unfortunately, the several testers do not produce the same results for essentially the same tablet. Studies found that operator variation, lack of calibration, spring fatigue, and manufacturer variation contribute a great deal to the lack of uniformity [144]. Even those testers designed to eliminate operator variability have been found to vary [149]. It is therefore very important that the formulator be aware of these variations, especially when the tablets are to be evaluated by other persons or in others labs. For accurate comparison, each instrument should be carefully calibrated against a known standard.

The hardness of a tablet is a function of many things all working together. The three factors that were noted in the preceding section as being sources of variation in tablet thickness may also produce variations in tablet hardness. Hardness is a function of the applied pressure and is therefore a function of those factors which cause the force to vary. As additional pressure is applied to make a tablet, the hardness values increase. This relationship holds up to a maximum value beyond which increases in pressure cause the tablet to laminate or cap, thus destroying the integrity of the tablet.

Factors that may alter tablet hardness in the course of a production run are substantial alterations in machine speed, a dirty or worn camtrack, and changes in the particle size distribution of the granulation during the course of the run, which alters the weights of the fill in the dies. Dies having a light fill (large particles, low density) will produce a softer tablet than dies that receive a heavy fill (small particles, high density).

It is the die fill/force relationship, using uniform tooling, that makes tablet hardness a very useful method of physically controlling tablet properties during a production operation, particularly when this measurement is combined with measurements of tablet thickness. The fill/force relationship is also the basis for instrumenting tablet machines.

Tablets generally are harder several hours after compression than they are immediately after compression. Lubricants can affect tablet hardness when used in too high a concentration or mixed for too long a period. The lubricants will coat the granulation particles and interfere with tablet bonding [150, 151]. Large tablets require a greater force to cause fracture and are therefore "harder" than small tablets. And for a given granulation, flat-faced tooling will produce a harder tablet than will a deep-cup tool.

A hardness of about 5 kg is probably minimal for uncoated tablets, although some chewable tablets may be somewhat softer. Tablet hardness is not an absolute indicator of strength, because some formulations, when compressed into very hard tablets, tend to "cap" on attrition, losing their crown portions. Similarly, an appropriate balance between a minimally acceptable tablet hardness to produce an adequate friability value and a maximally accepted tablet hardness to achieve adequate tablet dissolution may be required. Indeed, the influence of variations and compressive force on tablet hardness and drug dissolution should be established for all new potential formulations and may be a deciding factor in selecting an optimum formulation.

D. Color

Many pharmaceutical tablets use color as a vital means of rapid identification and consumer acceptance. It is therefore important that the color of a product be uniform: within a single tablet (nonuniformity is generally referred to as "mottling"), from tablet to tablet, and from lot to lot. Nonuniformity of coloring not only lacks aesthetic appeal but could be associated by the consumer with nonuniformity of content and general poor quality of the product [152].

The evaluation of color in tablets is usually a subjective test depending on the test person's ability to discriminate color differences visually. Because the eye is not an analytical instrument, it has shortcomings in the evaluation of surface color, and the storage of visually acquired data is very difficult. The eye cannot discriminate between small differences in color of two similar substances, nor can it precisely define color. In addition, the eye has limited memory-storage capacity for color. Therefore, people perceive the same color differently, and even one person will describe the same color differently at different times. Generally, visual comparisons require that a sample be compared against some standard. Color standards are subject to change with time, thus forcing frequent redefinition of standards, which can lead to a gradual and significant change in acceptable color [153].

Spectrophotometric techniques were used to analytically evaluate color uniformity between tablets as early as 1957 [154]. These techniques have used reflectance spectrophotometry [155-163], tristimulus colorimetric measurements [153, 163, 164], and the use of a microreflectance photometer to measure the color uniformity and gloss on a tablet surface [152].

A different approach was taken by Armstrong and March [165] to evaluate the problem of mottling. In their studies, photographs were taken of the mottled sample tablet surfaces. The photographic negatives were then scanned by a microdensitometer. This device was designed to produce a graphic record of the changes in absorbance along a path across the transparent negative.

E. Unique Identification Markings

In addition to color, companies producing tablets very often use some type of unique marking on the tablet to aid in the rapid identification of their product. These markings take the form of embossing, engraving, and printing. A look at the product identification section of the current Physician's Desk Reference [166] provides a quick reference to the multitude of variations that can be produced. While coated tablets are generally printed, engraved tablets have been successfully film-coated without obliterating the engraving.

The type of information placed on a tablet generally includes the company name or symbol, a product code such as that from the NDC number, the product name, or the potency. Of course, the more items compressed on the tablet surface, the greater the chance for the compression problems of sticking and picking. A great deal of care needs to be taken in the design, manufacture, and care of such intricate tooling.

In the future, these identifying marks, in conjunction with a greater diversity of sizes and shapes, may make up the sole means of identification of tablets if the pharmaceutical industry continues to lose the use of approved FDC colors.

XII. Feasibility Phase

Once the formulator has the conceptual requirements of the new tablet in mind, the first job is to see if a cohesive compact can be made to meet those requirements from the standpoint of weight, hardness, friability, general appearance, and disintegration.

A. Weight

As mentioned earlier, the dimensions of the tablet and the density of the mix will determine the weight of the tablet. In this phase, the formulator will have to determine whether a cohesive compact that will disintegrate can be produced within the size, shape, and thickness parameters wanted.

This feasibility work may influence the method of manufacture. For example, if a direct compression formula is preferred for a new tablet but the amount of binder required to make a cohesive compact exceeds the capacity of the die, a wet granulation technique may be required. The weight of the tablet will also determine the amount of weight variation allowed by the USP [167] within which the formulator will have to work later.

130 mg or less	10% difference
130 to 324 mg	7.5%
More than 324 mg	5%

Obviously, the weight of the tablet directly relates to the potency of the tablet once the tablet weight/tablet dimension relationship is defined.

B. General Appearance

The prototype tablet should have an aesthetic appearance that is free of the defects discussed in the preceding part of the chapter, which the formulator will have to evaluate visually.

C. Friability

Another measure of a tablet's strength is its friability. Friability is related to a tablet's ability to withstand both shock and abrasion without crumbling during the handling of manufacturing, packaging, shipment, and consumer use. Tablets that tend to powder, chip, and fragment when handled lack elegance, consumer acceptance, can create excessively dirty processes in such areas of manufacturing as coating and packaging, and can add to a tablet's weight variation or content uniformity problem. Historically, friability was subjectively measured by visually inspecting tablets after they had been shaken together for a few seconds in an operator's cupped hands. Tablets that did not cap or have excessively worn edges were acceptable. At one time, such measurements were made by field trials which involved shipping tablets in their usual containers and shipping cartons to various parts of the country. The difficulty with this approach is that it is uncontrolled, and at the conclusion of the study there is no indication of the actual exposures that the product may have been subjected to. As a result, a laboratory friability tester was developed, which is known as the Roche Friabilator [168].

This device subjects a number of tablets to the combined effects of abrasion and shock by utilizing a plastic chamber which revolves at 25 rpm, dropping the tablets a distance of 6 in. with each revolution. Normally, a preweighed tablet sample is placed in the Fribilator, which is then operated for 100 revolutions. The tablets are then dusted and reweighed. Conventional compressed tablets that lose less than 0.5 to 1.0% in weight are generally considered acceptable. Some chewable tablets and most effervescent tablets would have higher friability weight losses, which accounts for the special stack packaging that may be required for the latter system. When capping is observed during friability testing, the tablet should not be considered acceptable, regardless of what the percentage weight loss result is.

When concave, especially deep concave, punches are used in tableting, and especially if the punches are in poor condition or worn at their surface edges, the tablets produced will produce "whiskering" at the tablet edge. Such tablets will produce higher-than-normal friability values, because the "whiskers" will be removed in testing. Tablet friability may also be influenced by the moisture content of the tablet granulation in the finished tablets. A low but acceptable moisture level frequently serves to act as a binder. Very dry granulations that contain only fractional percentages of moisture will often produce more friable

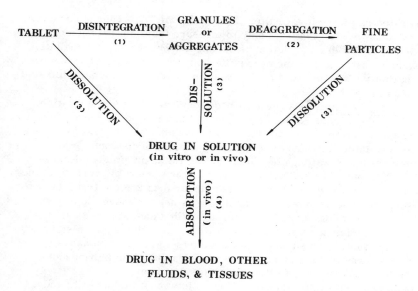

Figure 33. Processes involved when a tablet is exposed to fluid water under in vitro or in vivo conditions. (From Ref. 170.)

tablets than will granulations containing 2 to 4% moisture. It is for this reason that the manufacture of some hydrolyzable drugs into tablets having maximum chemical stability and mechanical soundness is very difficult.

D. Disintegration

It is generally accepted that in order for a drug to be available to the body, it has to be in solution. Figure 33 illustrates a scheme of the ways in which drugs formulated into a tablet become available to the body. For most tablets the first important step in the sequence is the breakdown of the tablet into smaller particles or granules. This process is known as disintegration. The time that it takes a tablet to disintegrate is measured in a device described in the United States Pharmacopeia [169]. Wagner [170] has written an excellent review of the disintegration test and the reader is referred to that reference for a more in-depth study.

It has been established that one should not expect a correlation between disintegration and dissolution [171]. However, since the dissolution of a drug from the fragmented tablet appears to partially or completely control the appearance of the drug in the blood, disintegration is still used as a guide to the formulator in the preparation of an optimum tablet formula and as an in-process control test to ensure lot-to-lot uniformity [172].

The measurement of the disintegration of a tablet has been attempted in several ways other than by the official test. Rubinstein and Wells [173] followed the disintegration of phenylbutazone tablets by the measurement of the surface

area of the generated particles in a Coulter Counter Model TA. Thermal analysis
has been used by Nakai et al. [174] not only to measure the disintegration of sugar-
coated tablets but to follow the dissolution of the sugar components, the inhibitive
action of the barrier coat, the release of the vitamins from the core, the reaction
of the calcium carbonate with the acid media, and the reaction of the ascorbic acid
with the metal ions in solution.

The United States Pharmacopeia has long had a device to test disintegration.
The device uses six glass tubes, 3 in. long, open at the top, and held against a
10-mesh screen at the bottom end of the basket rack assembly. To test for disintegration time, one tablet is placed in each tube, and the basket rack is positioned in a 1-liter beaker of water, simulated gastric fluid, or simulated intestinal fluid at 37 ± 2° C such that the tablets remain 2.5 cm below the surface of the
liquid on their upward movement and descent not closer than 2.5 cm from the bottom of the beaker. A standard motor-driven device is used to move the basket
assembly containing the tablets up and down through a distance of 5 to 6 cm at a
frequency of 28 to 32 cycles per minute. Perforated plastic disks may also be
used in the test. These are placed on top of the tablets and impart an abrasive
action to the tablets. The disks may or may not be meaningful or impart more
sensitivity to the test, but they are useful for tablets that float.

To be in compliance with USP standards, the tablets must disintegrate and all
particles pass through the 10-mesh screen in the time specified. If any residue
remains, it must have a soft mass with no palpably firm core. Procedures are
stated for running disintegration times for uncoated tablets, plain-coated tablets,
enteric-coated tablets, buccal tablets, and sublingual tablets. Uncoated USP tablets have disintegration-time standards as low as 5 min (aspirin tablets), but the
majority of the tablets have a maximum disintegration time of 30 min. Enteric-
coated tablets are to show no evidence of disintegration after 1 hr in simulated
gastric fluid. The same tablets are then tested in simulated intestinal fluid and
are to disintegrate in 2 hr plus the time specified in the monograph. If only the
enteric tablet is recognized in the USP, the disintegration in the simulated intestinal fluid must occur within the time specified in the monograph.

The formulator should be aware that the media used, the temperature of the
media, and the operator recording the results can have a significant effect on disintegration times [170]. In addition, many factors involved with a tablet's formula and method of manufacture can affect the disintegration. The nature of the
drug, the diluent used [175], the binder, the amount of binder, and the method
of incorporation can have an influence in tablet disintegration [170, 173]. The
type and amount of disintegrating agent can also have a profound effect on disintegration times [170]. The presence of excess amounts of lubricants or overly
mixed lubricated mixes can cause an increase in disintegration times. The compaction pressure used to make the tablets also influences the disintegration. In
general, disintegration times increase with an increase in pressure [175-178].

Madan [172] lists several design deficiencies of the USP apparatus that do
not allow the disintegration test to correlate better with in vivo conditions.

XIII. Development Phase

Once it has been decided that the new, desired tablet can be made within the conceptual specifications, the development efforts are directed toward designing the

final dosage form: a tablet formula that is stable, available, meets the conceptual specifications, and can be reproducibly made tablet to tablet and lot to lot. Whether this design of the final dosage form is carried out with the aid of mathematical optimization techniques [134, 135] or uses the expertise and experience of the development personnel, the tablet evaluations now performed are more sophisticated and are aimed at designing a tablet product that can be validated as to its safety, efficacy, and reliability.

A. Weight Variation

A tablet is designed to contain a specific amount of drug in a specific amount of tablet formula. To check that a tablet contains the proper amount of drug, the weight of the tablet being made is routinely measured. Composite samples of tablets (commonly 10) are taken and weighed throughout the compression process. This weight, however, is an average and contains the usual problems of average answers. Within the composite sample weighed, there could be tablets excessively overweight and tablets excessively underweight but with an average value that is acceptable. To help alleviate this problem, the United States Pharmacopeia [167] provides limits for the permissible variations in the weights of individual tablets as a percent of the average weight of the sample. The test is run by weighing 20 tablets individually, calculating the average weight, and comparing the individual tablet weights to the average. The tablets meet the USP weight variation test if no more than two tablets are outside the percentage limit and no tablet differs by more than twice the percentage limit. The weight variation tolerances for uncoated tablets differ depending on average tablet weight:

Average weight of tablets (mg)	Maximum percentage difference allowed
130 or less	10
130 to 324	7.5
More than 324	5

The Weight Variation Test is a satisfactory method of determining content uniformity of tablets if (1) the tablet is all-drug or essentially (90 to 95%) all-active-ingredient, or (2) the uniformity of drug distribution of the granulation or powder from which the tablets are made is perfect. For tablets such as aspirin tablets, which are usually 90% or more active ingredient, the ±5% weight variation should come very close to defining true potency and content uniformity (95 to 105% of label) if the average tablet weight is close to the theoretical average weight. The Weight Variation Test is not sufficient to assure uniform potency of tablets of moderate to low-dose drugs, in which excipients make up the bulk of the tablet weight [179-183].

The causes of weight variation can be separated into granulation problems and mechanical problems. The actual weight of the tablet is determined by the geometry of the die and the position of the lower punch in the die as dictated by the weight adjustment cam. If everything is working well mechanically, the weight can be caused to vary by a poorly flowing granulation, which causes a spasmodic filling of the dies. The improper mixing of the glidant into the granulation can influence the weight variation by not allowing for uniform flow. If the granulation particle size is too great for the die size, the dies will not be uniformly filled, causing weight variation [184]. Granulations that have a wide particle size distribution can have a localized nonuniformity of density in the granulation. With the geometry being fixed, nonuniform densities will cause varying amounts of granulation to fill the dies, causing variations in the resulting tablets' weights. A wide particle size distribution can also be produced when a granulation has not been thoroughly mixed or when the granulation has been stored in an area where vibrations were present to cause particle segregation which produced a wide particle size distribution. Ridgway and Williams [185] found for a uniform size granulation that as the particle shape became more angular, the weight variation increased.

Mechanical problems can cause weight variation with a good granulation. A set of lower punches of nonuniform length will cause weight variations, as will lower punches that are dirty enough to restrict their movement to their lowest point during die fill. A cupped lower punch that gets filled in with a sticking granulation will cause weight variation. And for a given granulation, Delonca et al. [184] found that as the tablet size itself increased, the weight variation also increased.

Advances in tablet machine technology have had several effects on tablet weight variation, and vice versa. Although tablet machines have been designed to operate at ever-increasing speeds and higher production rates (up to 10,000 to 15,000 tablets per minute theoretical maximum rate), the practical maximum production machine speed is often limited by tablet weight variation, caused by an inability to feed granulation to the rapidly circulating die cavities. When the demand for material by a tablet machine approaches or exceeds the flow capacity of the hopper or feed frame, tablet weight variation will increase greatly.

Induced-die feeding devices have been developed to permit higher production speed while achieving satisfactory weight variation control. Most recently, an automated tablet-weight-control device, the Thomas Tablet Sentinel,* has made improved weight variation control possible with high-speed equipment. The Sentinal is the commercial result of many studies of instrumented tablet machines. The Sentinel continuously measures the compression load using force transducers (strain gauges) and is capable of maintaining a preset compressive force by adjusting, as necessary, the machine's weight control setting, which is turned through a synchronous-drive motor. The motor is controlled by impulses from a "black box" according to the information sent from the force transducers. Such a controlled machine is termed an automated tablet machine (see Chap. 1, Vol. 3). Thus, if the particle size distribution of the granulation being compressed is reasonably consistent as it is fed from the hopper, the compressive load is a function of the volume of fill in the die cavity.

The automated tablet press has several advantages in addition to reducing tablet weight variation. Such machines continuously monitor tablet weight and provide assurance of total lot conformity. The Sentinel and similar units can be set to automatically turn a machine off and sound an alarm when it goes too far out of control or goes out of control too often.

---

*Thomas Engineering Inc., Hoffman Estates, Ill.

In addition, at high machine speeds, centrifugal effects may throw material to the outer die wall, and even throw some material from the dies. This is the current engineering limitation to maximum machine speed for horizontal-table rotary tablet machines. Other machine designs are currently in development which have the potential to overcome this limitation of engineering design.

Rapid and automatic weighing balances such as instruments available from Cahn* and Mettler† have greatly expedited tablet weight variation measurements. These instruments can also be coupled to a computer to provide various statistical control values as data printout. Ritschel [186] described such an installation and its application in automated tablet weight analysis and dosage accuracy calculation.

The potency of tablets is expressed in terms of grams, milligrams, or micrograms (for some very potent drugs) of drug per tablet, and is given as the label strength of the product. Compendial or other standards provide an acceptable potency range around the label potency. For very potent, low-dose drugs such as digitoxin, this range is usually not less than 90% and not more than 110% of the labeled amount. For most other drugs in tablet form, the official potency range that is permitted is not less than 95% and not more than 105% of the labeled amount. The usual method of determining the potency of tablet products (average assay content) involves taking 20 tablets, powdering them, taking an accurately weighed sample of the powder, analyzing that powder by an appropriate analytical technique, and calculating the average assay content of the product. For very potent drugs, 20 tablets may not provide an adequate sample for potency assay determination. For example, with digitoxin the monograph stipulates that a counted number of tablets be taken to represent about 5 mg of drug. The digitoxin assay goes on to specify that the tablets are finely powdered, and a powder sample representing about 2 mg of drug is taken for assay. The amount of powder required (and the number of tablets initially taken) will depend on the accuracy and precision of the analytical method and the amount of drugs thus required for accurate analytical measurement. For the 50-μg product, 100 tablets are thus required. The resultant assay results will disclose, on average, how close the tablets are to labeled potency and if they are within the specified potency range, on average. In the case of the digitoxin tablets, let us assume that the assay results indicate 1.9 rather than 2.0 mg in the powder sample—thus 4.75 mg in the total 100-tablet sample, or an average tablet potency of 47.5 μg. Since this monograph permits an average potency as low as 90% of label, or 45 μg, the product is within official potency assay limits on average. However, in such composite assays, resulting in an average content, individual discrepancies can be masked by the use of the blended, powdered samples.

In the hypothetical case of the digitoxin tablets, if 50 of the tablets averaged 42.5 μg, the overall average would be an acceptable 47.5 μg, yet half the tablets could be subpotent (less than 45 μg). Therefore, even though the average assay result looks acceptable, it could be the result of a wide variation in potency, with the result that a patient could be variably underdosed or overdosed. With a drug

---

*Cahn Instrument Div., Ventron Corp., Cerritos, Calif.
†Mettler Instrument Corp., Hightstown, N.J.

such as digitoxin, for which the safe and effective level and the toxic level is close (or even overlapping), exceeding the oficial or accepted potency range is not only undesirable but could be dangerous. It is for this reason that tablets are subjected to additional tests that relate to or quantify the range in potency from tablet to tablet.

B. Potency and Content Uniformity

Official potency analytical methods generally require that a composite sample be taken of the tablets, ground up, mixed, and analyzed to produce an average potency value. In composite assays, individual discrepancies can be masked by the use of the blended sample. As shown in the preceding part, the use of weight cannot be used as a potency indicator, except perhaps where the active ingredient is 90 to 95% of the total tablet weight. In tablets with smaller dosages, a good weight variation does not ensure good content uniformity, but a large weight variation precludes good content uniformity.

To assure uniform potency for tablets of low-dose drugs, a Content Uniformity Test is applied. In this test, 30 tablets are randomly selected for the sample and at least 10 of them are assayed individually. Nine of the 10 tablets must not contain less than 85% or more than 115% of the labeled drug content. The tenth tablet may not contain less than 75% or more than 125% of label. If these conditions are not met, the remaining tablets of the 30 must be assayed individually, and none may fall outside the 85 to 115% range. In evaluating a particular lot of tablets, several samples of tablets should be taken from various parts of the production run to satisfy statistical procedures.

What appears to be a wide acceptance range (85 to 115%) for content uniformity can be difficult to achieve for low-dose tablet formulations. Three factors can directly contribute to content uniformity problems in tablets: (1) nonuniform distribution of the drug substance throughout the powder mixture or granulation, (2) segregation of the powder mixture or granulation during the various manufacturing processes, and (3) tablet weight variation. The precision and variation of the assay used in the content uniformity test is also a factor that enters as a type of error in the determination of content uniformity.

The problem of nonuniform distribution is illustrated in Figure 34. The irregularly shaped drug particles are dispersed in irregularly shaped diluent particles of various sizes, and it is not difficult to comprehend why a perfect physical mixture never occurred geometrically (uniform physical placement of the drug particles) or statistically (equal probability that all sections of the mix will contain a certain number of drug particles). The squares drawn in the figure illustrate various possible random samples that might be drawn from the mixture and represent the amount of mixture required for one tablet. The squares contain as many as five particles and as few as one drug particle.

It is obvious that to achieve a reasonable content uniformity, there must be a larger number of drug particles in every sample taken. If there are only three particles, on the average, of drug in a particular weight sample, an error of plus or minus one particle will constitute an error of 33% in the dose. If, on the other hand, there are an average of 100 particles of drug in every sample taken, an error of plus or minus one particle per sample is only an error of 1%. Even 100 particles of drug per dosage unit might not be adequate in practice, however,

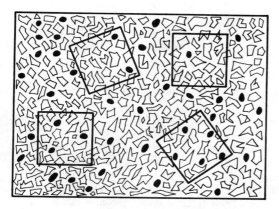

Figure 34. A powder mixture; angular open particles represent excipient; dark circles represent drug. The squares represent identical-size powder samples, which contain as few as one to as many as five drug particles. Solid dosage forms represent similar powder or granule "samples." The presence of a large number of drug particles per dose is critical to low-dose variation between tablets. [From G. S. Banker, in: Sprowl's American Pharmacy, 7th ed. (L. W. Ditlert, ed.). Lippincott, Philadelphia, 1974, p. 376.]

because statistical sampling might result in as many as 110 or as few as 90 particles much of the time. It would be more reasonable to have 1000 or more particles per dosage unit sample weight if acceptable content uniformity is to be achieved. Increasing the number of particles, however, requires a reduction in drug particle size, which is sometimes negated because of the increased electrostatic effects and potential for segregation.

The greatest potential for drug-diluent segregation in a tablet system occurs with powder or particulate mixtures intended for direct compression or with wet granulations in which drug migration is likely. In the first case, separation is promoted by vibration of the feed hopper or other parts of the machine, where differences in particle size and density of the drug and excipient will cause a consistent movement of the drug throughout the bulk of the mixture. In such a situation, denser and smaller particles will sift through the bulk of the granulation and move downward, while lighter or larger particles will tend to float to the top of the bed. In the case of wet granulations, segregation is most likely to occur if the drug is very soluble in the granulating fluid and if a static drying method is used. As the granulating fluid (drug solvent) evaporates, the drug tends to be carried to the surface of the drying granulation. This migration destroys the homogenous mix obtained prior to the drying step and reduces the changes of good content uniformity in the tablets, because the uniformity is now dependent on the mixing in the lubrication step [187].

Since the uniformity of drug distribution in tablets cannot generally be better than that of the granulation from which the tablets are made, it is advisable to determine the drug content uniformity of the granulation before compression, especially with new production runs of a product with which there is little experience or in tableting systems where uniformity problems are known to exist. Once the tablets are made, corrections such as grinding and recompressing a tablet batch may not be possible if the manufactured tablets are found to be outside the specification limits. Corrective steps that are taken before compression are simpler; less expensive; less likely to have a deleterious effect on tablet properties, such as the dissolution rate or in vivo drug availability; and are more likely to be permitted by a product's NDA.

In addition to the potency and content uniformity of solid pharmaceutical dosage forms, the pharmaceutical scientist should recognize a new concept, and that is the effective drug content of the product. This is not the amount of drug that is in the product and determinable by assay. The effective drug content is the amount of drug in the product that is present in an absorbable or bioavailable form. Many controlled studies in humans [188-195] indicate that the effective drug content of solid dosage forms is frequently not 100% of the assayable drug content of the product but may be as low as 50% or less of the labeled and assayed drug content. In addition, if certain manufacturing variables such as compressive load influence bioavailability, the effective drug content and effective drug content uniformity of a batch of tablets may be dependent upon both the actual drug content per tablet and the processing method and its variables employed to make that particular batch of product. The variation in effective drug content uniformity is undoubtedly much greater in certain cases than the chemical content uniformity indicates. To further complicate the matter, we now know that drugs which are subject to reduced effective drug content, and which may be further influenced by manufacturing methodology, are often critical in low-dose drugs such as the anticoagulants. Obviously, extreme care in production control operations is required when manufacturing products of this type. Where the effective content of a drug may be appreciably different than its labeled content, at some time in the future we may see a label indication of the effective bioavailable content on such products. Such labeling would help physicians and pharmacists to establish dosage regimens, provided that the effective bioavailable content did not vary widely from subject to subject, in which case such labeling could improve the safety of use of these drugs.

The purity of official tablets is usually assured by utilizing raw materials, both active drug and all excipients, which meet official or other rigid specifications. Extraneous substances present in a raw material or a drug which are not specifically allowed by compendial specifications or well-defined manufacturer's specifications may render the product unacceptable for pharmaceutical use. These extraneous substances may be toxic on acute or long-term use or may have an unpredictable or deleterious effect on product stability or efficacy. Certain well-defined impurities will often appear in the specification of raw materials or drug substances, or if they are the product of unavoidable decomposition of the drug, may be listed with an upper tolerance limit. For example, Aspirin Tablets, USP, may contain no more than 0.15% of free salicylic acid relative to the amount of aspirin present.

C. Special Film-Coating Tests

The development of a film coating for tablets could bring about an investigation concerning the adhesion of the polymeric film to the tablet surface and an adhesion prediction measurement. The actual adhesive force has been measured using a tensile-strength measuring device to measure either the peel strength [196, 197] or the actual adhesive force [198]. Using these force-measuring devices, several parameters were investigated as possible predictive measures: surface tension of the film-coating solution, contact angle of the film-coating solution placed on the tablet surface [196, 197], surface roughness of the tablet [197, 199, 202] and the porosity of the tablet [199, 200]. Rowe [202] concluded that there are direct relationships between porosity and roughness of the tablet surface, between porosity and adhesion, and between roughness and adhesion [197]. Rowe [202] therefore argues that a measurement of the average surface roughness is the measure to be used in optimizing film coatings for adhesion.

D. Dissolution

In our earlier discussion of disintegration, a scheme was presented to show how a drug in a solid dosage form is absorbed. It was pointed out that the original rationale for using tablet disintegration tests was the fact that as the tablet broke down into small particles, it offered a greater surface area to the dissolving media and therefore must be related to the availability of the drug to the body. However, the disintegration tests offer no assurance that the formulation will release the drug, even in the form of small particles.

Since a drug must normally be in solution before absorption can take place, orally administered tablets must have their drugs dissolved in the contents of the gastrointestinal tract before the absorption of the drug can occur. Often, the rate of drug absorption is determined by the rate of drug dissolution from the tablet. Therefore, if it is important to achieve peak blood levels for a drug quickly, it will usually be important to obtain rapid drug dissolution from the tablet. For drugs that are absorbed high in the gastrointestinal tract (i.e., acidic drugs), which have a large dose and a low solubility, rapid dissolution may be especially important. The design of the tablet and the dissolution profile for such drugs may determine the total amount of drug absorbed as well as its rate of absorption. Thus, the rate of dissolution may be directly related to the efficacy of the tablet product as well as bioavailability differences between formulations. It is therefore important to evaluate whether a tablet releases its drug contents when placed into the environment of the gastrointestinal tract. The most direct assessment of the drug's release would be in vivo bioavailability tests. However, there are several reasons that restrict the use of in vivo studies: length of time required, highly skilled personnel required especially for human studies, low precision of the measurements, inadequate discrimination between products, and a correlation with the diseased state might have to be made with healthy human subjects or with animals.

The utility of using in vitro results has been presented in the literature for the past 15-20 years. Only a brief introduction to dissolution testing will be presented in this section; the reader is referred to the literature for a more in-depth study [203-206].

The objectives of an in vitro dissolution test should be to show that (1) the release of the drug from the tablet is as close to 100% as possible, and that (2) the rate of the release is uniform batch to batch and is the same as the release rate from those batches proven to be bioavailable and clinically effective.

In designing a dissolution test, several requirements should be kept in mind. The dissolution test should be designed to be suitable for use with a wide range of drugs and dosage forms. The test should be able to meaningfully discriminate between formulations. There should be a reliable and reproducible assay for the drug being tested. The test should be simple to do, reproducible, and easily converted to an automatic system. Many different dissolution test apparatus have been reported on in the literature. This section, however, will restrict itself to a discussion concerning the USP Apparatus 1 and Apparatus 2 [207].

Various parameters of the dissolution testing apparatus can affect the results. Water has been used as the preferred dissolution medium by some but is hardly the universal medium because of solubility restrictions and pH changes as the drug dissolves. In the latter case, the addition of appropriate buffers can remedy the problem. The pH of the medium is important regarding the solubility and stability of some drugs and formulations. It is also important when trying to make the medium of dissolution reflect the medium at the site of absorption or above it in the gastrointestinal tract. For example, acidic drugs should be tested in an acidic medium, since for best absorption, they must dissolve in the stomach or upper small intestine. Dissolution testing of such drugs in a medium of pH 7.4, such as simulated intestinal fluid, would serve little purpose, since the acidic drugs would be nearly completely ionized and the absorption would be inhibited at that pH.

The volume of the dissolution medium, in theory, should be sufficient to maintain sink conditions throughout the test. To maintain sink conditions, it has been suggested that the volume of the medium used be four to five times the saturation volume. For low-solubility drugs, this volume could conceivably be several liters. In practice, however, the volume of medium used is usually determined by the apparatus used. This then forces the use of hydroalcoholic or mixed-solvent systems for the dissolution medium.

The temperature of the medium is generally $37 \pm 0.5°$ C maintained throughcut the test. Those performing the test should allow enough time for the medium to warm up to the proper temperature, which in some instances could take 2 to 3 hr. Both the dissolution vessel and the water bath used to warm the dissolution vessel should be covered to minimize the losses of heat and evaporation. In some instances the removal of dissolved gases from the medium may be required. For example, in the use of Method 1, the basket can become covered with air bubbles and thus retard the dissolution test.

The agitation of the medium should be widely variable but highly controlled. Both high and low agitation speeds can cause problems in dissolution testing. High-speed agitation may cause excessive agitation and dissolution rates, incompatible with a correlation with in vivo availability. Low-speed agitation could produce a very discriminating dissolution test but could also reduce the agitation to a point where homogenous mixing is lost. Without homogenous mixing, areas of differing drug concentration can be developed in the dissolution vessel, thus making the position from which the sample is drawn for assay very important in obtaining meaningful data. The stirring motors should be checked on a regular basis for speed uniformity and speed calibration. In addition, many motors should be warmed up prior to use to eliminate any speed variations or increases during the test itself.

The dissolution test apparatus is to be constructed such that "no part of the assembly, including the environment in which the assembly is placed, contributes significant motion, agitation or vibration beyond that due to the smoothly rotating stirring element" [207]. This extra agitation can cause differences in mean dissolution rates and increase the differences between dissolution vessels. The vibrations can come from the dissolution test equipment itself, such as the water bath and its agitator/pump, and from external sources, such as equipment operating on the same benchtop as the dissolution test equipment or even from heavy machinery operating in close proximity. Another source of extra medium agitation or movement can come from currents set up by the sampling pump in an automatic dissolution test apparatus.

The dissolution apparatus should permit a convenient method of placing a tablet into the dissolution medium and holding it there for the duration of the test while retaining the ability to observe the tablet throughout the test procedure. The dissolution vessel itself must be exactly specified as to its dimensions, especially with multivessel test apparatus. Significant differences in dissolution rates have been found for products tested in different vessels [208].

Dissolution samples removed for assay are filtered to remove solid particles of drug present and to remove tablet excipients that might otherwise interfere with the assay. Care must be used to choose a filter which does not release elements that can interfere with the assay or adsorb the drug from solution.

Dissolution testing may employ intermittent sampling or continuous analysis of the dissolution medium. When intermittent sampling is employed, corrections may be necessary to account for the volume and drug content of the samples removed for analysis or for dilution resulting from the addition of fresh medium to maintain volume. When the dissolution medium is continuously analyzed, these corrections are usually unnecessary, since the medium is returned to the apparatus after it is analyzed. However, as mentioned before, the sampling pump should not induce additional agitation by setting up currents inside the vessel. One of the main problems of automated intermittant sampling and analysis lies in the fact that the sample probe, lines, spectrophotometer flow cells, and so on, contain a certain volume of medium. This volume mixes with the next sample aliquot, giving an apparent reading that is higher or lower than the real one. This effect can be minimized by using suitable flow rates and short runs of small-diameter tubing. Important in any dissolution test is that the analytical method be highly reliable and reproducible. The simple direct analytical methods are preferred and care must be used to make sure that tablet excipients do not interfere with the assay method.

Equally important as running the dissolution test properly is proper interpretation of the resulting data. Dissolution results may be expressed in terms of the concentration of drug in the dissolution medium versus time, the amount of drug released from the dosage form versus time, or the amount of drug remaining unreleased from the dosage form versus time. Most commonly, the results are expressed in terms of the time required to release some percentage of the labeled amount of drug from the dosage form. For example, the USP specifies that 60% of the labeled amount of hydrochlorothiazide shall dissolve from Hydrochlorothiazide Tablets, USP, in not more than 30 min. Such expressions of dissolution and release characteristics suffer from the disadvantage that they do not account for the portion of the drug remaining unreleased. For example, it is entirely possible that 60% of the labeled amount of hydrochlorothiazide could be released from a given tablet in 5 min and also that 10% or more would never be released from the same tablet. Alternatively, it is possible for 60% to be released rapidly and for the remaining 40% to be released very slowly. Thus, the description of a dissolution process in terms of a single point in time is inherently risky. Such expressions are useful, however, for quality control purposes once the dissolution characteristics of a drug and dosage form are well understood. For tablet dosage form design purposes and for critical product comparisons, the time required for substantially complete (80 to 90%) release or amount released versus time profiles are the most desired data.

E. Porosity

Since many of the traditionally measured physical characteristics of tablets probably relate to tablet porosity structure, and as the alterations in these physical characteristics result from alterations in pore structure, interest in porosity structure determination and characterization has been growing.

The major parameters associated with the porous nature of solids is the volume of the void space, designated as the porosity or pore volume; the size of the pores, characterized by their diameters; and the distribution of the pore sizes [209]. Measurement of the pore size can be measured by air permeametry [210-212], adsorption isotherms [213, 214], and mercury intrusion [215-218].

Higuchi et al. [219] stated in 1952 that "it seems reasonable to assume that the volume of void space in a given tablet would greatly influence its disintegrating property." Taking this lead, several investigators have used a measure of porosity in an attempt to determine the effects of porosity on tablet disintegration and to study the mechanism of disintegrant action [217, 220].

Stanley-Wood and Johansson [214] evaluated the surface area, pore size, and total voidage in an effort to get an insight into the mechanisms of compaction. By evaluating the contact areas between particles, the authors were able to show particle rearrangement or plastic flow bonding.

From the standpoint of tablet stability, especially when dealing with hydrolyzable drugs, a physical description of the porous state of tablets may be of fundamental importance if the porosity and pore size distribution affect the accessibility of water and water vapor into the pore system of the tablet.

Gucluyildiz et al. [216], using the mercury intrusion technique for porosity determinations, found that the stability of aspirin tablets increased when the porosity of the tablets was decreased by the addition of silicon dioxide. The increase in stability was explained in terms of the silicon dioxide reducing the porosity by reducing the size and volume of the coarser pores, thereby reducing the accessibility of water vapor to the aspirin component of the tablet.

The correlation between the more basic tablet physical properties and tablet pore structure and between the chemical stability and the tablet pore structure remains to be fully illustrated. It is predicted, however, that in the future, fundamental studies of tablet properties and performance will be based on an examination of tablet porosity and structure and changes in these properties with time.

F. Physical Stability

Stability is important not only from the standpoint of aesthetics and customer acceptance but also important in maintaining uniform drug strength, identity, quality, and purity, as exemplified by the inclusion of a stability section in the Current Good Manufacturing Practices (21CFR, Part 211, Section 211.166) and a section of "Stability Considerations In Dispensing Practice" in the United States Pharmacopeia [221].

It is now recognized that the physical characteristics of tablets may have a stability profile just as do chemical characteristics. Since some of the physical properties of tablets may have a profound influence on drug dissolution and release, including bioavailability, changes of these physical properties on aging may produce corresponding changes, usually resulting in a reduction in bioavailability. In establishing expiry dates for solid dosage forms, it is essential that the physical characteristics and the bioavailability properties be given equal consideration with the chemical characteristics, since all of these properties may change with product age and with product exposure. Therefore, many of the physical parameters, such as hardness, disintegration, and dissolution, are routinely tested within the framework of the tablet's chemical stability program.

One aspect of a tablet's stability, that of color, has been investigated in an effort to produce an accelerated means of determining the light stability of colored products. Lachman et al. [155, 157-159] described a series of color-stability tests using a light-stability cabinet. More recently, Turi et al. [222] described the use of a fadeometer in doing accelerated color-stability work. The fadeometer proved to be 50 to 100 times faster than a light cabinet in obtaining results. A 24-hr exposure in the fadeometer was found sufficient to compare the fading behavior of tablets and to predict color stability under normal environmental conditions.

XIV. Finalization Phase

Sometime during the final design of the tablet formulation, a new tablet should be tested as to its durability during the handling associated with such operations as coating, printing, packaging, and shipping. The traditional evaluations performed on tablets involve only a small sample of tablets. How the tablets will withstand the mechanical shocks of a production environment is a function of the large number of tablets involved, production equipment, and production personnel. Rough-handling tests can be performed to give an indication of how well the new tablet will hold up in its specified package and shipping container during shipment. Rough-handling tests generally include a vibration test, a drop test, and an inclined-plane impact test [223-225]. Some investigators have actually shipped bottled product across the country and back again to get an idea of the strength of the new tablet product in shipment.

Problems can and do arise with new tablets in the packaging operation. Tablets undergo a number of mechanical shocks during the packaging operation, such as dumping into the packaging machine hopper, rectification into the filling slats (Merrill[*] filler), dropping into bottles (especially glass bottles), compression by the cottoning operation, and squeezing by the labeling operation (plastic bottles). Probably the best way to test a new tablet is to allow the packaging personnel to

---

[*]Merrill Div., Pennwalt Corp., Chicago, Ill.

package a large number of tablets under normal operating conditions, to evaluate the tablet's performance in comparison to how other tablets run under the same conditions. This same approach should be carried out with the printing of coated tablets by letting the production people comment on how the new tablet functions under normal production conditions.

XV. Production/Release Phase

The majority of in-process tests performed by production and the release tests performed by quality assurance are tests used by the formulator to develop the new tablet. In fact, data supplied by the formulator is generally acted on by quality assurance to establish the product/release specifications.

As additional checks for identity, strength, quality, and purity, several other evaluations can be made during and after tablet production. Many companies are using automatic force/weight monitoring devices with automatic weight control feedback mechanisms to reduce tablet weight variation. Metal-detection devices have been experimented with for on-line metal detection in tablets. Coated tablets are mechanically sorted or visually inspected to eliminate out-of-size tablets, tablets with poor printing, or tablets with other defects. Some quality assurance release specifications include microbial contamination tests and a test for penicillin contamination.

XVI. Summary

As noted earlier in the chapter, the quality of pharmaceutical tablets can be no higher than the quality of the granulation from which the tablets are made. It is for this reason that a fairly detailed section was included on the characterization of granulations. An oft-repeated axiom in pharmaceutical research, development, and manufacture is that quality must be built into a product; it cannot be assayed in. This is certainly true in tablet product design and manufacture. A critical element in building quality into tablet products is thus in the design of the granulation or direct compression systems from which tablets are made. The quality of the tablets can, of course, be much lower than the quality of the granulation source, depending on processing conditions, the equipment used, and the skills of the personnel employed in the tablet manufacturing step.

Tablets are the most widely used and most frequently used of all dosage-form classes. They are, however, heterogeneous systems, and as such they are one of the most complex classes of drug products from a physical sense. They have a range of mechanical properties not seen in other dosage forms because they are compressed systems. Achieving satisfactory drug dissolution profiles is more difficult from tablets than from any other class or oral dosage form. It is increasingly recognized that the physical and mechanical properties of tablets may undergo change on aging or on exposure to environmental stresses, thus having a stability profile that affects bioavailability and other fundamental tablet properties. Thus, it can be seen that the physical and mechanical properties stability profile can be as important as, if not more important than, the chemical stability of a tablet product. It is also becoming apparent that attempts at optimizing tablet dosage forms can only be as successful as the accuracy and adequacy of the physical methods used in product evaluation. This chapter has attempted not only to provide comprehensive listings and descriptions (with full reference to the literature) of test methods for granulations and tablets, but has developed the tablet evaluation section in a sequential manner in accordance with the typical steps in a product development activity.

References

1. Barlow, C. G., Chem. Eng. (Lond.)., 220:196 (1968).
2. Pilpel, N., Chem. Process Eng., 50:67 (July 1969).
3. Leuenberger, H., Bier, H., and Sucuer, H., Phar. Tech., 3:61 (June 1979).
4. Mehta, A., Adams, K., Zoglio, M. A., and Carstensen, J. T., J. Pharm. Sci., 66:1462 (1977).
5. Hunter, B. M., and Ganderton, D., J. Pharm. Pharmacol., 25:71P (1973).
6. Ganderton, D., and Hunter, B. M., J. Pharm. Pharmacol., 23:1S (1971).
7. Newton, J. M., Manuf. Chem. Aerosol News, 37:33 (Apr. 1966).
8. Kanig, J. L., J. Pharm. Sci., 53:188 (1964).
9. Fonner, D. E., Banker, G. S., and Swarbrick, J., J. Pharm. Sci., 55:181 (1966).
10. Irani, R. R., and Callis, C. F., Particle Size: Measurement, Interpretation, and Application. Wiley, New York, 1963.
11. Herdan, G., Small Particle Statistics. Elsevier, New York, 1953.
12. Dallavalle, J. M., Micromeretics. Pitman, New York, 1948.
13. Edmundson, I. C., in: Advances in Pharmaceutical Sciences, Vol. 2 (H. S. Bean, A. H. Beckett, and J. E. Carless, eds.). Academic Press, New York, 1967, pp. 95-129
14. Heywood, H., J. Pharm. Pharmacol., 15:56T (1963).
15. Wilks, S. S., Elementary Statistical Analysis. Princeton University Press, Princeton, N.J., 1961.
16. Smith, J. E., and Jordan, M. L., J. Colloid Sci., 19:549 (1964).
17. Aitchison, J., and Brown, J. A. C., The Log-Normal Distribution. Cambridge University Press, Cambridge, 1957.
18. Kottler, F., J. Franklin Inst., 250:339, 419 (1950).
19. Ames, D. P., Irani, R. R., and Callis, C. F., J. Phys. Chem., 63:531 (1959).
20. Hatch, T., J. Franklin Inst., 215:27 (1933).
21. Fonner, D. E., Banker, G. S., and Swarbrick, J., J. Pharm. Sci., 55:576 (1966).
22. Hatch, T., and Choate, S. P., J. Franklin Inst., 207:369 (1929).
23. Opankunle, W. O., Bhutani, B. R., and Bhatia, V. N., J. Pharm. Sci., 64:1023 (1975).
24. Whitby, K. T., ASTM Spec. Tech. Publ. No. 234 (1958).
25. Shergold, F. A., J. Soc. Chem. Ind., 65:245 (1946).
26. Davis, R. F., Trans. Inst. Chem. Eng., 18:76 (1940).
27. Kluge, W., Quarry Manager's J., p. 506 (Mar. 1953).
28. Wolff, E. R., Ind. Eng. Chem., 46:1778 (1954).
29. Roberts, T. A., and Beddow, J. K., Powder Technol., 2:121 (1968/1969).

30. Jansen, M. L., and Glastonbury, J. R., Powder Technol., 1:334 (1967/1968).
31. Lapple, C. E., Chem. Eng., 75:149 (May 1968).
32. Laws, E. Q., Analyst, 88:156 (1963).
33. Arambulo, A. S., and Deardorff, D. L., J. Am. Pharm. Assoc., Sci. Ed., 42:690 (1953).
34. Marks, A. M., and Sciarra, J. J., J. Pharm. Sci., 57:497 (1968).
35. Forlano, A. J., and Chavkin, L., J. Am. Pharm. Assoc., Sci. Ed., 49:67 (1960).
36. Pitkin, C., and Carstensen, J., J. Pharm. Sci., 62:1215 (1973).
37. Chalmers, A. A., and Elworthy, P. H., J. Pharm. Pharmacol., 28:228 (1976).
38. Chalmers, A. A., and Elworthy, P. H., J. Pharm. Pharmacol., 28:234 (1976).
39. Chalmers, A. A., and Elworthy, P. H., J. Pharm. Pharmacol., 28:239 (1976).
40. Davies, W. L., and Gloor, W. T., J. Pharm. Sci., 60:1869 (1971).
41. Davies, W. L., and Gloor, W. T., J. Pharm. Sci., 61:618 (1972).
42. Davies, W. L., and Gloor, W. T., J. Pharm. Sci., 62:170 (1973).
43. Ridgway, K., and Rupp, R., J. Pharm. Pharmacol., 21:30S (1969).
44. Shotton, E., and Obiorah, B. A., J. Pharm. Sci., 64:1213 (1975).
45. Rose, H. E., The Measurement of Particle Size in Very Fine Powders. Chemical Publishing Co., New York, 1954.
46. Fair, G. M., and Hatch, L. P., J. Am. Water Works Assoc., 25:1551 (1933).
47. Rupp, R., Boll. Chim. Farm., 116:251 (1977).
48. Ridgway, K., and Shotton, J. B., J. Pharm. Pharmacol., 22:24S (1970).
49. Pahl, M. H., Shadel, G., and Rumpf, H., Aufbereit. Tech., 14:Secs. 5, 10, 11 (1973).
50. Davies, R., Powder Technol., 12:111 (1975).
51. Martin, A. N., Swarbrick, J., and Cammarata, A., Physical Pharmacy. Lea & Febiger, Philadelphia, 1969.
52. Fries, J., The Determination of Particle Size by Adsorption Methods, ASTM Spec. Tech. Publ. No. 234 (1958).
53. Shaw, D. J., Introduction to Colloid and Surface Chemistry. Butterworths, Washington, D.C., 1966.
54. Adamson, A. W., Physical Chemistry of Surfaces. Interscience, New York, 1960.
55. Rigden, P. J., J. Soc. Chem. Ind., 66:130 (1947).
56. Carman, P. C., J. Soc. Chem. Ind., 57:225 (1938).
57. Carman, P. C., Flow of Gases Through Porous Media. Butterworths, Washington, D.C., 1956.
58. Strickland, W. A., Busse, L. W., and Higuchi, T., J. Am. Pharm. Assoc., Sci. Ed., 45:482 (1956).
59. Weissberger, A., Techniques of Organic Chemistry: Physical Methods, Part 1, 3rd ed., Interscience, New York, 1959.
60. Armstrong, N. A., and March, G. A., J. Pharm. Sci., 65:198 (1976).
61. Hunter, B. M., and Ganderton, D., J. Pharm. Pharmacol., 24:17P (1972).
62. Graton, L. C., and Fraser, H. J., J. Geol., 43:785 (1935).

63. Heywood, H., J. Imp. Coll. Chem. Eng. Soc., 2:9 (1946).
64. Neumann, B. S., in: Flow Properties of Disperse Systems (J. J. Hermans, ed.). North-Holland, Amsterdam, 1953, Chap. 10.
65. Butler, Q. A., and Ramsey, J. C., Drug Stand., 20:217 (1952).
66. Neumann, B. S., in: Advances in Pharmaceutical Sciences, Vol. 2 (H. S. Bean, A. H. Beckett, and J. E. Carless, eds.). Academic Press, New York, 1967, pp. 182-221
67. Carr, R. L., Chem. Eng., 72:163 (Jan. 1965).
68. Harwood, C. F., and Pilpel, N., J. Pharm. Sci., 57:478 (1968).
69. Eaves, T., and Jones, T. M., J. Pharm. Pharmacol., 25:729 (1973).
70. Arthur, J. R. F., and Dunstan, T., Nature (Lond.), 223:464 (1969).
71. Arthur, J. R. F., and Dunstan, T., Powder Technol., 3:195 (1969/1970).
72. Gold, G., Duvall, R. N., Palermo, B. T., and Hurtle, R. L., J. Pharm. Sci., 60:922 (1971).
73. Mehta, A., Zoglio, M. A., and Carstensen, J. T., J. Pharm. Sci., 67:905 (1978).
74. Ridgway, K., and Rubinstein, M. H., J. Pharm. Pharmacol., 23:11S (1971).
75. Ganderton, D., and Selkirk, A. A., J. Pharm. Pharmacol., 22:345 (1970).
76. Jaiyeoba, K. T., and Spring, M. S., J. Pharm. Pharmacol., 31:192 (1978).
77. Hill, P. M., J. Pharm. Sci., 65:313 (1976).
78. Milosovich, G., Drug Cosmet. Ind., 92:557 (1963).
79. Pilpel, N., J. Pharm. Pharmacol., 16:705 (1964).
80. Gold, G., and Palermo, B. T., J. Pharm. Sci., 54:310 (1965).
81. Ridge, W. A. D., Philos. Mag., 25:481 (1913).
82. Boning, P., Z. Tech. Phys., 8:385 (1927).
83. Kunkel, W. B., J. Appl. Phys., 21:820, 833 (1950).
84. Jefimenko, O., Am. J. Phys., 27:604 (1959).
85. Harper, W. R., Adv. Phys. (Suppl. to Philos. Mag.), 6:365 (1957).
86. Harper, W. R., Soc. Chem. Ind. (Lond.), Monogr. 14:115 (1961).
87. Krupp, H., Adv. Colloid Interface Sci., 1:111 (1967).
88. Hiestand, E. N., J. Pharm. Sci., 55:1325 (1966).
89. Gold, G., and Palermo, B. T., J. Pharm. Sci., 54:1517 (1965).
90. Gold, G., Duvall, R. N., and Palermo, B. T., J. Pharm. Sci., 55:1133 (1966).
91. Lachman, L., and Lin, S., J. Pharm. Sci., 57:504 (1968).
92. Pilpel, N., Br. Chem. Eng., 11:699 (1966).
93. Zenz, F. A., and Othmer, D. F., Fluidization and Fluid Particle Systems. Reinhold, New York, 1960.
94. Train, D., J. Pharm. Pharmacol., 10:127T (1958).
95. Pathirana, W. K., and Gupta, B. K., Can. J. Pharm. Sci., 11:30 (1976).
96. Lowes, T. M., Fuel Soc. J. Univ. Sheffield, 16:35 (1965).
97. Lowes, T. M., and Perry, M. G., Rheol. Acta, 4:166 (1965).
98. Pilpel, N., in: Advances in Pharmaceutical Sciences, Vol. 3 (H. S. Bean, A. H. Beckett, and J. E. Carless, eds.), Academic Press, New York, 1971, pp. 173-219.
99. Danish, F. Q., and Parrott, E. L., J. Pharm. Sci., 60:548 (1971).
100. Nelson, E., J. Am. Pharm. Assoc., Sci. Ed., 44:435 (1955).
101. Kelley, J. J., J. Soc. Cosmet. Chem., 21:37 (1970).
102. Jones, T. M., and Pilpel, N., J. Pharm. Pharmacol., 18:182S (1966).

103. Jones, T. M., and Pilpel, N., J. Pharm. Pharmacol., 17:440 (1965).
104. Craik, D. J., J. Pharm. Pharmacol., 10:73 (1958).
105. Craik, D. J., and Miller, B. F., J. Pharm. Pharmacol., 10:136T (1958).
106. York, P., J. Pharm. Sci., 64:1216 (1975).
107. Tawashi, R., Drug Cosmet. Ind., 106:46 (1970).
108. Gold, G., Duvall, R. N., Palermo, B. T., and Slater, J. G., J. Pharm. Sci., 55:1291 (1966).
109. Nash, J. H., Leiter, G. G., and Johnson, A. P., Ind. Chem. Prod. Res. Dev., 4:140 (1965).
110. Awada, E., Nakajima, E., Morioka, T., Ikegami, Y., and Yoshizumi, M., J. Pharm. Soc. Jap., 80:1657 (1960).
111. Dawes, J. G., Min. Fuel Power (Br.) Safety Mines Res. Estab., No. 36 (1952).
112. Carstensen, J. T., and Chan, P. C., J. Pharm. Sci., 66:1235 (1977).
113. Fowler, R. T., and Wyatt, F. A., Aust. J. Chem., 1:5 (June 1960).
114. Johanson, J. R., Chem. Eng., 85:9 (Oct. 30, 1978).
115. Jenike, A. W., Elsey, P. J., and Wooley, R. H., Proc. ASTM, 60:1168 (1960).
116. Jenike, A. W., Utah Eng. Exp. Sta. Bull. No. 108, Univ. Utah (1961).
117. Jenike, A. W., Trans. Inst. Chem. Eng., 40:264 (1962).
118. Jenike, A. W., Utah Eng. Exp. Sta. Bull. No. 123, Univ. Utah (1964).
119. Williams, J. C., Chem. Process Eng., 46(4):173 (1965).
120. Carr, J. F., and Walker, D. M., Powder Technol., 1:369 (1967/1968).
121. Heistand, E. N., Valvani, S. C., Peot, C. B., Strazelinski, E. P., and Glasscock, J. F., J. Pharm. Sci., 62:1513 (1973).
122. Williams, J. C., and Birks, A. H., Powder Technol., 1:199 (1967).
123. Hiestand, E. N., and Peot, C. B., J. Pharm. Sci., 63:605 (1974).
124. Peleg, M., and Mannheim, C. H., Powder Technol., 7:45 (1973).
125. Kurup, T. R. R., and Pilpel, N., Powder Technol., 14:115 (1976).
126. Farley, R., and Valentin, F. H. H., Powder Technol., 1:344 (1967/1968).
127. Gold, G., Duvall, R. N., Palermo, B. T., and Slater, J. G., J. Pharm. Sci., 57:667 (1968).
128. Gold, G., Duvall, R. N., Palermo, B. T., and Slater, J. G., J. Pharm. Sci., 57:2153 (1968).
129. Jones, T. M., J. Soc. Cosmet. Chem., 21:483 (1970).
130. Hiestand, E. N., Wells, J. E., Peot, C. B., and Ochs, J. F., J. Pharm. Sci., 66:510 (1977).
131. Train, D., J. Pharm. Pharmacol., 8:45T (1956).
132. Higuchi, T., Rao, A. N., Busse, L. W., and Swintosky, J. V., J. Am. Pharm. Assoc., Sci. Ed., 42:194 (1953).
133. Rubinstein, M. H., J. Pharm. Sci., 65:376 (1976).
134. Hiestand, E. N., paper presented at International Conference on Powder Technology and Pharmacy, Basel, Switzerland, 1978.
135. Buck, J. R., Peck, G. E., and Banker, G. S., Drug Dev. Commun., 1(2):89 (1974/1975).
136. Fonner, D. E., Banker, G. S., and Buck, J. R., J. Pharm. Sci., 59:1587 (1970).
137. Ling, W. C., J. Pharm. Sci., 62:2007 (1973).
138. IPT Standard Specifications for Tableting Tools, Tableting Specification Manual. Academy of Pharmaceutical Sciences, Washington, D.C., 1971.

139. Gunsel, W. C., and Kanig, J. L., in: The Theory and Practice of Industrial Pharmacy, 2nd ed. (L. Lachman, H. A. Lieberman, and J. L. Kanig, eds.). Lea & Febiger, Philadelphia, 1976, p. 347.

140. Smith, F. D., and Grosch, D., U.S. Patent 2,041,869 (1936).

141. Albrecht, R., U.S. Patent 2,645,936 (1953).

142. Michel, F., U.S. Patent 2,975,630 (1961).

143. Brook, D. B., and Marshall, K., J. Pharm. Sci., 57:481 (1968).

144. Goodhart, F. W., Draper, J. R., Dancz, D., and Ninger, F. C., J. Pharm. Sci., 62:297 (1973).

145. Nystrom, C., Alex, W., and Malmquist, K., Acta Pharm. Suec., 14:317 (1977).

146. Rees, P. J., and Richardson, S. C., J. Pharm. Pharmacol., 29:38P (1977).

147. Hiestand, E. N., Bane, J. M., and Strzelinski, E. P., J. Pharm. Sci., 60:758 (1971).

148. Bhata, R. P., and Lordi, N. G., J. Pharm. Sci., 68:898 (1979).

149. Newton, J. M., and Stanley, P., J. Pharm. Pharmacol., 29:41P (1977).

150. Lerk, C. F., and Bolhuis, G. K., Pharm. Acta Helv., 52:39 (1977).

151. Shah, A. C., and Mlodozeniec, A. R., J. Pharm. Sci., 66:1377 (1977).

152. Matthews, B. A., Matsumota, S., and Shibata, M., Drug Dev. Commun., 1:303 (1974/1975).

153. Bogdansky, F. M., J. Pharm. Sci., 64:323 (1975).

154. McKeehan, C. W., and Christian, J. E., J. Am. Pharm. Assoc., Sci. Ed., 46:631 (1957).

155. Lachman, L., and Cooper, J., J. Am. Pharm. Assoc., Sci. Ed., 48:226 (1959).

156. Urbanyi, T., Swartz, C. J., and Lachman, L., J. Am. Pharm. Assoc., Sci. Ed., 49:163 (1960).

157. Lachman, L., Swartz, C. J., Urbanyi, T., and Cooper, J., J. Am. Pharm. Assoc., Sci. Ed., 49:165 (1960).

158. Lachman, L., Swartz, C. J., and Cooper, J., J. Am. Pharm. Assoc., Sci. Ed., 49:213 (1960).

159. Lachman, L., Weinstein, S., Swartz, C. J., Urbanyi, T., and Cooper, J., J. Pharm. Sci., 50:141 (1961).

160. Swartz, C. J., Lachman, L., Urbanyi, T., and Cooper, J., J. Pharm. Sci., 50:145 (1961).

161. Swartz, C. J., Lachman, L., Urbanyi, T., Weinstein, S., and Cooper, J., J. Pharm. Sci., 51:326 (1962).

162. Everhard, M. E., and Goodhart, F. W., J. Pharm. Sci., 52:281 (1963).

163. Goodhart, F. W., Everhard, M. E., and Dickcius, D. A., J. Pharm. Sci., 53:338 (1964).

164. Goodhart, F. W., Lieberman, H. A., Mody, D. S., and Nimger, F. C., J. Pharm. Sci., 56:63 (1967).

165. Armstrong, N. A., and March, G. A., J. Pharm. Sci., 63:126 (1974).

166. Physician's Desk Reference, 33rd ed. Medical Economics, Oradell, N.J., 1979, p. 402.

167. The United States Pharmacopeia, 20th rev. Mack, Easton, Pa., 1980, p. 990.

168. Shafer, E. G. E., Wollish, E. G., and Engel, C. E., J. Am. Pharm. Assoc., Sci. Ed., 45:114 (1956).

169. The United States Pharmacopeia, 20th rev. Mack, Easton, Pa., 1980, pp. 958-959

170. Wagner, J. G., Biopharmaceutics and Relevant Pharmacokinetics. Drug
     Intelligence Publications, Hamilton, Ill., 1971, pp. 64-97.
171. Alam, and Parrott, E. L., J. Pharm. Sci., 60:795 (1971).
172. Madan, P. L., Can. J. Pharm. Sci., 13:12 (1978).
173. Rubinstein, M. H., and Wells, J. I., J. Pharm. Pharmacol., 29:363 (1977).
174. Nakai, Y., Nakajima, S., and Kakizawa, H., Chem. Pharm. Bull., 22:2910
     (1974).
175. Lerk, C. F., Bolhuis, G. K., and DeBoer, A. H., Pharm. Weekbl., 109:945
     (1974).
176. Kitazawa, S., Johno, I., Ito, Y., Teramura, S., and Okada, J., J. Pharm.
     Pharmacol., 27:765 (1975).
177. Suren, G., Acta Pharm. Suec., 7:483 (1970).
178. Bolhuis, G. K., and Lerk, C. F., Pharm. Weekbl., 108:469 (1973).
179. Breunig, H. L., and King, E. P., J. Pharm. Sci., 51:1187 (1962).
180. Brochmann-Hanssen, E., and Medina, J. C., J. Pharm. Sci., 52:630 (1963).
181. Garrett, E. R., J. Pharm. Sci., 51:672 (1962).
182. Garrett, E. R., and Olson, E. C., J. Pharm. Sci., 51:764 (1962).
183. Ingram, J. T., and Lowenthal, W., J. Pharm. Sci., 57:187 (1968).
184. Delonca, H., Puech, A., Youakin, Y., and Segura, G., Pharm. Acta Helv.,
     44:464 (1969).
185. Ridgway, K., and Williams, I. E., J. Pharm. Pharmacol., 29:57P (1977).
186. Ritschel, W. A., Pharm. Ind., 26:757 (1964).
187. Warren, Jr., J. W., and Price, J. C., J. Pharm. Sci., 66:1409 (1977).
188. Caminetsky, S., Can. Med. Assoc. J., 88:950 (1963).
189. Campagna, F. A., Cureton, G., Mirigian, R. A., and Nelson, E.,
     J. Pharm. Sci., 52:605 (1963).
190. Catz, B., Ginsberg, E., and Salenger, S., N. Engl. J. Med., 266:136
     (1962).
191. Engle, G. B., Australas. J. Pharm., 47(Suppl. 39):S22 (1966).
192. Glasko, A. J., Kinkel, A. W., Alegnani, W., and Holmes, E. L., Clin.
     Pharmacol. Ther., 9:472 (1968).
193. Levy, G., Hall, N., and Nelson, E., Am. J. Hosp. Pharm., 21:402 (1964).
194. Lozinski, E., Can. Med. Assoc. J., 83:177 (1960).
195. Searl, R., and Pernarowski, M., Can. Med. Assoc. J., 96:1513 (1967).
196. Wood, J. A., and Harder, S. W., Can. J. Pharm. Sci., 5:18 (1970).
197. Nadkarni, P. D., Kildsig, D. O., Kramer, P. A., and Banker, G. S.,
     J. Pharm. Sci., 64:1554 (1975).
198. Fisher, D. G., and Rowe, R. C., J. Pharm. Pharmacol., 28:886 (1976).
199. Rowe, R. C., J. Pharm. Pharmacol., 29:723 (1977).
200. Rowe, R. C., J. Pharm. Pharmacol., 30:343 (1978).
201. Rowe, R. C., J. Pharm. Pharmacol., 30:669 (1978).
202. Rowe, R. C., J. Pharm. Pharmacol., 31:473 (1979).
203. Hersey, J. A., Manuf. Chem. Aerosol News, 40:32 (1969).
204. Wagner, J. G., Biopharmaceutics and Relevant Pharmacokinetics. Drug
     Intelligence Publications, Hamilton, Ill., 1971, pp. 98-147.
205. Cooper, J., and Rees, J. E., J. Pharm. Sci., 61:1511, 1972.
206. Leeson, L. J., and Carstensen, J. T., eds., Dissolution Technology. In-
     dustrial Pharmaceutical Technology Section, Academy of Pharmaceutical
     Sciences, Washington, D.C., 1974.

207. The United States Pharmacopeia, 20th rev. Mack, Easton, Pa., 1980, pp. 959-960.

208. Cox, D. C., Doyle, C. C., Furman, W. B., Kirchoeffer, R. D., Wyrick, J. W., and Wells, C. C., Pharm. Technol., 2:41 (1978).

209. Swartz, J. B., J. Pharm. Sci., 63:774 (1974).

210. Nogami, H., Fukusawa, H., and Nakai, Y., Chem. Pharm. Bull., 11:1389 (1963).

211. Lowenthal, W., and Burruss, R. A., J. Pharm. Sci., 60:1325 (1971).

212. Rispin, W. T., Selkirk, A. B., and Stones, P. W., J. Pharm. Pharmacol., 23(Suppl.):215S (1971).

213. Matusmaru, H., Yakugaku Zasshi, 78:1198 (1958).

214. Stanley-Wood, N. G., and Johansson, M. E., Drug Dev. Ind. Pharm., 4:69 (1978).

215. Selkirk, A. B., and Ganderton, D., J. Pharm. Pharmacol., 22(Suppl.):79S (1970).

216. Gucluyildiz, H., Banker, G. S., and Peck, G. E., J. Pharm. Sci., 66:407 (1977).

217. Dees, P. J., Jr., Dubois, F. L., Oomen, J. J. J., and Polderman, J., Pharm. Weekbl., 113:1297 (1978).

218. Lowenthal, W., J. Pharm. Sci., 61:303 (1972).

219. Higuchi, T., Arnold, R. D., Tucker, S. J., and Busse, L. W., J. Am. Pharm. Assoc., Sci. Ed., 41:93 (1952).

220. Lowenthal, W., J. Pharm. Sci., 61:1695 (1972).

221. The United States Pharmacopeia, 20th rev. Mack, Easton, Pa., pp. 1035-1037.

222. Turi, P., Brusco, D., Maulding, H. V., Tausendfreund, R. A., and Michaelis, A. F., J. Pharm. Sci., 61:1811 (1972).

223. Drop Test for Shipping Containers, D775, Annual Book of ASTM Standards, Part 20. American Society for Testing and Materials, Philadelphia, 1978, pp. 180-187.

224. Incline Impact Test for Shipping Containers, D880, Annual Book of ASTM Standards, Part 20. American Society for Testing and Materials, Philadelphia, 1978, pp. 229-233.

225. Vibration Testing of Shipping Containers, D999, Annual Book of ASTM Standards, Part 20. American Society for Testing and Materials, Philadelphia, 1978, pp. 282-285.

6

Bioavailability in Tablet Technology

James W. McGinity, Salomon A. Stavchansky, and Alfred Martin

Drug Dynamics Institute
College of Pharmacy
University of Texas at Austin
Austin, Texas

I. General Considerations

Drugs are administered locally for protective action, antisepsis, local anesthetic, and antibiotic effects, and they are given systemically for action on the cells and organs of the body or to counter the effects of invading organisms. Figure 1 depicts the many parts of the body where drugs are absorbed, biotransformed, and eliminated. A number of physiological and chemical factors are important in the absorption, distribution, and elimination of drugs in the body. Some of the properties of the buccal cavity, stomach, and small and large intestines that influence drug therapy are found in Tables 1 and 2.

When drugs are given for systemic action, a number of routes are available, including oral, rectal, parenteral, sublingual, and inhalation. After absorption into the body, a drug is distributed by the blood and lymphatic system and passes into the extracellular fluids of various tissues. The drug molecules may enter cells immediately and exert their pharmacological action in this way or be stored as a reservoir in muscle and fatty tissue for prolonged action. The drug may also be bound to albumin and other components of the plasma, altering tissue distribution and elimination from the body.

Drugs are metabolized by enzyme systems of the body, and this process is given the general term "biotransformation." The net effect may be inactivation or detoxification of the compound, or the drug may be converted from an inactive or prodrug form into the pharmacologically active species. For example, the azo dye Prontosil is reduced in the body to sulfanilamide, and the discovery of this conversion led to the development and use of sulfonamides as medicinal agents. Biotransformation is mainly handled in the liver, but the process also occurs in the kidneys, intestines, muscles, and blood.

Whether biotransformed or not, the drug molecules must finally be eliminated from the body. The kidneys are the principal organs of excretion, but foreign compounds may be eliminated from the lungs or in bile, saliva, and sweat. The

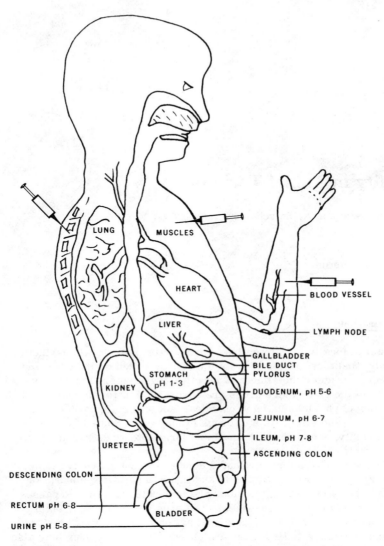

Figure 1. Parts of body involved in absorption, distribution, metabolism, and
elimination of drugs.

kidney (Fig. 2) is composed of millions of units consisting of a filtering capsule or
glomerulus. The liquid, which contains soluble excrement that is filtered through
the glomerulus into the kidney tubules, is referred to as the glomerular filtrate.
The tubules are surrounded by capillaries, and some solute molecules present in
the glomerular filtrate may be reabsorbed and returned to the bloodstream. Molecules of physiological importance, such as glucose, water, chloride, potassium,
and sodium ions, are reabsorbed at various segments of the tubules. Some drugs,

Table 1

Physiological and Chemical Characteristics of Gastrointestinal Fluids in the Gastrointestinal Tract

Factors	Stomach	Small intestine
Properties of fluids[a]		
pH value	1–3	5–8
Volume of fluid available (ml)	50–250	25–125
Surface tension (dyn cm^{-1})	35–50	32–45
Viscosity (cP)	0.8–2.5	0.7–1.2
Buffer capacity[b]		
β (NaOH)	30–60	4–8
β (HCl)	600	8–16
Δt (° C)	0.3–0.8	0.62
Density	1.01	1.01
Water (%)	98	98
Juice secretion (liter day^{-1})	2–4	0.2–0.8
Water circulation (liter day^{-1})	1–5	1.5–5
Enzymes and electrolytes	Variable	Variable

[a] Fasting subjects, temperature 37°C.
[b] = mmol NaOH or HCl/liter × ΔpH × pH (stomach fluid 1.5 ± 0.1).
Source: Modified from Ref. 110.

Table 2

Buccal, Gastric, and Intestinal Fluids

	Daily volume (ml)	pH
Saliva	1200	6.0–7.0
Gastric secretion	2000	1.0–3.5
Pancreatic secretion	1200	8.0–8.3
Bile	700	7.8
Succus entericus	2000	7.8–8.0
Brunner's gland secretion	50	8.0–8.9
Larger intestinal secretion	60	7.5–8.0

Source: Modified from Ref. 110.

KIDNEY

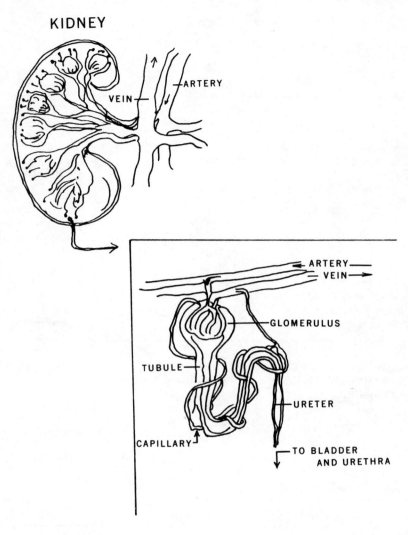

Figure 2. Schematic diagram of kidney. A glomerulus and associated structure are enlarged and shown in the insert.

such as penicillin G, do not pass through the glomerular apparatus but rather are actively transported from capillaries directly to the tubules where they are excreted in the urine. Thus, owing to pH, active transport mechanisms, solubility, and ionic characteristics, drug molecules may be eliminated in the glomerular filtrate or directly absorbed into the tubules and excreted, and may be reabsorbed from the tubules into the systemic circulation for recycling through the body. The

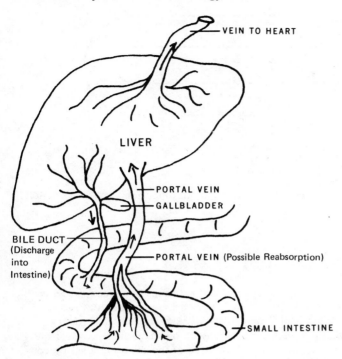

Figure 3. Liver, portal vein, gallbladder, and bile duct in relation to small intestine.

excretion of weakly acidic and basic drugs is influenced by the pH of the urine, and elimination of these compounds may be altered by controlling urinary pH. Alkalinizing the urine results in reabsorption of quinidine and may result in sufficiently high plasma levels of the drug as to manifest toxicity.

Biliary excretion has been found to be an important elimination route for some drugs (see Fig. 3). The drug present in the bile is discharged into the intestines and may be eliminated in the feces or into the vascular system from a region lower in the intestinal tract. Thus, as in kidney excretion, biliary passage may involve a cycle of elimination and reabsorption. This process, which occurs with morphine, penicillins, and a number of dyes, is called enterohepatic circulation; the process tends to promote higher and prolonged concentrations of the drug and its metabolites in the body than would be expected were the recycling process not involved. However, repeated passage through the liver may lead to significant metabolism of the drug. The reader should refer to first pass effect described in Section I.G.

The processes of diffusion and the partitioning of drug molecules across membranes as a function of pH, pK_a, and other factors will be discussed in later sections of this chapter.

The kinetics of absorption, distribution, and excretion of drugs following administration was first set forth by Teorell [1] in 1937 (Fig. 4).

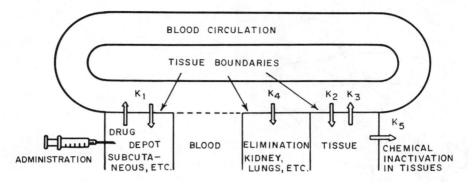

Figure 4. Schematic description of drug absorption, distribution, and elimination. (After Ref. 1.)

A. Biopharmaceutics and Pharmacokinetics

A drug administered as a tablet or another dosage form must be released and reach its site of action in an active state before it can exert a pharmacological response. The physical chemical properties of the drug, the characteristics of the dosage form in which the drug is administered, and the physiological factors controlling absorption, distribution, metabolism, and elimination of the drug must all be considered in order to formulate and manufacture effective and safe therapeutic agents. This wide range of considerations comprise the subject called biopharmaceutics.

Pharmacokinetics is a branch of biopharmaceutics and encompasses in a quantitative way the kinetics of absorption, distribution, metabolism, and excretion, often called ADME, of therapeutic agents and related chemical substances. The time course of passage of intact drugs and metabolites in various body tissues and fluids and the models constructed to interpret these data, which comprise the subjects of pharmacokinetics, will be introduced as elementary mathematical expressions and graphs of data early in the chapter and elaborated upon in later sections. The final part of the chapter considers the elements of pharmacokinetics in some detail. The subject is presented step by step with worked examples, so that a reader with a background in pharmacy, chemistry, or biology but minimal grounding in mathematics can follow the treatment with relative ease.

At the beginning it is well to define some of the terms to be used throughout the chapter, particularly the words biopharmaceutics, pharmacokinetics, and bioequivalency. Some of the terms, as defined in the 1977 Bioequivalence Requirements and In Vitro Bioavailability Procedures of the FDA [2], are found in Table 3.

B. Bioequivalence

The forces that have led in the last decade to the concept of bioavailability were principally those due to the generic equivalence (bioequivalence) issue. Specifically, it is of the utmost importance to be assured that chemically equivalent drug products from different manufacturers result in essentially the same degree of therapeutic action.

Table 3

Definition of Terms Dealing with Bioavailability and Bioequivalence

Drug	Active therapeutic moiety.
Drug product	Delivery system, tablet, capsule, suspension (e.g., containing the therapeutic moiety), generally but not necessarily in association with inactive ingredients.
Bioavailability	The rate and extent to which the active drug ingredient or therapeutic moiety is absorbed from a drug product and becomes available at the site of action.
Bioequivalent drug products	Pharmaceutical equivalents or alternatives whose rate and extent of absorption are not significantly different when administered to humans at the same molar dose under similar conditions.
Pharmaceutical equivalents	Drug products identical in amount of active drug ingredient and dosage form, and meeting compendial or other standards for identity, strength, quality, and purity. They may not be identical in terms of inactive ingredients. An example is erythromycin stearate tablets (Brand X and Brand Y).
Pharmaceutical alternatives	Drug products that contain the identical therapeutic moiety or its precursor but not necessarily in the same amount or dosage form and not necessarily as the same salt or ester. Examples are erythromycin stearate versus erythromycin ester; chlorpheniramine maleate chewable tablets versus chlorpheniramine maleate capsules.
Bioequivalence requirements	A requirement imposed by the FDA for in vitro and/or in vivo testing of specified drug products which must be satisfied as a condition of marketing.

An examination of the definitions as outlined in Table 3 above shows that emphasis has been placed on the ability of two or more drug products to produce essentially identical blood levels in the same individual. The dosage form is a drug delivery system; it can be a good one or a poor one in its role of releasing the drug efficiently for absorption into the systemic circulation or site of action. Thus, appropriate testing of generic products must be conducted. These tests are not done only through clinical trials of efficacy since it is ordinarily not

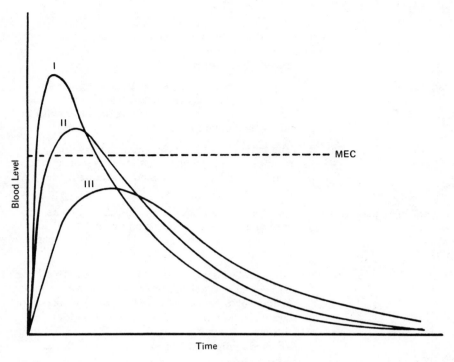

Figure 5. Blood levels from three products, illustrating differences in the rate of absorption but not in the total amount of drug absorbed.

the drug that is in question but the dosage form; the latter primarily influencing the absorption step. It is the absorption process or factors connected with the delivery system that must be studied to assure proper bioavailability of the drug and bioequivalence of products from one manufacturer to another and from batch to batch.

A number of studies of marketed drug products containing the same chemical ingredient have revealed differences in bioavailability. Examples of problems with chemically equivalent drug products include tetracycline [3, 4], chloramphenicol [5], digoxin [6, 7], phenylbutazone [8, 9], and oxytetracycline [10, 11]. In addition, variations in bioavailability of different batches of digoxin from the same company have been demonstrated [7]. In one report, a thyroid preparation that met compendial standards was found to be therapeutically inactive [12]. Since lack of bioequivalence in these examples involves marketed products, it can be concluded that neither standards for testing the finished product nor specifications for materials, manufacturing processes, and controls are presently adequate to ensure that drug products are bioequivalent. Good Laboratory Practice and Good Manufacturing Practice regulations promulgated by the U.S. Food and Drug Administration (FDA) will assist in correcting the problem, but specific actions regarding bioavailability must be taken to assure equivalent marketed products. In most instances it is concluded that therapeutic inequivalence is a result of variations in the bioavailability of drug products.

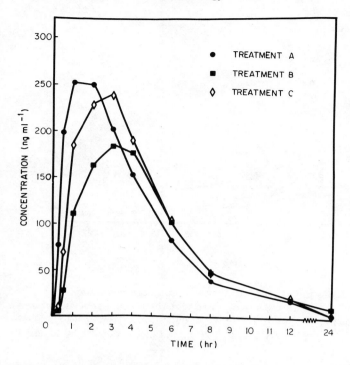

Figure 6. Average plasma levels of prednisone in nine adult volunteers following oral administration of 10 mg of prednisone (as two 5-mg tablets). (From Ref. 13.)

C. Relative Bioavailability and Drug Performance

If a drug is administered at a dosage level that does not greatly exceed the minimum effective blood concentration (MEC) required, the availability of the drug from the dosage form may greatly influence the drug's performance. Figure 5 schematically illustrates this case. In curve I the product formulation causes the drug to have a good therapeutic response. In curve II, because of a delayed rate of absorption, the effective response is more transient. The slow absorption process of curve III leads to a lack of pharmacological response, even though the amount absorbed as determined by the total area under the curve is equal to the other two. This example illustrates that although the amount of drug absorbed may not differ, the rate of absorption of three products may be quite different, leading to variations in therapeutic action. A real example is presented in Figure 6, illustrating the work by Sullivan et al. [13]. It shows average plasma levels of prednisone obtained in nine adult volunteers in a three-way crossover study when a 10-mg dose of prednisone was administered as two 5-mg tablets made by three different manufacturers. Treatment A gave the fastest absorption and highest plasma levels. Treatments B and C were two generic prednisone tablets that had a history of clinical failure and did not pass the USP tablet dissolution test. Treatment A passed all compendial tests in the laboratories of the FDA. In this case the rate of

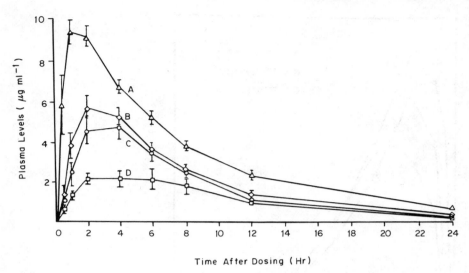

Figure 7. Mean plasma levels for groups of 10 human subjects receiving single
0.5-g oral doses of chloramphenicol capsules. Vertical lines represent one standard error on either side of the mean. Capsule A, Δ; capsule B, ◇; capsule C, O;
capsule D, □. (From Ref. 5; reproduced with permission of the copyright owner.)

appearance of prednisone in plasma was different for the three tablets, although
the average areas under the plasma concentration-time curves of individual subjects did not differ significantly. This is a case in which documented evidence of
clinical failure with generic tablets can be related to differences in rates of absorption.

    Figure 7 illustrates the results obtained by Glazko et al. [5] when testing four
capsules of chloramphenicol in human subjects. Here the principal difference, as
indicated by the area under the curve, is that the four products differ in the total
amount of chloramphenicol absorbed. Product A gave an excellent blood level
curve in subjects, whereas the other three formulations gave poor plasma levels.
Because of these data, the FDA had products B, C, and D recalled and reformulated, and then instituted requirements that have brought the problem of chloramphenicol products under control. The significance of this finding is that all the
products were chemically equivalent. That is, they contained the correct amount
of chloramphenicol, and the particle size of the drug in each of the products was
similar. Figure 8 illustrates the results obtained by Aguiar, showing that the disintegration rates of the four products differed greatly [14]. Product A, the one
that produced the highest plasma level in the study of Glazko, had excellent disintegration characteristics, whereas products B and C showed poor rates, and
product D, the product having the poorest plasma level in patients, exhibited the
poorest disintegration rate. In fact, product D had such poor disintegration properties that the powder mass maintained its capsule shape in simulated gastric
fluid after the gelatin capsule had dissolved. The results in Figure 9 demonstrate
the performance of the four products in a dissolution rate test. When product A

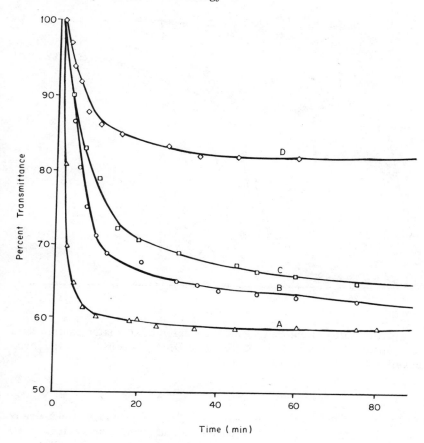

Figure 8. Relative disintegration rates of chloramphenicol capsules in simulated gastric fluid. Capsule A, Δ; capsule B, O, capsule C, □, capsule D, ◇. (From Ref. 14; reproduced with permission of the copyright owner.)

was placed in simulated gastric fluid, it dissolved rapidly, whereas products B, C, And D showed greater lag times prior to dissolution, principally because of the time required for deaggregation [14].

Dissolution tests and disintegration tests in some cases have been shown to correlate well with human bioavailability tests, as evidenced by the previous example. Lindenbaum's work on digoxin is another example of in vivo/in vitro correlations [7].

The FDA, in its bioequivalence preamble, stated [2]:

Advances in pharmaceutical technology have made bioequivalence a most precise and reproducible method for determining drug product variability. These bioequivalence techniques are not inadequately defined or reachless concepts. They are scientifically valid methods of comparing different drug products as well as different batches of the same drug products.

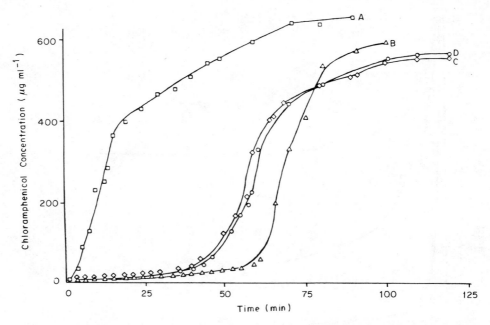

Figure 9. Dissolution rates of chloramphenicol capsules in simulated gastric fluid. Capsule A, □, capsule B, Δ; capsule C, ◇, capsule D, O. (From Ref. 14; reproduced with permission of the copyright owner.)

It is indeed fortunate that dissolution methodology frequently provides a measure of variability among drug dosage forms. The conclusion that can be drawn from the bioequivalence requirements and in vivo bioavailability procedures of the FDA, published in the Federal Register of January 1977, is that dissolution testing will more than likely become the most frequently used means of testing and assuring bioequivalence [2]. Although it will probably not be the only criterion for obtaining marketing approval, the FDA report states that "a dissolution test may constitute a proper element in reaching the decision to approve an NDA or supplemental application for a drug product with a bioequivalence problem." In another section of this chapter we discuss some of the methodology presently available for dissolution testing.

The digoxin tablet problem is an example of a situation that led to establishment by the FDA of a dissolution rate certification requirement and adoption of a dissolution specification by the USP. Digoxin is a drug in which the effective blood level is close to the toxic concentration. Product formulation may greatly influence the rate and extent of absorption, and consequently the therapeutic activity and toxicity of digoxin.

D. Federal Regulations Covering Bioavailability and Bioequivalence

In the Federal Register of January 1973 [15], the FDA published proposed bioavailability requirements for new drugs and for generic drug products. These proposals become regulations as published in the Federal Register of January 1977

[2], with appropriate modifications as suggested by various individuals and groups. The regulations clearly establish that studies must be undertaken with new drugs or new dosage forms to assure that optimal absorption characteristics are achieved.

The selection of the reference material (standard drug sample) as stated by the FDA is an important consideration. It depends upon the scientific questions to be answered, the data needed to establish comparability with a currently marketed drug product, and the data needed to establish dosage regimens. The reference material should be taken from a current batch of a drug product that is the subject of an approved new drug application and that contains the same active drug ingredient or therapeutic moiety. Thus, tetracycline hydrochloride cannot be the reference product for tetracycline phosphate; salts cannot be compared against esters; capsules cannot be compared with tablets.

In the report of the Office of Technology Assessment (OTA), Drug Bioequivalence Study Panel [16], it was concluded that studies on bioavailability are neither feasible nor desirable for all drugs or drug products. According to OTA, certain classes of drug should be identified for which evidence of bioequivalence is critical. Selection of these classes would be based on clinical importance, ratio of therapeutic to toxic concentration in blood, and certain pharmaceutical characteristics. The panel believed, however, that bioavailability studies should be required for products if the active ingredient in the product had not yet been introduced into the market.

A large number of drug products are available on the market, and for only a few of these are there adequate data documenting bioavailability in humans. Thus, many bioavailability studies would be required; this involves large numbers of human volunteers and the expense of clinical investigators and other scientific personnel. Consequently, it is not feasible and justifiable to carry out studies of bioavailability in humans for all drug products. In asserting that studies of bioavailability will not be required for all drug products, it becomes important to set general criteria to guide the selection of those products whose bioavailability should be documented by testing in humans, those requiring no testing, and those few in which in vitro methodology would be deemed adequate. The report of the OTA study panel concluded that for drugs with a wide therapeutic range, moderate differences in drug blood levels, owing to differences in bioavailability of chemically equivalent products, would be tolerated. Conversely, drugs that have a relatively narrow therapeutic range would be candidates for testing of bioavailability on human subjects. Examples of drugs that fall into this category include cardioactive agents (digitalis glycosides), anticonvulsants (diphenylhydantoin), some corticosteroids, and certain antibiotics (chloramphenicol and cephalosporins). In summary, drug products will be considered candidates for human bioavailability studies if they:

are used for treatment or prevention of serious illness;
have steep dose-response curves or unfavorable therapeutic indices;
contain active ingredients that are relatively insoluble or are converted to insoluble forms in the gastrointestinal fluids.

In the Federal Register of January 1977, the FDA [2] published criteria for waiver of evidence of bioavailability. The requirement for the submission of in vivo bioavailability data will be waived if:

1. The drug product meets both of the following conditions:
   a. It is a solution intended solely for intravenous administration.

    b.   It contains an active drug ingredient or therapeutic moiety in the same solvent and concentration as an intravenous solution that is the subject of an approved full new drug application.

2.   The drug product is a topically applied preparation (e.g., a cream, ointment, or gel) intended for local therapeutic effect.

3.   The drug product is an oral dosage form that is not intended to be absorbed (e.g., an antacid or a radiopaque medium).

4.   The drug product meets both of the following conditions:

    a.   It is an oral solution, elixir, syrup, tincture, or similar other solubilized form.

    b.   It contains an active drug ingredient or therapeutic moiety in the same concentration as a drug product that is the subject of an approved full new drug application.

    c.   It contains no inactive ingredient that is known to significantly affect absorption of the active drug ingredient or therapeutic moiety.

The regulations proceed to list drugs for which in vivo bioavailability data of solid oral dosage forms need not be submitted to the FDA.

For certain drug products, bioavailability may be demonstrated by evidence obtained in vitro in lieu of in vivo data. The FDA waives the requirements for the submission of evidence obtained in vivo demonstrating the bioavailability of the drug product if the drug product meets one of the following criteria:

1.   The drug product is subjected to the bioequivalence requirement established by the Food and Drug Administration under Subpart C of this part that specifies only an in vitro testing requirement.

2.   The drug product is in the same dosage form, but in a different strength, and is proportionally similar in its active and inactive ingredients to another drug product made by the same manufacturer and the following conditions are met:

    a.   The bioavailability of this other drug product has been demonstrated.

    b.   Both drug products meet an appropriate in vitro test approved by the Food and Drug Administration.

    c.   The applicant submits evidence showing that both drug products are proportionally similar in their active and inactive ingredients.

3.   The drug product is, on the basis of scientific evidence submitted in the application, shown to meet an in vitro test that assures bioavailability (i.e., an in vitro test that has been correlated with in vivo data).

4.   The drug product is a reformulated product that is identical, except for color, flavor, or preservative, to another drug product made by the same manufacturer and both of the following conditions are met:

    a.   The bioavailability of the other product has been demonstrated.

    b.   Both drug products meet an appropriate in vitro test approved by the Food and Drug Administration.

5.   The drug product contains the same active drug ingredient or therapeutic moiety and is in the same strength and dosage form as a drug product that is the subject of an approved full or abbreviated new drug application, and both drug products meet an appropriate in vitro test that has been approved by the Food and Drug Administration.

The FDA, for good cause, may defer or waive a requirement for the submission of evidence of in vivo bioavailability if deferral or waiver is compatible with the protection of the public health.

E. In Vitro Indexes of Bioavailability

In view of these regulations, additional research aimed at improving the assessment and prediction of bioequivalence is needed. It is important that this research include efforts to develop in vitro tests that will be valid predictors of bioavailability in humans. If in vitro dissolution properties for a drug are found to serve as a useful index of in vivo absorption, the time, expense, and difficulties of clinical studies may be reduced or eliminated. Levy et al. [17] and Wagner [18] have shown in several cases that correlations exist between in vitro testing and in vivo absorption.

In vitro dissolution rate screening has been used [19] as a sensitive quality control measure to show changes in drug release for products undergoing variable storage conditions. It is also used to warn of poor bioavailability of drugs from dosage forms that show erratic release patterns in comparative studies.

An early investigation by Nelson [20] demonstrated a correlation between in vitro dissolution rate and the speed at which tetracycline in four different dosage forms was excreted in vivo. Levy [21] showed a linear correlation between salicylate excretion following oral administration of two aspirin tablets and rate of in vitro dissolution. Levy went on to demonstrate a correlation between percent of drug absorbed and rate of dissolution. MacDonald et al. [22] found differences in in vivo availability among tetracycline capsules from various sources and attempted to correlate these differences by an in vitro method using an automated dissolution apparatus. The authors reported that they were partially successful in their goal. Bergan et al. [23] determined the in vitro dissolution rates of two tetracycline and seven oxytetracycline preparations and compared them with absorption characteristics as obtained by a crossover study on 10 volunteers. The products showed marked variations in bioavailability. The rate of dissolution was found to correlate well with absorption characteristics for some products but not for others.

Other workers [24, 25] have found good correlation between dissolution rate and drug plasma levels. However, correlations cannot always be expected between in vivo and in vitro results. The failure of good correlation is the result of a number of factors, including improper in vitro stirring rate, variable gastric emptying time, rapid versus slow absorbers, failure of dissolution to be the rate-limiting step in vivo, and other problems.

F. Methodology for Conducting Bioavailability Studies

In 1972, the Academy of Pharmaceutical Sciences [26] published Guidelines for Biopharmaceutical Studies in Man. This monograph presents a systematic approach to the conduct of bioavailability studies based on analytical determination of drug in blood and/or urine.

In January 1977, the FDA [2] published in the <u>Federal Register</u> the Characteristics of good analytical methodology for an in vivo bioavailability study. They stated that the method for

metabolite(s), in body fluids or excretory products, or the method used to measure an acute pharmacological effect shall be demonstrated to be accurate and of sufficient sensitivity to measure, with appropriate precision, the actual concentration of the active drug ingredient or therapeutic moiety, or its metabolite(s), achieved in the body.

In addition, when the analytical method is not sensitive enough to measure accurately the concentration of the active drug ingredient or therapeutic moiety, or its "metabolite(s), in body fluids or excretory products produced by a single dose of the test product, two or more single doses may be given together to produce higher concentration."

It is interesting that the regulations were not more specific in their analytical requirements. For example, no distinction is made between chemical, radioactive, microbiological, and other methods. Radioactive methods are used extensively today in drug development, and the investigators must be careful to verify that the measured radioactivity is contained in the intact compound separated from its metabolites. It is also important to recognize that the dosage form containing the radioactive drug to be tested possess physical and chemical properties identical to those of the unlabeled dosage form.

The 1977 monograph of the FDA [2] listed the following general approaches for determining bioavailability:

1. Bioavailability is usually determined by measurement of:
   a. The concentration of the active drug ingredient or therapeutic moiety, or its metabolite(s), in biological fluids as a function of time; or
   b. The urinary excretion of the therapeutic moiety or its metabolite(s) as a function of time; or
   c. An appropriate acute pharmacological effect.
2. Bioavailability may be determined by several direct or indirect in vivo methods, generally involving testing in humans. The selection of the method depends upon the purpose of the study, the analytical method available, and the nature of the drug product. These limitations affect the degree to which precise pharmacokinetic studies can be applied and, in some cases, necessitate the use of other methods. Bioavailability testing shall be conducted using the most accurate, sensitive, and reproducible approach available among those set forth in paragraph (c) of this section.
3. The following in vivo approaches, in descending order of accuracy, sensitivity, and reproducibility, are acceptable for determining the bioavailability of a drug product:
   a. In vivo testing in humans in which the concentration of the active drug ingredient or therapeutic moiety or its metabolite(s), in whole blood, plasma, serum, or other appropriate biological fluid is measured as a function of time, or in which the urinary excretion of the therapeutic moiety, or its metabolite(s), is measured as a function of time. This approach is particularly applicable to dosage forms intended to deliver

the active drug ingredient or therapeutic moiety to the bloodstream for systemic distribution within the body (i.e., injectable drugs, most oral dosage forms, most suppositories, certain drugs administered by inhalation, and some drugs administered by local application to mucous membranes).

b. In vivo testing in humans in which an appropriate acute pharmacological effect of the active drug ingredient or therapeutic moiety, or metabolite(s), is measured as a function of time if such effect can be measured with sufficient accuracy, sensitivity, and reproducibility. This approach is applicable when appropriate methods are not available for measurement of the concentration of the active drug ingredient or therapeutic moiety, or its metabolite(s), in biological fluids or excretory products but a method is available for the measurement of an appropriate acute pharmacological effect. This approach is applicable to the same dosage forms listed in paragraph (3, a) of this section.

c. Well-controlled clinical trials in humans that establish the safety and effectiveness of the drug product. This approach is the least accurate, sensitive, and reproducible of the general approaches for determining in vivo bioavailability in humans. For dosage forms intended to deliver the active drug ingredient or therapeutic moiety to the bloodstream for systemic distribution within the body, this approach shall be considered as providing a sufficiently accurate estimate of in vivo bioavailability only when analytical methods are not available to permit use of one of the approaches outlined in paragraph (3, a and b) of this section. This approach shall also be considered as sufficiently accurate for determining the bioavailability of dosage forms intended to deliver the therapeutic moiety locally (e.g., topical preparations for the skin, eye, ear, mucous membranes); oral dosage forms not intended to be absorbed (e.g., an antacid or a radiopaque medium); and bronchodilators administered by inhalation if the onset and duration of pharmacological activity are defined.

d. Any other in vivo approach approved by the Food and Drug Administration intended for special situations should include those circumstances where the in vivo bioavailability of a drug product might be determined in a suitable animal model rather than in humans or by using a radioactive or nonradioactive isotopically labeled drug product.

When a drug dosage form is administered to humans and/or animals and serial blood samples are obtained and quantified for drug content, data are obtained as a function of time. This enables one to graphically represent the results as illustrated in Figure 10. The curve can be mathematically analyzed and pharmacokinetic parameters obtained as discussed in Section IV. However, it should be noted that there are three important parameters necessary for the interpretation of bioavailability studies. These include the peak height concentration, the time of the peak concentration, and the area under the plasma concentration–time curve. The peak height is important because it gives an indication of the intensity, and in conjunction with the minimum effective concentration (MEC), provides an indication of duration of action. The time for the peak to occur is important because it is related to the rate of absorption of the drug from dosage form after oral

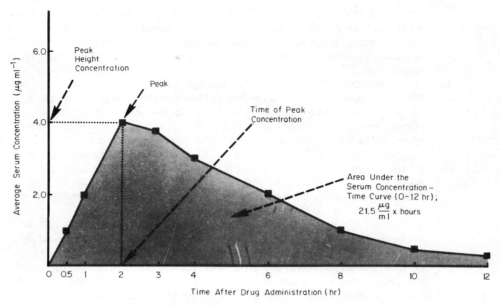

Figure 10. Serum concentration-time curve following a single dose of a drug that shows an absorption phase and an elimination phase. (From Ref. 30; reproduced with permission of the copyright owner.)

administration. It should only be considered as a simple measurement of rate of absorption. The area under the curve is perhaps one of the most important parameters. It represents, in this case, the amount of drug absorbed following a single administration of the drug.

Several integration techniques may be used to determine the area under the curve, and the accuracy of the value obtained will vary depending on the integration technique selected. The following integration methods (in decreasing order of accuracy) have been employed [27]:

1. Milne fifth-order predictor-corrector
2. Runge-Kutta fourth order
3. Adams second order
4. Simpson's rule
5. Trapezoidal rule
6. Rectangular rule

The trapezoid rule has gained popularity, although it is not the most accurate method. It is described in a later section, where the trapezoidal rule is used in a sample calculation.

Let us assume that a bioavailability study is conducted with the purpose of comparing two different formulations containing the same therapeutic moiety. The results of these studies are graphically illustrated in Figure 11. It can be seen that disparities exist between both formulations in regard to peak height

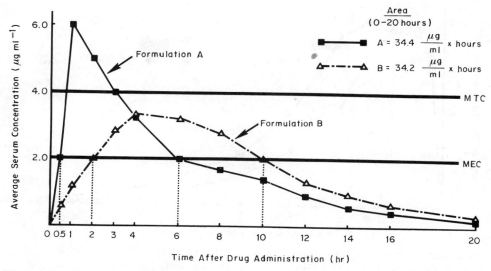

Figure 11. Serum concentration-time curves obtained for two different formulations of the same drug given at the same dose. The relationship of the curves to the minimum toxic concentration (MTC) and minimum effective concentration (MEC) is shown. (From Ref. 30; reproduced with permission of the copyright owner.)

concentration and time to peak. The area under the concentration-time curve for each formulation is the same, indicating that the extent (amount) of drug absorption is the same for both formulations. However, since disparities exist with regard to peak height and time to peak, these formulations cannot be considered to be bioequivalent. Consequently, they may not perform equivalently in terms of efficacy and toxicity. It should be emphasized that differences between formulations are reflected in rate of absorption and not in extent of absorption. Figure 12 illustrates an example in which the rate of absorption is the same for both formulations, as observed by the same time to peak and peak concentration, but the extent of drug absorption as reflected by the areas under the respective concentration curves is different. In neither of the cases can the formulations be considered bioequivalent; these are clear examples of inequivalence in bioavailability. Wagner [28] summarized the different types of comparative bioavailability studies.

Figures 13 to 15 depict methods of estimating bioavailability based on studies in humans where blood levels, urinary excretion, or acute pharmacological response are measured. The methods can be classified depending on the measurement that is made: Figure 13 considers measurement of unchanged drug, Figure 14 a metabolite of a drug, and Figure 15, the total drug, that is, metabolite(s) plus unchanged drug. The symbol τ represents the dosing interval.

The quantitative aspects of biopharmaceutics and pharmacokinetics and associated methods are presented in later sections of the chapter. But before we can study the absorption kinetics of a drug, we should become familiar with the preparation of protocols for comparative bioavailability testing, and then examine various factors, both physiological and physical chemical, which influence the release of a drug from its dosage form and absorption into the systemic circulation.

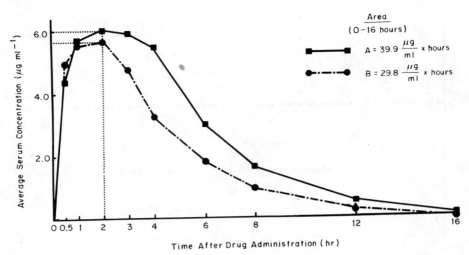

Figure 12. Serum concentration-time curves obtained for two formulations of the same drug given at the same dose, showing similar peak heights and times, but significantly different areas under the curve. (From Ref. 30; reproduced with permission of the copyright owner.)

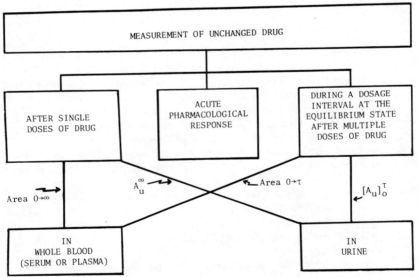

Figure 13. Measurement of unchanged drug for the estimation of bioavailability. (From Ref. 28.)

Area $0 \to \infty$ = area under concentration curve from zero to infinite time.

Area $0 \to \tau$ = area under concentration curve within a dosage interval τ.

A_μ^∞ = amount of unchanged drug excreted in the urine in infinite time after a single dose.

$[A_\mu]_o^\tau$ = amount of unchanged drug excreted in the urine during a dosage interval τ. (From Ref. 28 and reproduced with the permission of the copyright owner.)

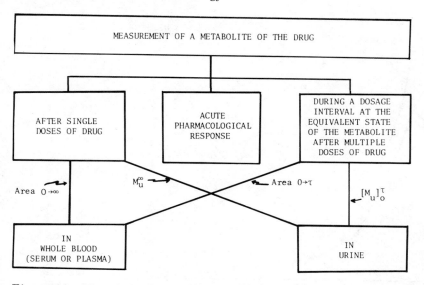

Figure 14. Measurement of a drug metabolite for the estimation of bioavailability. M_{μ}^{∞} = the amount of a metabolite excreted in the urine in infinite time. $[M_{\mu}]_{0}^{\tau}$ = the amount of metabolite excreted in the urine in a dosage interval τ. (From Ref. 28 and reproduced with permission of the copyright owner.)

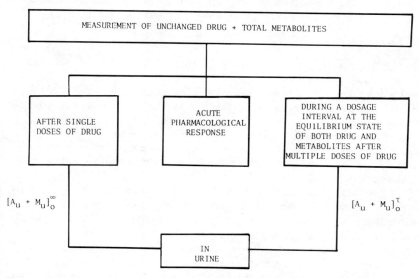

Figure 15. Measurement of unchanged drug and total metabolites for the estimation of bioavailability.
$[A_{\mu} + M_{\mu}]_{0}^{\infty}$ = total amount of unchanged drug and all metabolites excreted in the urine in infinite time.
$[A_{\mu} + M_{\mu}]_{0}^{\tau}$ = total amount of unchanged drug and all metabolites excreted in the urine during a dosage interval τ.
(From Ref. 28 and reproduced with the permission of the copyright owner.)

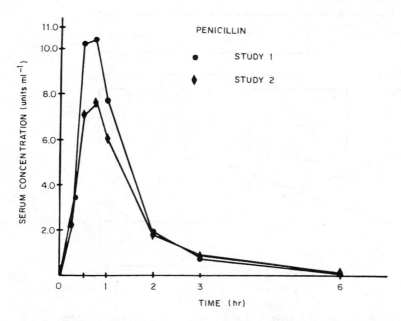

Figure 16. Average serum concentrations obtained after a single oral 500-mg dose of penicillin using the same lot of penicillin tablets in two different subject populations. (From Ref. 30; reproduced with permission of the copyright owner.)

G. Protocols for Comparative Bioavailability Trials

The success of any experiment lies in its design. For this reason, protocols for bioavailability studies are of extreme importance. At the 13th Annual International Industrial Pharmacy Conference at Lakeway, Texas, Skelly [29] discussed the elements of a good protocol. His intent was to make it easier for the FDA and the applicant to recognize and resolve differences of opinion before a study got under way rather than after, in order to expedite the review of drugs where bioavailability is a critical requirement for approval.

The protocol guidelines for ANDA and NDA submissions as suggested by Skelly [29] include information on the drug and its clinical use; clinical facilities to be used and investigators responsible for the study; a plan of experimentation including reference to subjects involved; drugs to be administered; the treatment plan; sample collection; chemical, pharmacological, and/or clinical end points; assay methodology; and data analysis. Appendices to the protocol should include the consent form, precautions for the subject regarding possible adverse reactions, subject instruction sheet, clinical chemistry form, and an insert describing the characteristics of the drug. The reader should refer to the original paper [29] for a detailed outline of the proposed protocol.

H. Common Pitfalls in Evaluating Bioavailability Data

Dittert and DiSanto [30] have discussed common pitfalls in evaluating bioavailability data. They indicated that perhaps the single most common error made in

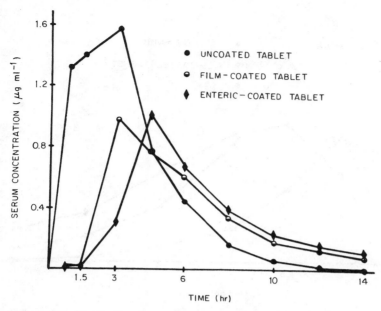

Figure 17. Serum level-time profiles of an acid-labile antibiotic administered in equal doses but as three different tablet dosage forms. The single oral dose consisted of two 250-mg tablets. Results are for 21 normal adults who fasted overnight. (From Ref. 30; reproduced with permission of the copyright owner.)

interpreting bioavailability data is that of "cross-study comparison." This occurs when the blood concentration-time curve of a drug product in one study is compared with the blood-concentration-time curve of that drug product in another study. They stated three reasons why such cross-study comparisons are dangerous and can lead to false conclusions. The following examples used to illustrate the three points are taken from actual bioavailability data.

1. <u>Different Subject Populations</u>: Figure 16 shows serum concentration-time curves for the same lot of penicillin tablets in two subject populations. Both studies were performed with the same protocol. Study 1 was done with hospital employees, while study 2 was done with prison volunteers. There is approximately a 25% difference in both peak concentration and area (0 to 6 hr) under the serum concentration-time curve. This apparent difference in the bioavailability of the same lot of tablets conducted with identical protocols and assayed by the same technique can be attributed to the different subjects used in these studies.

2. <u>Different Study Conditions</u>: Parameters such as the food intake of the subjects before and after drug administration can have dramatic effects on the absorption of certain drugs. Figure 17 shows the results of a three-way crossover test where the subjects were fasted 12 hr overnight and 2 hr after drug administration of (a) an uncoated tablet, (b) a film-coated tablet, and (c) an enteric-coated tablet of an acid-labile antibiotic. The results of this study suggest that the unprotected tablet is superior to both the film-coated and enteric-coated tablet in terms of blood level performance. These results also suggest that neither film coating nor

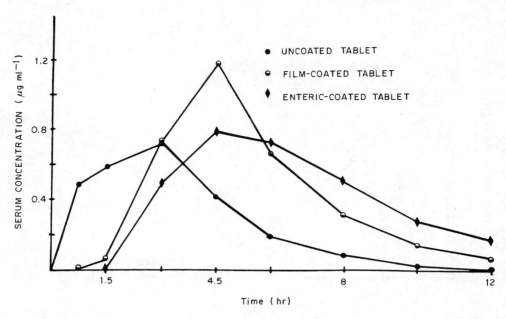

Figure 18. Serum level-time profiles of an acid-labile antibiotic administered in equal doses but as three different tablet dosage forms. The single oral dose consisted of two 250-mg tablets. Results are for 12 normal adults with only a 2-hr preadministration fast. (From Ref. 30; reproduced with permission of the copyright owner.)

enteric coating is necessary for optimal blood level performance. Figure 18 shows results with the same tablets when the study conditions were changed to only a 2-hr preadministration fast with 2 hr of fasting postadministration. In this case, the blood levels of the uncoated tablet were markedly depressed, whereas the film-coated and enteric-coated tablets showed relatively little difference in blood levels. From this second study, it might be concluded that film coating appears to impart the same degree of acid stability as does an enteric coating. This might be acceptable if only one dose of the antibiotic were required. However, Figure 19 shows the results of a multiple-dose study in which the enteric-coated tablet and the film-coated tablet were administered four times a day immediately after meals. The results show that the film coating indeed does not impart the degree of acid stability that the enteric coating does when the tablets are administered immediately after food in a typical clinical situation.

3. Different Assay Methodology: Depending on the drug under study, more than one assay method may be available. For example, some steroids can be assayed by a radioimmunoassay, competitive protein binding, gas-liquid chromatography, or indirectly by a 17-hydroxycorticosteroid assay. Figure 20 shows the results of a comparison of steroid tablets using a competitive protein binding method and a radioimmunoassay, respectively. Obviously, the wrong conclusion would have

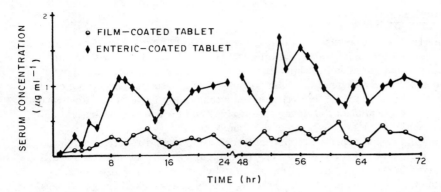

Figure 19. Average serum level-time curves for an acid-labile antibiotic administered in two different tablet dosage forms. In each case the oral tablets were tested in 24 normal adults each of whom received the medication q.i.d., with meals and at bedtime. (From Ref. 30; reproduced with permission of the copyright owner.)

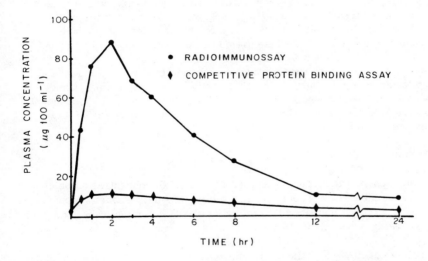

Figure 20. Average plasma level curves for a steroid administered as single oral doses to 24 normal adults. In one case plasma levels were determined by a competitive protein binding assay and in the other case by a radioimmunoassay. (From Ref. 30; reproduced with permission of the copyright owner.)

been reached if one product had been assayed by one method and the other product by the second method and the results had been compared. Even in cases where only one assay method is employed, there are numerous modifications with respect to technique among laboratories which could make direct comparisons hazardous.

II. Drug Absorption

A drug must transverse several biological membranes before it reaches its site of action irrespective of the route of administration. In the oral cavity there are two regions, buccal and sublingual, where the membranes are very thin and have a copious blood supply. Sublingual administration of a drug entails the placing of the drug in its dosage form (e.g., tablet) under the tongue for its ultimate absorption into the systemic circulation. Buccal administration of a drug is ordinarily accomplished by placing the drug between the cheek and the gums.

Drugs administered orally, and probably rectally, pass directly through the liver on their circulation through the body (see Figure 3). If the drug is readily biotransformed in the liver, this initial passage by way of the hepatic route can result in considerable metabolism of the drug before it arrives at the peripheral circulation. This loss of drug on first passage through the liver is called the first pass effect. Drugs given by intravenous, intramuscular, subcutaneous, sublingual, and buccal administration, on the other hand, enter the circulation directly and are carried to body tissues before passage through the liver, where they might be broken down. Sublingual and buccal tablets are therefore ideal for potent, low-dose drugs.

Venous drainage from the oral cavity goes directly to the heart, which makes it an excellent route for treating angina with nitroglycerin. On the other hand, toxic drugs such as nicotine also pass directly to the heart without any chance of detoxication. Once widely used as an insecticide, nicotine produced an environmental hazard because of its great toxicity.

The transport or passage of drugs across membranes in various parts of the body depends to a large degree on the selectivity and characteristics of the membrane. Pore size, membrane composition, and the presence of energy-dependent carriers may all affect drug absorption; however, most drugs pass across biological membranes by simple or passive diffusion.

A. Passive Membrane Diffusion

Passive diffusion happens when drug molecules exist in high concentration on one side of a membrane and lower concentration on the other side. Diffusion occurs in an effort to equalize drug concentration on both sides of the membrane, the rate of transport being proportional to the concentration gradient across the membrane.

When the volume of fluids are fixed, the movement of drug across a membrane can be described in terms of Fick's laws. Fick's first law states that the rate of diffusion or transport across a membrane is directly proportional to the surface area of the membrane and to the concentration gradient, and is inversely proportional to the thickness of the membrane. The expression for Fick's first law is

$$\frac{dm}{dt} = -DA \frac{dc}{dx} \tag{1}$$

where m is the quantity of drug or solute diffusing in time t, dm/dt the rate of diffusion, D the diffusion constant, A the cross-sectional area of the membrane, dc the change in concentration, and dx the thickness of the membrane. A change in any of these variables will alter the rate of transport of drug into the blood. The value of the diffusion coefficient is dependent on the chemical nature of the drug and, in particular, its degree of lipophilicity, which can be evaluated approximately from the oil-water partition coefficient. Diffusion can also be influenced by temperature, pressure, and by the nature of the solvent. Faster absorption occurs in the small intestine rather than the stomach because of the high surface area provided by villi and microvilli found in the small intestine. Drugs are rapidly absorbed through very thin membranes (e.g., the alveolar membrane of the lungs). This explains why inhaled medication is more rapid acting than drugs in oral dosage forms. The driving force for passive diffusion in Equation (1) is the concentration gradient between drug in the gut and drug in the blood. According to Fick's law, the rate of diffusion is proportional to the concentration gradient. Therefore, the rate of change of concentration is proportional to the concentration, and since the concentration of drug in the blood is negligible compared to that in the gut:

$$\frac{dc}{dt} = -kc \tag{2}$$

The negative sign in this first-order equation indicates that concentration decreases with time.

If the concentration of drug at the absorption site is c_0 at $t = 0$, then at some later time t, the concentration of drug remaining unabsorbed may be designated as c. Integration of Equation (2),

$$\int_{c_0}^{c} \frac{dc}{c} = -k \int_{0}^{t} dt \tag{3}$$

yields the equation

$$\ln \frac{c}{c_0} = -kt \tag{4}$$

or

$$\log \frac{c}{c_0} = \frac{-kt}{2.303} \tag{5}$$

A plot of c/c_0 on a logarithmic scale against time on a rectangular scale should produce a straight line with a negative slope representing the absorption rate constant k, as seen in Figure 21. The half-life for drug absorption is the time required for the concentration of drug in the gut, c, to be reduced to one-half its initial value, and for a first-order process can be calculated by using the expression

$$t_{1/2} = \frac{0.693}{k} \tag{6}$$

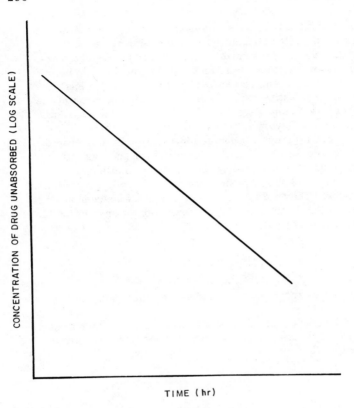

Figure 21. Concentration of drug remaining in the gastrointestinal tract, as a function of time.

B. Active Membrane Transport

Drugs absorbed via an active transport mechanism may pass from areas of lower concentration to areas of higher concentration. The transfer is thought to be mediated by a "carrier," and in contrast to passive diffusion, chemical energy expended by the body is required for active transport to occur. The carrier system may consist of an enzyme or other substance in the gastrointestinal wall. The carrier combines with the drug and accompanies it through the membrane to be discharged on the other side. The carrier-drug complex is considered to have a higher permeability through the membrane of the gut than the drug alone. The process is depicted in Figure 22. Active transport of drugs is site-specific, and the greatest absorption occurs in locations of the gastrointestinal tract, where carrier concentration is highest. At low concentrations, the rate of drug absorption by active transport is proportional to drug concentration in the gut. At higher levels of drug, the carrier system eventually becomes saturated and the absorption levels off at a fixed maximum rate. Therefore, the absorption rate

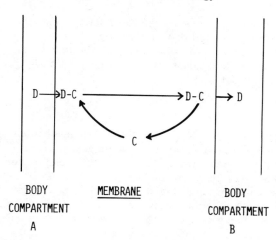

Figure 22. Action of carrier C, which facilitates passage of drug molecule D across a membrane. C combines with the drug at the surface of compartment A and releases the drug at compartment B. Carrier C returns to ferry the next drug molecule across the membrane.

for substances absorbed via active transport will not increase as the dose increases, once the carrier mechanism has been saturated. Several body nutrients and vitamins, such as amino acids, thiamine, niacin, and riboflavin, are absorbed via active transport [31, 32]. Where the structure of a drug resembles that of an actively absorbed material, a strong possibility exists for the drug to pass into the blood via active transport. A number of organic compounds, including penicillin and phenol red, are secreted in the proximal renal tubules by active transport. Other examples include the transport of sodium ions from the gut lumen into the blood, and the secretion of hydrogen ions into the stomach [33]. Some antitumor drugs are thought to be transported actively, and these include 5-fluorouracil [34] and the serine and threonine derivatives of nitrogen mustard [35].

Facilitated diffusion is a special form of carrier transport (Fig. 22) that has many of the characteristics of active transport, but the substrate does not move against a concentration gradient. The uptake of glucose by cells is an example of facilitated diffusion. As with active transport, facilitated diffusion is mediated via a carrier molecule in the mucosa, is selective, saturable, and can be "poisoned" or inhibited by certain electrolytes (e.g., fluoride, and organic dinitrophenols). The main difference between active transport and facilitated diffusion is that there is no energy expenditure by the body for the latter process to occur.

Other mechanisms of absorption include pinocytosis and ion-pair absorption. Pinocytosis literally means "cell drinking" and is a process whereby the cell surface invaginates and takes in a small vacuole of liquid containing the solute or drug. It is an important transport mechanism for proteins, but its significance in drug absorption is not entirely clear. The ion-pair absorption mechanism was postulated by Higuchi [36] to explain the absorption of large ionized compounds (e.g., quaternary amines and sulfonic acids), where absorption cannot be explained by the pH/partition theory. The authors postulated that the organic ion combined with a large ion of opposite charge to form an nonionized species. The increased lipoidal nature of the resulting molecule would account for rapid passage through the mucous membranes of the gastrointestinal tract.

C. The pH-Partition Hypothesis

Passive diffusion through a membrane is probably the most common mechanism of drug absorption in the body regardless of the location of the membrane. Therefore, the greater the lipid solubility of the nonionized moiety, the faster and easier a drug will pass through the membrane. The pH-partition hypothesis was developed by Brodie et al. [37-40] to explain the absorption of ionized and nonionized drugs. The pK_a and oil/water partition ratio are two important parameters involved in the pH-partition theory of drug absorption. For a particular pH in the gastrointestinal tract, these parameters dictate the degree of ionization and lipoid solubility of a drug, which, in turn, determine the rate of absorption of drugs and transport through cellular membranes in the body. The pH of the human stomach varies from 1 to 3.5, although higher values have been recorded. Disease and the presence of food or antacids may drastically increase gastric pH. The duodenal pH is generally in the range 5 to 6 and the lower ileum may approach a pH of 8. Theoretical calculations and predictions as to the amounts and sites of absorption of weakly acidic and basic drugs have been made using the Henderson-Hasselbalch equations and the pH-partition principle.

For acids:

$$pH = pK_a + \log \frac{[\text{ionized form}]}{[\text{nonionized acid}]} \tag{7}$$

For bases:

$$pH = pK_a + \log \frac{[\text{nonionized base}]}{[\text{ionized form}]} \tag{8}$$

From the equations, one might expect acidic drugs or very weakly basic drugs to be absorbed predominantly from the stomach and basic drugs or very weakly acidic drugs to be absorbed from regions of higher pH in the intestines. These expectations are based on the premise, following the pH partition theory, that the primary mode of drug absorption is via passive diffusion of the uncharged species. Thus, the Henderson-Hasselbalch equation can be used to calculate the relative amounts of charged and neutral forms from the pK_a of the drug and the pH of the environment.

The percent ionized is given by

$$\% \text{ Ionized} = \frac{I \times 100}{I + U} \tag{9}$$

where I is the concentration of a species in the ionized conjugate form and U the concentration of unionized species. Equation (7) may be rearranged to give

$$\frac{U}{I} = \text{antilog} (pK_a - pH) \tag{10}$$

Table 4

Percentages of Morphine in Ionized (I) and Un-
ionized (U) Forms at Various pH Values

pH	Percent I	Percent U
2.0	100	0.00
4.0	99.99	0.01
6.0	98.67	1.33
7.0	88.11	11.89
7.5	70.10	29.90
8.0	42.57	57.43
8.5	19.00	81.00
9.0	6.90	93.10
10.0	0.74	99.26
13.0	0.00	100.00

for a weak acid so that Equation (9) becomes

$$\% \text{ Ionized} = \frac{100}{1 + \text{antilog } (pK_a - pH)} \tag{11}$$

where pK_a is the dissociation constant for the neutral or nonionized acid. For a weak base, such as atropine or morphine, the comparable expression is

$$\% \text{ Ionized} = \frac{100}{1 + \text{antilog } (pH - pK_a)} \tag{12}$$

where pK_a is the dissociation constant for the cationic acid conjugate to the molecular base.

As an example, if one considers morphine, in which the pK_a of its cationic acid form (morphine H)$^+$ is 7.87 at 25% C, the percentage ionization of morphine at a pH of 7.50 can be calculated using Equation (12):

$$\% \text{ Ionized} = \frac{100}{1 + \text{antilog } (7.50 - 7.87)} = \frac{100}{1 + \text{antilog } (-0.37)}$$

$$= \frac{100}{1 + 0.427} = 70.10$$

The percentages of ionic (I) and molecular (U) forms of morphine ($pK_a = 7.87$) at various pH values are shown in Table 4. As observed in Figure 23, nonionized drug will distribute across the membrane so that the concentration of nonionized in fluid A will equal nonionized in fluid B. It is assumed that the ionized form of the drug cannot pass through the membrane. The pH of the fluids and the pK_a of the drug will then determine the ratio of nonionized to ionized drug in the two fluids, as seen in Figure 24. The relationship between pK_a and pH at the absorption site has been demonstrated for a variety of acids and bases. Table 5 shows the absorption of drugs from the rat stomach. The acidity of the stomach ensures that weak acids are but slightly ionized. The exceptions are relatively strong acids, such as phenol red, which is highly ionized even at pH 1.

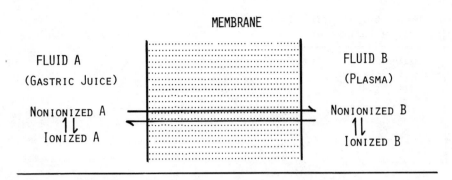

Figure 23. Partitioning of drug between gastric fluid and plasma.

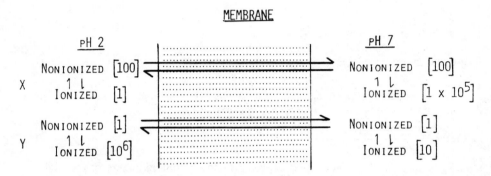

Figure 24. X, Nonionized and ionized concentrations of a weakly acidic drug with a pK_a of 4 in fluids with a pH of 2 and 7 separated by a membrane; Y, nonionized and ionized concentrations of a weakly basic drug with a pK_a of 8, under the same conditions as X.

The poor absorption of barbital illustrates that pK_a is not the only limiting factor, the lipid solubility of the nonionized form also being important. Very weak bases such as caffeine are well absorbed in the stomach, since these bases exist predominantely in a nonionized form, even at acid pH. The varying degrees of absorption of three barbiturates has been shown by Schanker [41] to be related to the lipid-water partition coefficient, as shown in Table 6. The three barbiturates have very similar pK_a values but differ in lipid solubility, which apparently controls the degree of absorption.

The absorption of weak acids and weak bases from the rat intestine at varying pHs is shown in Table 7. As the pH of the solution in the intestinal lumen increased, the absorption of weak acids was found to decrease. The opposite was seen for weak bases: as the pH increased, the percent drug absorbed increased.

Table 5

Absorption of Drugs from the Rat Stomach

Drug	pK	Absorption (%)
Acid		
5–Sulphosalicylic	Strong	0
Phenol red	Strong	2
Salicylic	3.0	61
Thiopental	7.6	46
Barbital	7.8	4
Quinalbarbitone	7.9	30
Phenol	9.9	40
Base		
Acetanilide	0.3	36
Caffeine	0.8	24
Aniline	4.6	6
Dextromethorphan	9.2	0
Mecamylamine	11.2	0
Mepipophenidol	Strong	0
Tetraethylammonium	Strong	0

Source: From Ref. 39; reproduced with the permission of the copyright owner.

Table 6

Gastric Absorption of Barbiturates Compared with Their pK_a Values and Lipid-Water Partition Coefficients

Barbiturate	pK_a	Absorption (%)	$K = \dfrac{[CHCl_3]}{[H_2O]}$
Barbital	7.8	4	0.7
Secobarbital	7.9	30	23.3
Thiopental	7.6	46	100.0

Source: Reprinted with permission from Schanker, L. S., J. Med. Chem.; 2:343 (1960). Copyright by the American Chemical Society.

Table 7

Comparison of Intestinal Absorption in the Rat at Several pH Values

Substance	pK_a	Percent absorbed at:			
		pH 4	pH 5	pH 7	pH 8
Acid					
5-Nitrosalicylic	2.3	40	27	0	0
Salicylic	3.0	64	35	30	10
Acetylsalicylic	3.5	41	27	–	–
Benzoic	4.2	62	36	35	5
Base					
Aniline	4.6	40	48	58	61
Amidopyrine	5.0	21	35	48	52
p-Toluidine	5.3	30	42	65	64
Quinine	8.4	9	11	41	54

Source: From Ref. 42; reproduced with the permission of the copyright owner.

It is important to realize that information in Table 4 was obtained from experiments conducted on animals under special conditions and that, as such, the data are highly idealized. Hogben et al. [38] postulated that the distribution across the gut with weak acids or bases is dependent on the "virtual" pH of the mucosal solution (i.e., the pH of a narrow microclimate adjacent to the mucosal surface rather than the pH of the bulk solution in the lumen of the gut). They pointed out that such a microclimate of fluid with a low pH calculated to be 5.3 would lead to a relatively high concentration of nonionized acid next to the mucosa, as compared to the concentration of nonionized species in the bulk mucosal solution at a higher pH, normally 6.6. The high concentration of the un-ionized species would lead to increased mucosal to serosal movement of the acid by a passive diffusion of the nonionic form. Values greater than 1 for the steady-state concentration ratio C_{plasma}/C_{gut} of a weak acid could be explained by this mechanism without postulating specific active transport.

   For weak acids, ratios of C_{plasma}/C_{gut} are much higher for the stomach than for the intestine, which accounts for the generalization that weak acids are best absorbed from the stomach. The steady-state or equilibrium conditions employed by Brodie are not present in the intact animals and do not take into account the rate of absorption, which is a better determinant for the optimal absorption site than is the equilibrium ratio of C_{plasma}/C_{gut}. For weak acids the large surface area of the intestines results in a higher rate of absorption than in the stomach, and this is more important than the less favorable pH of the intestine.

Suzuki et al. [43, 44] have used theoretical models to study drug transport and absorption phenomena and have shown that pH-partition theory is a special limiting case of a more general approach. These investigators tested their models using the experimental data of Kakemi et al. [45-48]. These data included the in situ results in rats for intestinal, gastric, and rectal absorption of sulfonamides and barbituric acid derivatives. The correlations of in situ data using the models proved to be generally satisfactory, and pointed out the various diffusional coefficients and constants that should be accounted for in the study of absorption of drugs through living membranes.

D. Gastric Emptying Rate: Influence of Food and Other Factors

When a medicinal agent is preferentially absorbed in the stomach or intestine, and when absorption is site-specific in the gastrointestinal tract, the presence of food can have a profound influence on drug bioavailability. Food will slow tablet disintegration, decrease the dissolution rate of the active ingredient, and decrease intestinal absorption by reducing gastric emptying. An increase in the gut residual of certain drugs may result in several toxic side effects to the patient. Alteration in the normal microbiologic flora of the stomach by broad-spectrum antibiotics results in malabsorption of essential nutrients. The change in flora may cause infections in the tract because of the presence of foreign organisms that are usually kept under control by the natural flora. The ulcerogenic potential of potassium chloride and antiinflammatory agents, both steroidal and nonsteroidal, may be increased by lengthening gut residence time.

Among the several factors [49] that influence gastric emptying are the types of food ingested, volume, pH, temperature, osmotic pressure, and viscosity of stomach contents. The age, health, and position of the patient are also important. Davenport [49] reported that cold meals increase and hot meals decrease the emptying time of gastric contents. Levy and Jusko [50] have shown that an increase in the viscosity of the gastrointestinal fluids can decrease the absorption rate of certain drugs by retarding the diffusion of drug molecules to the absorbing membrane. However, Okuda [51] showed that a delay in gastric emptying due to high viscosity results in enhanced absorption of certain drugs (e.g., vitamin B_{12} and other vitamins).

A surfactant may also exert a specific pharmacologic effect on the gastrointestinal tract which influences drug absorption. Lish [52] reported that dioctyl sodium sulfosuccinate inhibits the propulsion of a test meal in the rat, owing to the formation of an inhibitory compound when the surface-active agent came in contact with the intestinal mucosa. Gastric motility in the dog was also found to be inhibited following the introduction of certain detergents into the gastric pouch [53].

The coadministration of a number of drugs, such as anticholinergics [54], narcotic analgesics [55], nonnarcotic analgesics [56], and certain tricylic antidepressants [57], also cause delayed stomach emptying. Studies in humans have been reported correlating drug availability and stomach emptying with L-dopa [58] and digitoxin [59].

Jaffee et al. [60] demonstrated that the type of food can influence absorption. In studies with acetaminophen, carbohydrates were found to decrease absorption, whereas proteins did not. A recent report [61] related to the effects of food on nitrofurantoin absorption in humans indicated that the presence of food in the stomach appreciably delayed gastric emptying. A marked enhancement in the bioavailability of both macro- and microcrystalline nitrofurantoin from commercial solid dosage forms in nonfasting as compared to fasting subjects was also observed. These findings are consistent with the argument that a significant fraction of drug from both dosage forms dissolves in the stomach prior to being emptied into the duodenal region of the small intestine, where absorption is optimal [62]. Penicillin [63], lincomycin [64], tetracycline [65], and erythromycin [66] have all shown reduced absorption efficiency when given with meals. Meals containing a high content of fats have been shown to increase the absorption of griseofulvin [67].

Drug absorption and excretion in some instances may be influenced by the quantity of fluid intake. Nogami et al. [68] followed the disintegration in vivo of calcium p-aminosalicylate tablets by X-ray. The tablets disintegrated more rapidly when ingested with water than without water. Human studies with digoxin have employed volumes of 240 ml [6] and 100 ml [7] of water administered to the patient. The effect of such gross differences in the quantity of water utilized in bioavailability studies has not been extensively studied. The influence of the type of beverage administered with drugs has been studied by Levy et al. [69-71]. Theophylline absorption in the rat [69] was enhanced when administered in hydroalcoholic solutions containing 5 or 15% ethanol. Absorption was significantly decreased when theophylline was administered in 20% ethanolic solutions, as seen in Figure 25. When tested in several normal subjects, there was no significant difference in the average plasma concentrations of theophylline produced by these two solutions [70]. However, three subjects (all female) experienced nausea after taking the aqueous solution, whereas none became nauseous after taking theophylline in the hydroalcoholic solution.

A recent study [72] in humans showed that caffeine contained in a proprietary carbonated beverage (Coca-Cola) was absorbed much more slowly from this beverage than from coffee or tea. The sucrose and phosphoric acid contained in carbonated beverages have been shown to inhibit gastric emptying [73, 74]. On the other hand, a more recent paper by Houston and Levy [71] reported that compared to water, the carbonated beverage increased the bioavailability of riboflavin-5'-phosphate and significantly altered the metabolic rate of salicylamide when administered to healthy human adults. Sodium and calcium cyclamates have been reported to interfere markedly with the absorption of lincomycin [75]. The interference occurs both when the sweetening agent was mixed in solution and then ingested, and when the antibiotic was ingested and the sweetening agent was coadministered as a diet beverage.

E. Drug Interactions with Components of the Gastrointestinal Tract

Bile salts, present in the biliary secretions of the small intestine, act as surface-active agents. The influence of orally administered bile salts on the enhancement of drug absorption has been reviewed by Gibaldi and Feldmann [76]. It was suggested that the wetting action of these salts would promote the dissolution of hydrophobic and poorly soluble drugs, resulting in a faster rate of absorption. The dissolution rate of griseofulvin and hexestrol was, in fact, increased in solutions of bile salts [77]. Since the administration of a fatty meal stimulates bile production

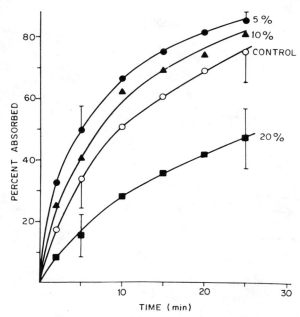

Figure 25. Effect of 0, 5, 10, and 20% (v/v) ethanol on the absorption of theophylline from a 50 mg% solution instilled into a cannulated segment of the small intestine of anesthetized rats (average of six animals per group). Vertical bars indicate one standard deviation in each direction. (From Ref. 69; reproduced with permission of the copyright owner.)

in the body, the high blood levels of griseofulvin in Figure 26 following such a meal can readily be explained [65].

However, other investigators have shown that bile salts do not enhance drug efficacy in all cases. The formation of insoluble nonabsorbable complexes have been demonstrated with neomycin and kanamycin [78]. More recent studies by Thompson et al. [79] demonstrated by analyses of aspirated intestinal content that ionized fatty acids, bile salts, and labeled cholesterol administered in a test meal were precipitated by neomycin. The precipitation of micellar lipids by the polymeric antibiotic provides an explanation for the hypocholesterolemia induced by this compound. Neomycin had no effect on the lipase concentration in the mixed pancrease and lipases, which is called pancreatin. Neomycin was found to have no effect on the pH of intestinal contents. The loss of activity of antibacterial and antimycotic agents has been reported by Scheierson and Amsterdam [80].

Other components in the gastrointestinal tract that may influence drug activity include enzymes and proteins plus the mucopolysaccharide material called mucin, which lines the mucosal surfaces of the stomach and intestine. Enzymes found in the gastrointestinal tract transform the inactive drug moieties, chloramphenicol palmitate [81] and the acetoxymethyl ester of benzylpenicillin [82] to their active parent compounds. The binding of large quantities of dihydrostreptomycin and streptomycin [83] and quaternary ammonium compounds [84] to mucin has been suggested to explain the poor absorption seen with these compounds.

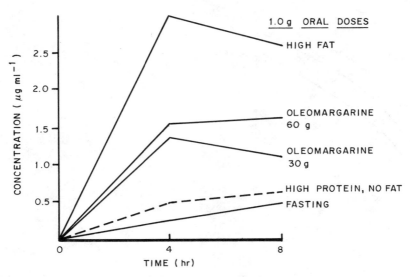

Figure 26. Effects of different types of food intake on the serum griseofulvin levels following a 1-g oral dose. (From Ref. 67; reprinted with permission of the copyright owner.)

F. Cigarette Smoking and Drug Absorption

Recent studies have shown that the clinical efficacy and toxicity of benzodiazepine [85], propoxyphene [86], and chlorpromazine [87] may be influenced by cigarette smoking. An increase in the metabolism of these drugs by stimulated microsomal systems has been postulated as a possible mechanism. An increase in the rate of biotransformation of pentazocaine [88], phenacetin [89], and nicotine [90] has been demonstrated, and the effect of smoking on the disposition of theophylline was recently examined [91]. The results showed that the plasma half-life of theophylline (administered as aminophylline) in smokers was nearly half (mean value 4.3 hr) that found in nonsmokers (mean value 7.0 hr) and that the apparent volume of distribution of theophylline was larger in smokers than in nonsmokers. The authors suggested that the increase in theophylline clearance caused by smoking was probably the result of induction of drug-metabolizing enzymes, and that these enzymes do not normalize after cessation of smoking for 3 months.

G. Patient Characteristics

Considerable difference in patterns of drug absorption for some drugs have been found. Riegelman [92] and Levy [93] have reported that bioavailabilities of a drug from the same product can differ in the same person from one day to another or with the time of day. In addition, the age, posture, activity, stress, temperature, gastrointestinal pH, mobility, mucosal perfusion, gut flora, and disease state may all influence drug absorption. Drug-induced changes in portal blood flow or in hepatic function would alter the degree of biotransformation of a drug during its passage through the liver in the portal venous blood. Achlorhydria, biliary disorders, malabsorption syndromes [94], and reconstructive gastrointestinal surgery [95] can appreciably impair drug bioavailability. The drugs most influenced by patient factors are those whose bioavailability is quite incomplete under the best of circumstances.

III. Physicochemical Properties of Drug and Dosage Form

Of prime concern to the pharmaceutical scientist involved in preformulation and dosage form design is a knowledge of the various properties of dosage forms that influence the biological effectiveness of medicinal agents.

A. Release of Drug from its Dosage Form

When a drug is administered orally in tablet dosage form, the rate of absorption is often controlled by the slowest step in the sequence [96] shown in Figure 27.

Drug must be released from the tablet into the gastrointestinal fluids for absorption to occur. The tableting of a medicinal substance allows the introduction of several variables during the manufacture of the dosage form. Process and formulation variables can be adjusted to assure bioequivalence of generic dosage forms produced by different manufacturers but may also result in bioinequivalence, and this subject will be addressed later in the chapter. The introduction of direct compression excipients in tablet formulations has circumvented many of the problems of wet granulation associated with the granulating and drying stages. However, drug stability and physical tablet properties, such as color, shape, size, weight, hardness, and dissolution profile, must all be maintained within narrow limits for direct-compressed tablets. In addition to these properties, the characteristics and processing of tablets that influence disintegration and drug release include:

Nature of diluents
Process of mixing
Granule size and distribution
Nature of disintegrant
Nature and concentration of lubricant
Age of finished tablets
Presence or absence of surface-active agent
Physical properties of the drug
Flow of granulation through hopper and into dies
Compressional force in production

It is evident from this list that the formulation of a stable and bioavailable product requires a thorough study of the physiochemical properties of drug and tablet to ensure efficacy.

The search for an apparatus that will afford reliable and reproducible information concerning the dissolution of pharmaceutical dosage forms continues. Unfortunately, there appear to be as many varieties of dissolution apparatus as there are investigators studying dissolution phenomena. The aim is essentially to develop an apparatus that enables correlation between in vitro data and in vivo results. In a comprehensive review [97], Wagner avers that an apparatus cannot be devised to simulate the human intestinal tract because of the complexity of the physiological environment. More will be said about in vitro apparatus and in vitro/in vivo correlation later in this chapter.

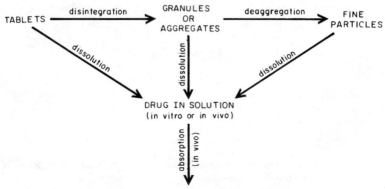

Figure 27. Drug dissolution from a tablet dosage form followed by absorption into the bloodstream. (From Ref. 96.)

B. Dissolution: Theory and Practice

To be absorbed through the gastrointestinal membrane, a drug must first pass into solution. Drugs with poor solubility are absorbed with difficulty, and with such compounds the rate of dissolution in gastrointestinal fluids is generally the rate-controlling step for absorption.

According to Higuchi [98], there are three processes (see Fig. 28) which either alone or in combination describe dissolution-rate mechanisms: the diffusion layer model, the interfacial barrier model, and Danckwert's model. Dissolution by the diffusion layer model (Fig. 28A) is diffusion-limited and consists of two stages: (1) interaction between the solvent with the surface of the drug, resulting in the hydration and solution of the drug to form a layer of saturated solution around the drug particle; and (2) the diffusion of drug molecules into the bulk of the system. The diffusion of drug away from the saturated layer is regarded as the rate-determining step. Therefore, this model regards the rate of dissolution as being diffusion-limited. Once the molecules of solute pass the liquid film/bulk interface, rapid mixing will destroy the concentration gradient. In the interfacial barrier model (Fig. 28B), it is proposed that all collisions of solvent molecules with the solid surface do not result in release of solute molecules because of high free energy of activation requirements. Danckwert's model (Fig. 28C) postulates that removal of solute from the solid is achieved by macroscopic packets of solvent being carried right up to the solid-liquid interface by eddy currents. Goyan [99] used Danckwert's model to study the dissolution of spherical particles.

1. Noyes and Whitney's Equation

Noyes and Whitney [100] proposed the following relationship, which applies under standard conditions of agitation and temperature to the dissolution rate process for solids:

$$\frac{dw}{dt} = kS(c_s - c_t) \tag{13}$$

The loss of weight of a particle per unit time dw/dt is proportional to the surface area of the solid S and to the difference between the concentration at saturation c_s and the concentration of the solid at a given time, c_t. The rate of dissolution $dw/dt(1/S)$ is the amount dissolved per unit area per unit time and for most solids can be expressed in units of g cm^{-2} sec^{-1}.

When c_t is less than 15% of the saturation solubility c_s, c_t has a negligible influence on the dissolution rate of the solid. Under such circumstances, the dissolution of the solid is said to be occurring under "sink" conditions and Equation (13) will reduce to

$$\frac{dw}{dt} = kSc_s \tag{14}$$

In general, the surface area S is not constant except when the quantity of material present exceeds the saturation solubility, or initially when only small quantities of drug have dissolved. As an example of the Noyes-Whitney equation used under sink conditions, consider a drug weighing 2.5 g and having a total particle surface area of 0.5 m^2 g^{-1}. When this drug was added to 2000 ml of water, 600 mg of drug dissolved after 1 min. If the dissolution rate constant k is 7.5×10^{-5} cm sec^{-1}, calculate the saturation solubility c_s and the dissolution rate dw/dt of the drug during the first minute. Is the experiment conducted under sink conditions?

The surface area is $2.5 \times 0.5 \times 10^4$ cm^2 (i.e., 1.25×10^4 cm^2). [Note: 1 m^2 = $(100)^2$ cm^2 = 10^4 cm^2.] Using Equation (14) yields

$$\frac{600}{60} = 7.5 \times 10^{-5} \times 1.25 \times 10^4 \times c_s$$

$$c_s = 10.67 \text{ mg cm}^{-3}$$

$$\text{Rate of dissolution} = \frac{dw}{dt} = \frac{600}{60} = 10 \text{ mg sec}^{-1}$$

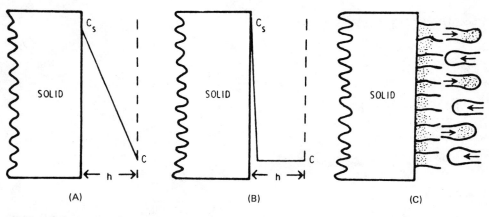

(A)   (B)   (C)

Figure 28. Mechanisms of dissolution. (A) Diffusion layer model, (B) interfacial barrier model, (C) Danckwert's model. (From Ref. 98; reproduced with permission of the copyright owner.)

Now $c_t = 2.5$ g per 2000 cm^3 (i.e., $c_t = 0.3$ mg cm^{-3}), so

$$\frac{c_t}{c_s} = \frac{0.3}{10.67}$$

$$= 0.028$$

$$\frac{c_t}{c_s} \times 100 = 2.8\%$$

Therefore, sink conditions are in effect.

2. Hixson and Crowell's Cube-Root Equation

As a solid dissolves, the surface area S changes with time. The Hixson and Crowell cube-root equation for dissolution kinetics is based on the assumption that:

1. Dissolution occurs normal to the surface of the solute particle.
2. Agitation is uniform over all exposed surfaces and there is no stagnation.
3. The particle of solute retains its geometric shape.

For a monodisperse powder with spherical particles of radius r, the surface area S of N particles at time t is

$$S = N \times 4\pi r^2 \, dr \tag{15}$$

The change in volume of the particle or the volume of particle dissolved over an infinitesimally small time increment dt is

$$dV = -N \times 4\pi r^2 \, dr \tag{16}$$

Since $dw/dt = kSc_s$, according to the Noyes-Whitney equation,

$$dw = \rho \, dV = kSc_s \, dt \tag{17}$$

or

$$-N\rho \times 4\pi r^2 \frac{dr}{dt} = kN \times 4\pi r^2 c_s \tag{18}$$

which reduces to

$$-\rho \frac{dr}{dt} = kc_s \tag{19}$$

Integration gives

$$r = r_0 - \frac{kc_s}{\rho} t \tag{20}$$

or

$$d = d_0 - \frac{2kc_s}{\rho} t \tag{21}$$

Table 8

Dissolution of a Sulfonamide as a Function of Time

Time (min)	Concentration (mg cc^{-1})	Weight undissolved (g)	$w_0^{1/3} - w^{1/3}$	K
0	0	0.500	0	–
10	0.240	0.260	0.150	0.0150
20	0.392	0.108	0.310	0.0155
30	0.471	0.029	0.487	0.0162
40	0.4940	0.006	0.612	0.0153
50	0.4999	0.0001	0.744	0.0149

$$\Sigma K = 0.0769$$

$$K \text{ (average)} = \frac{\Sigma K}{5} = 0.0153$$

where d is the diameter of the particle and d_0 the diameter at $t = $ zero. The weight of a spherical particle is related to its diameter by

$$w = N\rho \frac{\pi}{6} d^3 \tag{22}$$

or

$$w^{1/3} = \left(\frac{N\rho\pi}{6}\right)^{1/3} d \tag{23}$$

The dissolution equation then becomes

$$w_0^{1/3} - w^{1/3} = Kt \tag{24}$$

where

$$K = w_0^{1/3} \frac{2kc_s}{\rho d_0} \tag{25}$$

Equation (24) is the Hixson-Crowell cube-root dissolution law and K is the cube-root dissolution-rate constant.

As an example of the use of the cube-root law, consider a sample of essentially spherical particles of a sulfonamide powder having an initial weight of 500 mg, dissolved in 1000 cm^3 of water. The results obtained when samples were withdrawn at various times and analyzed for drug content appear in Table 8. From Table 8 the average cube-root dissolution rate constant obtained from these data is 0.0153 g$^{1/3}$ min^{-1}.

It will be recalled that Fick's first law [Eq. (1)] involves a diffusion coefficient D (cm^2 sec^{-1}) and a term h (cm) for the thickness of the liquid film. These may be combined and expressed as the intrinsic dissolution rate constant, k:

$$k = \frac{D}{h} \times cm\ sec^{-1} \tag{26}$$

In the example above,

$$k = \frac{D}{h} = K \frac{\rho d_0}{2c_s w_0^{1/3}} \tag{27}$$

If the original particle diameter of the drug (assumed spherical) is 32 µm, the density is 1.33 g cc^{-1}, and solubility 1.0 g $liter^{-1}$, the intrinsic dissolution rate constant can be calculated as follows:

$$k = 0.0153 \times \frac{(1.33)\ (32 \times 10^{-4})}{2(1 \times 10^{-3})\ (0.500)^{1/3}}$$

$$= \frac{0.0153 \times 1.33 \times 32 \times 10^{-4}}{2 \times 10^{-3} \times 0.7937}$$

$$= 4.102 \times 10^{-2}\ cm\ sec^{-1}$$

In a well-written and clearly presented monograph on solid dosage forms, Carstensen [101] differentiated between the dissolution of directly compressed tablets and those manufactured by the wet granulation process. Equations and examples are provided here to illustrate these two cases

3. Dissolution of Direct-Compressed Tablets

When tablets prepared by direct compression or slugging disintegrate into the primary particles within a reasonable time period, dissolution follows the cube-root law (see Fig. 29). The portion AB of the curve can be represented by the Hixson-Crowell cube-root law:

$$w_0^{1/3} - w^{1/3} = K(t - t_1) \tag{28}$$

where t_1 is the disintegration time and

$$K = \frac{2kc_s}{\rho d_0} w_0^{1/3} \tag{25}$$

The term c_s is the solubility of the drug in g cm^{-3}, ρ the true density of the drug in g cm^{-3}, k the intrinsic dissolution rate constant in cm sec^{-1}, w_0 the original mass of drug in the tablet, and d_0 the original diameter of the particles. If the diameters

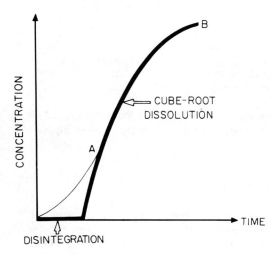

Figure 29. Dissolution-rate curve for a directly compressed or slugged tablet. (From Ref. 101; reprinted with permission of the copyright owner.)

of the particles have increased during compression due to agglomeration, then the size is greater than d_0 of the primary particle. The dissolution process is occurring concomitantly with disintegration, so early in the process the curve does not show a sharp break at t_1 but rather has a smooth curvature AB. A plot of $w_0^{1/3} - w^{1/3}$ versus time is seen in Figure 29, and extrapolation to the horizontal axis will give a good measure of the disintegration time t_1.

As an example of the use of Equation (28) for the disintegration of tablets into granules and liberation of drug into the bulk liquid, consider an aspirin tablet that disintegrates in 2 min in aqueous medium. If the tablet contains 325 mg of acetylsalicylic acid and 60% of the drug is released in a dissolution test in the first 10 min, what is the time required for 90% of the drug to be released?

Forty percent of 325 mg, or 130 mg, of aspirin remains after 10 min. Equation (28) gives

$$(325)^{1/3} - (130)^{1/3} = K(10 - 2)$$

$$K = 0.226 \text{ mg}^{1/3} \text{ min}^{-1}$$

At the time desired, $t_{10\%}$, w = 32.5 mg, since 90% of the aspirin has dissolved in the medium.

$$(325)^{1/3} - (32.5)^{1/3} = 0.226(t - 2)$$

$$t_{10\%} = 18.32 \text{ min}$$

Thus, it requires 18.3 min for 90% of the aspirin in this tablet to be released from the granule and pass into solution.

4. Dissolution of Wet Granulated Tablets

When tablets are manufactured by wet granulation techniques, they first disintegrate into various size granules containing drug and excipients, rather than into primary drug particles, as in the case of directly compressed tablets. Two cases may be considered: tablets can disintegrate into porous or into relatively nonporous granules.

First, for the disintegration of tablets into porous granules and diffusion of drug from the granules into the bulk solution, Carstensen [101] gives the equation

$$\ln \frac{W}{V} - C = -k' (t - t_1 - t_2) + \ln \frac{W}{V} \tag{29}$$

where W is the amount of drug in the dose being dissolved, C the concentration of drug in the solution, t the time, t_1 the disintegration time of the tablet into granules, t_2 the time required for penetration of liquid into the porous granule, and t_3 or $(t - t_1 - t_2)$ the time for the drug to diffuse into the bulk solution (see Fig. 30).

If, in the second case, the granules contain insoluble material and are relatively nonporous, the time for penetration of the liquid into the granule may be rate-determining rather than the process of drug diffusion into the bulk solution.

In this case the drug is released from the granules according to the equation

$$Q = (K'B\epsilon t)^{1/2} \tag{30}$$

where Q is the amount of drug dissolved per unit area of surface, B the fraction of drug in the tablet or granule, ϵ the porosity of the granules or dosage form mass, and t the time. K' is a constant equal to $2Dc_s$, where D is the diffusion coefficient of drug in the dissolving medium and c_s the solubility of drug in the medium. This equation is a form of the Higuchi square-root law [102]. Equation (30) is also applicable to the release of a drug from a capsule containing hydrophobic excipients such as talc and magnesium stearate. The dissolving liquid penetrates this mass only with difficulty, and the time for penetration is therefore the rate-determining step.

The dissolution-rate constant K' is calculated as follows. A tablet of nonporous granules contains 200 mg of drug and 150 mg of excipients, both of density 1.6 g cc^{-1}. The tablet has a surface area of 1.22 cm^2 and a volume of 0.25 cm^3. Calculate the dissolution rate constant K' and obtain Q, the amount of drug dissolved per unit area of tablet surface after 25 min. Experimentally, it is found that 180 mg of the drug has been released from the tablet after 5.0 min.

The total amount of drug and excipient is 0.35 g. The volume taken up by this mass is 0.35 g/1.6 (g/cc^{-1}) or 0.219 cc of drug plus excipient. Since the volume of the tablet is 0.230 cc, the air space in the tablet is 0.230 cc minus 0.219 cc, or 0.011 cc. This amounts to a porosity of 0.011/0.230 = 0.048, or 4.8%.

1. Using Equation (30), we obtain for Q of 180 mg, at a t of 5 min and B = 200/350, the following:

$$180 \text{ mg cm}^{-2} = \left[K' \frac{200}{350} (0.048) (5.0 \text{ min}) \right]^{1/2}$$

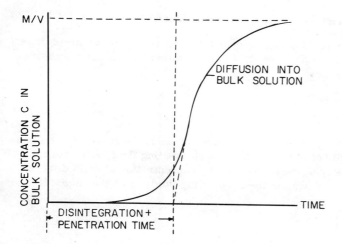

Figure 30. Dissolution-rate curve for a wet granulated tablet. (From Ref. 101.)

$$K'^{1/2} = \frac{180 \text{ mg}}{0.370} = 486.1$$

$$K' = 236,250 \text{ mg}^2 \text{ cm}^{-4} \text{ min}^{-1}$$

2. After 25 min, the amount of drug dissolved is

$$Q = \left[236,250 \left(\frac{200}{350}\right)(0.048) \ (25) \right]^{1/2}$$

$$= 403 \text{ mg cm}^{-2}$$

5. Dissolution of Coated Tablets

Tablets may be film-coated to seal the ingredients from moisture and to inhibit photolytic degradation of the active constituents. Tablets and pellets are also coated to produce a sustained release product or provide enteric properties, thus protecting acid-sensitive drugs from decomposition in the gastric fluids. Ideally, a sustained-release preparation should provide part of the drug quickly at the absorption site to achieve sufficient absorption and produce a rapid therapeutic response. The balance of the drug should be provided at a sufficient rate to maintain pharmacological activity over an extended time. In the simplest case (i.e., a one-compartment open model with essentially 100% absorption and total urinary excretion via first-order kinetics), the drug should be provided to the blood at a rate equal to the rate loss from the compartment [103].

As in other cases previously described, liquid must penetrate the film of the tablet or pellet and enter the dosage matrix in order for the drug to be released and diffused into the bulk solution. Barriers such as polymeric coatings and wax matrices, used in timed-release medication, can function to prolong therapeutic activity; however, such dosage forms suffer the inherent problem of possible drug nonavailability and must be carefully formulated so that they provide a uniform drug release over the desired time interval.

The dissolution of phenylpropanolamine hydrochloride from a wax matrix timed-release tablet was shown by Goodhart et al. [104] to follow the diffusion equation proposed by Higuchi [102]:

$$Q = \left[\frac{D\epsilon}{\tau} (2A - \epsilon c_s) c_s t \right]^{1/2} \tag{31}$$

Here Q is the amount of drug released per unit area of the tablet exposed to the solvent, D the diffusion coefficient of the drug in the permeating fluid, ϵ the porosity of the matrix, τ the tortuosity of the matrix, A the concentration of solid drug in the matrix, c_s the solubility of drug in the permeating fluid, and t the time. If

$$K'' = \left[\frac{D\epsilon}{\tau} (2A - \epsilon c_s) c_s \right]^{1/2} \tag{32}$$

then

$$Q = K'' t^{1/2} \tag{33}$$

For a diffusion-controlled mechanism as postulated in Equation (31), a plot of the amount released per unit area versus the square root of time should be linear, as predicted by Equation (33), and the slope of the line would equal K''. Goodhart et al. [104] showed that after 1 hr, a drug release from the tablet matrix followed Higuchi's equation and that different tablet thickness and hardness caused less than 10% variation in drug release at any particular time interval. As seen in Figure 31, wax matrix tablets are slowly permeated by the dissolution media as a function of time.

The percentage volume penetration of dissolution fluid was proportional to $t^{1/2}$. In the earlier time period, drug release lagged about 1 hr behind fluid penetration. This lag time increased at later time periods. The authors found from extrapolation of the curves that 7 hr was required for complete penetration and 11.5 hr for complete drug release.

C. Dissolution Apparatus

Taking into consideration the considerable amount of work done to date on dissolution of tablet dosage forms, it is not surprising that more than 100 different apparatuses have been proposed for the measurement of in vitro drug release from solid dosage forms. Pernarowski [105] cited 100 published methods, and Lettir [106], Hersey [107], and Baun and Walker [108] described the technology in detail. It is not our intention to review the apparatus and methods in detail, but rather to highlight official methods, together with others that have gained popularity.

Swarbrick [109] classified the various techniques of dissolution from a consideration of their associated hydrodynamics. Hersey [107] classified dissolution methods on the basis not only of the type of agitation but also whether the dissolution process occurs under sink or nonsink conditions. Stricker [110] divided the dissolution methods into three groups: closed-compartment systems,

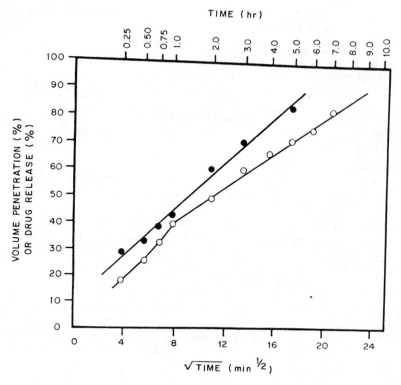

Figure 31. Comparison of fluid penetration and percent drug release from a phenyl-propanolamine hydrochloride 150-mg wax matrix tablet. Compression force was 544.3 kg. ●, Percent volume penetration of dissolution fluid; O, percent drug release. (From Ref. 105; reproduced with permission of the copyright owner.)

open-flow-through chambers, and dialysis and diffusion models. Table 9 illustrates this classification. In diffusion models, dissolved substance passes through a membrane or dividing layer into a second compartment. Closed-compartment systems usually employ large volumes of dissolution solvent. Open flow-through chambers also use large volumes of solvent, but only a small amount, similar to the volume present in the gastrointestinal tract, is actually active in the dissolution process at any point in time.

The types of apparatus, as indicated by Barr [19], differ in a number of respects. These differences involve the type of agitation; the intensity of agitation; the dispersion of the particles; the abrasion of the intact tablet or particles; the volume and rate of exchange of the dissolving medium; the flexibility of the system to vary volumes or agitation intensities; the reproducibility of the system from run to run; the reproducibility of the system in different laboratories, which depends on the availability of standardized components; the container; the stirrer; the volume and rate of exchange of the dissolving fluid relative to the solubility of the drug tested; and experience and documentation available for the method.

Wagner [111] indicated that a dissolution rate apparatus suitable for both research and quality control purposes should meet certain criteria:

1. The apparatus should be economically practical. Ideally, the apparatus should be capable of being fashioned from standard laboratory equipment.
2. The apparatus should be scientifically realistic. The inherent variability in the apparatus should be less than the inherent variability in the products being tested.
3. The apparatus must be flexible in providing an effective degree of agitation. That is, one must be able to alter the effective degree of agitation by altering stirring rate or some similar parameter.

Shah et al. [112] suggested additional criteria:

1. Dissolution rates evaluated by the apparatus under appropriate physiological test conditions should correlate with the in vivo dissolution rate-controlled drug absorption process.

2. The equipment must provide a convenient means for introducing a test sample (tablet, capsule, etc.) into the dissolution medium and holding it at a set position such that the sample is completely immersed in the fluid medium. During the dissolution process, the test sample must be subjected to minimal mechanical impacts, abrasion, and wear in order to retain its microenvironment.

3. The dissolution fluid container must be closed to prevent solvent evaporation, thermostated to regulate fluid temperature, and preferably transparent to permit visual observation of the disintegration characteristics of the test sample and fluid flow conditions during dissolution. It should be possible to maintain solvent sink conditions by employing either a relatively large volume of dissolution fluid or other convenient means, such as continuous flow dilution of the bulk fluid with fresh solvent.

4. Withdrawal of representative fluid sample of the bulk medium for analysis, either by manual or automated methods, must be possible without interrupting solution agitation. As an automated system, it should be possible to conduct continuous filtration of the fluid samples efficiently without encountering operational or analytical problems.

5. The apparatus must be applicable for the evaluation of disintegrating, nondisintegrating, dense, or "floating" tablets and capsules; finely powdered drugs; and all other types of solid drug forms.

1. USP XIX Apparatus

The apparatus for dissolution testing was described in the USP XIX in detail and the flask and rotating basket are shown in Figure 32. The description of the apparatus and method in the USP XIX are as follows: It consists of a covered, 1000-ml vessel made of glass or other inert, transparent material; a variable-speed motor; and a cylindrical stainless steel basket fabricated from Type 316 stainless steel throughout. The whole assembly is immersed in a suitable water bath of any convenient size that permits keeping the water constantly in motion and holding the temperature at $37 \pm 0.5°$ C throughout the test. The vessel (A) is cylindrical, with a slightly concave bottom. It is 16 cm high, and is 10 cm in inside diameter, and its nominal capacity is 1000 ml. Its sides are flanged near the top to accept a fitted cover (B) that has four ports, one of which is centered. The shaft of the motor (C) is placed in the center port, and one of the outer ports may be used for insertion of a thermometer. Samples may be removed for analysis and dissolution

Table 9

In Vitro Methods for the Study of Drug Dissolution

Closed-compartment systems	Open flow-through systems	Dialysis and diffusion models	Other methods
Rotating basket USP XIX	Pernarowski et al. [132]	Marlow and Shangraw [149]	Tape method (Goldberg et al. [152])
NF XIV Method II	Striker [110]		
Hanging pellet (Nelson [20])			
Rotating disk (Nelson and Levy [42])			
Rotating bottle (Souder and Ellenbogen [143])	Langenbucher [147]	Barzilay and Hersey [150]	Coulter Counter (Edmundson and Lees [153])
Oscillating tube (Vleit [144])	Marshall and Brook [148]		
Beaker method (Levy and Hayes [123])		Northern et al. [151]	Simultaneous dissolution and partition rates (Niebergall et al. [155])
Static disk (Levy [124])			
Stationary basket (Cook et al. [145])	Shah and Ochs [134]		
Rocking apparatus (MacDonald et al. [22])			
Rotating flask (Gibaldi and Weintraub [25])			
Circulating flow-through cell (Baun and Walker [108])			
Paddle method (Poole [131])			
Sintered filter (Cook [146])	Tingstad and Riegelman [154]		
Spin filter (Shah et al. [112, 134])			

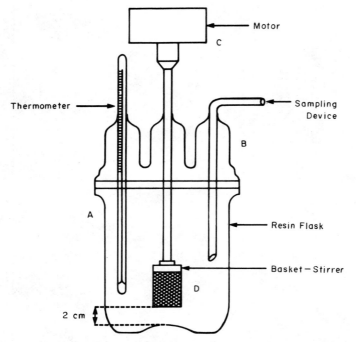

Figure 32. USP dissolution apparatus. (See the text for a description.) (From USP XIX.*)

medium replaced as needed through the other two ports. The motor is fitted with a speed-regulating device that allows the motor speed to be varied between 25 and 200 rpm and to be maintained at the rate specified in the individual monograph, within ±5%. The motor is suspended above the vessel in such a way that it may be raised or lowered to position the basket (D). The shaft is 6 mm in diameter and about 30 cm in length. It is centered so that the basket rotates smoothly and without perceptible wobble. The basket consists of two parts, one of which, the top, is attached to the shaft. It is of solid metal except for a 2-mm vent, and it is fitted with three spring clips that allow removal of the lower part, or the basket proper, to admit the test sample. The USP no longer shows a diagram of the dissolution apparatus, but rather, suggests three types of equipment, the one to be used being indicated in each particular tablet or capsule monograph. The multiple spindle apparatus as described on page 99 can be adapted for both the basket and paddle methods which are the methods of choice in the USP XX.

2. National Formulary XIV Apparatus

   The National Formulary describes two different methods for dissolution. Method I consists of an apparatus practically equivalent to the USP apparatus. Method II uses an apparatus and a basket-rack assembly as described for tablet disintegration

*The use of portions of the text of USP XX–NF XV and USP XIX is by permission of the USP Convention. The Convention is not responsible for any inaccuracy of quotation or for any false or misleading implication that may arise from separation of excerpts from the original context or by obsolescence resulting from publication of a supplement.

testing. The following modifications to the apparatus have to be made when running dissolution studies:

1. Replace the 10-mesh stainless steel cloth in the basket-rack assembly with a 40-mesh stainless steel cloth (of Type 316). A 40-mesh stainless steel cloth should be affixed to the top of the basket-rack assembly, if necessary, to provide for immersion in the dissolution fluid of tablets or capsules which otherwise would float on the surface of the dissolution fluid.
2. Adjust the apparatus so that it descends to 1 to 0.1 cm from the bottom of the vessel on the downward stroke.
3. The disks are not used in this method. The apparatus consists of a basket rack assembly, a suitable vessel for the immersion fluid (preferably a 1-liter beaker), a thermostatic arrangement for heating the fluid between 35 and 39°C, and a device for raising and lowering the basket in the immersion fluid at a constant frequency rate between 28 and 32 cycles per minute through a distance of not less than 5 cm and not more than 6 cm. The volume of the fluid in the vessel is such that at the highest point of the upward stroke the wire mesh remains at least 2.5 cm below the surface of the water and descends to not less than 2.5 cm from the bottom of the vessel on the downward stroke.

Basket-Rack Assembly

The basket-rack assembly consists of six open-end glass tubes, each 7.75 ± 0.25 cm in length and having an inside diameter of approximately 21.5 mm and a wall approximately 2 mm in thickness; the tubes are held in a vertical position by two plastic plates, each about 9 cm in diameter and 6 mm in thickness, with six holes, each about 24 mm in diameter, equidistant from the center of the plate and equally spaced from one another. Attached by screws to the undersurface of the lower plate is 10-mesh No. 23 (0.65 mm) W. and M. gage woven (stainless steel)-wire cloth. The glass tubes and the upper plastic plate are secured in position at the top by means of a stainless steel plate, about 9 cm in diameter and 1 mm in thickness, having six perforations, each about 20 mm in diameter, which coincide with those of the upper plastic plate and the upper open ends of the glass tubes. A central shaft about 8 cm in length, the upper end of which terminates in an eye through which a string or wire may be inserted, is attached to the stainless steel plate. The parts of the apparatus are assembled and rigidly held by means of three bolts passing through the two plastic plates and the steel plate.

The design of the basket-rack assembly may be varied somewhat provided that the specifications for the glass tubes and the screen mesh size are maintained.

Disks

Each tube is provided with a slotted and perforated cylindrical disk 9.5 ± 0.15 mm in thickness and 20.7 ± 0.15 mm in diameter. The disk is made of a suitable transparent or translucent plastic material having a specific gravity between 1.18 and 1.20. Five 2-mm holes extend between the ends of the cylinder, one of the holes being through the cylinder, one of the holes being through the cylinder axis, and the others being parallel with it equally spaced on a 6-mm radius from it. Equally spaced on the sides of the cylinder are four notches that form V-shaped

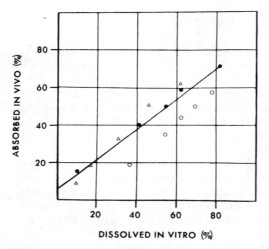

Figure 33. Percent of dose of aspirin absorbed to time T after drug administration, versus percent dissolved in vitro at time T. O, Conventional tablets; ●, buffered tablets; Δ, timed-release tablets. (From Ref. 25; reproduced with permission of the copyright owner.)

planes that are perpendicular to the ends of the cylinder. The dimensions of each notch are such that the openings on the bottom of the cylinder are 1.60 mm square and those on the top are 9.5 mm in width and 2.55 mm in depth. All surfaces of the disk are smooth.

Hanson Research Corporation (Northridge, California) offers a multiple-spindle drive apparatus (Model 72) which was redesigned to reduce vibration levels. Preliminary results of their investigations [113] indicate that vibration significantly decreases dissolution times on a linear basis when it is measured at the resin flask and the displacements are in excess of 0.2 ml. Significant changes were noticeable at lower speeds (25 rpm) but were not significant at speeds of 100 rpm or above. The dissolution apparatus previously discussed is based upon the apparatus designed by Gershberg and Stoll [114]. Huber et al. [115], Kaplan [116], Schroeter and Hamlin [117], Schroeter and Wagner [118], and Lazarus et al. [119] have used modifications of the USP-NF tablet disintegration apparatus for drug dissolution studies.

3. Rotating Flask Dissolution Apparatus

This equipment, as introduced by Gibaldi and Wintraub [25], permitted an absolute quantitative correlation between absorption and in vitro dissolution of aspirin from three dosage forms, as illustrated in Figure 33. Figure 34 shows a schematic diagram of the rotating flask apparatus used by them to determine the rate of release of drug. It consists of a spherical glass flask suspended in a constant-temperature bath. The globe is supported by glass rods, fused to its sides, which form the horizontal axis of the sphere. One support rod is coupled

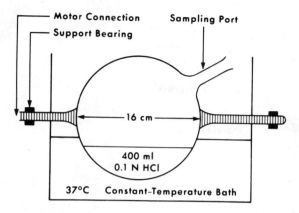

Figure 34. Schematic diagram of rotating flask dissolution apparatus. (From Ref. 25; reproduced with permission of the copyright owner.)

to a constant-speed motor, which provides rotation about the horizontal axis. A sampling port is molded into the sphere to permit introduction of the dosage form and periodic withdrawal of samples. The volume of the dissolution medium (in this case, 400 ml) and the position of the sampling port are such that fluid does not enter the port, regardless of the position of the flask as it proceeds through a revolution. These measures prevent the accumulation of undissolved solid in the port. The port is stoppered to prevent loss of the dissolution medium to the water bath. This method is based on experience with the apparatus described by Simoons [120]. The hydrodynamics of the two pieces of equipment are similar.

4. Beaker Methods

Parrott et al. [121] reported the use of a 2-liter, three-neck round-bottom flask to follow the dissolution of nondisintegrating spherical tablets. They used a stirring rate of 550 rpm, causing the tablets to rotate freely in the liquid rather than remaining on the bottom of the flask. Nelson [122] described a dissolution apparatus in which a nondisintegrating drug pellet was mounted on a glass slide so that only the upper face was exposed. The mounted pellet was placed at the bottom of a 600-ml beaker in such a manner that it could not rotate. The stirring rate was 500 rpm.

Levy and Hayes [123] were the first to use less intense agitation (80 to 60 rpm); their procedure is one of the simplest yet most widely used techniques. The dissolution assembly consists of a 400-ml Pyrex Griffin beaker immersed in a constant-temperature bath adjusted to $37 \pm 0.1°C$. A three-blade 5-cm-diameter polyethylene stirrer is attached to an electronically controlled stirring motor affording precision speed control. The stirrer is immersed in the dissolution medium to a depth of 27 mm and accurately centered by means of a girdle. Stirring rates of 30 to 60 rpm are usually used. The stirring speed is sufficient to obtain a homogenous solution for sampling purposes, but at the same time it is low enough so that the solids of the disintegrated tablet remain at the bottom of the

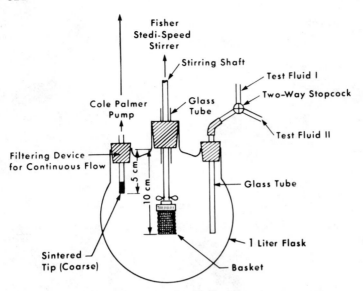

Figure 35. Continuous-flow dissolution apparatus. Rotating basket. (From Ref. 132; reproduced with permission of the copyright owner.)

beakers. Typically, the circular flow of the dissolution medium causes the pow-dered drug to aggregate at the center of the bottom of the beaker within an area of 1 or 2 cm^2.

This method has been successfully utilized by Levy [21, 124] and by Levy and Procknal [125]. Modifications to the Levy-Hayes method have been performed by Campagna et al. [126], Niebergall and Goyan [127], Gibaldi and Feldman [128], Castello et al. [129], and Paikoff and Drumm [130].

5. Paddle Method of Poole [131]

The basic features of this procedure are the use of a three-neck round-bottom flask as the dissolution vessel and a standard Teflon stirring paddle located in a standard position relative to the bottom of the flask and maintained at a constant speed by electronically controlled stirrers. The dissolution vessel is immersed in a temperature-controlled water bath maintained constant at 37° C. The solu-tion is pumped from the dissolution vessel through Tygon tubing to a spectro-photometer by means of a peristaltic pump. The dissolution vessel is either a 1- or 2-liter three-neck round-bottom flask. This enables use of from 500 to 2000 ml of solvent media in the test procedure. The stirring paddle is a 7.6-cm-diameter Teflon paddle and is positioned 2.5 cm from the bottom of the flask. The stirring rate is maintained at 15 rpm by means of an electronically controlled stirrer. The dosage form is introduced through one opening of the three-neck flask. In cases where tablets are the dosage form being evaluated, the dosage unit positions itself at the bottom of the round flask directly under the paddle. In cases where capsules are the formulation under investigation, a wire spiral

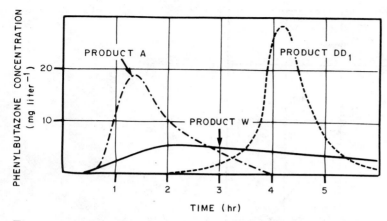

Figure 36. Dissolution profiles for three brands of phenylbutazone tablets. (From Ref. 105; reprinted with permission of the copyright owner.)

around the capsule is utilized as a sinker and is employed to position the capsule at the bottom of the flask under the paddle in essentially the same position that the tablet assumes.

Wagner [111] used this type of dissolution assembly with silicone rubber tubing and directly pumped the solution through a flow cell using a peristaltic pump. He has obtained a good correlation of in vitro results with absorption rates.

Hanson Research Corporation (Northridge, California) has modified this apparatus and offers a vibration-free apparatus with Teflon shafts and stirrers.

6. Rotating Basket Method

The NF XIV dissolution method is based on the rotating basket method introduced by Pernarowski et al. [132]. Figure 35 illustrates the continuous-flow dissolution rotating basket apparatus. The dissolution container is a 1-liter, three-neck flask. The main neck is 35 mm in diameter; the secondary necks are 20 mm in diameter. The total volume of the container is slightly more than 1 liter. If fluid flow or changeover is necessary, the container is connected (via a suitable filtering device and short lengths of latex tubing) to a Cole-Parmer series A-76910 or similar pump. Flow rates of up to 70 ml min^{-1} have been used. Test fluids may be circulated through a 1-cm flow cell in a spectrophotometer. Dissolution profiles are graphed externally on a previously calibrated recorder. Figure 36 shows the dissolution profile for three brands of phenylbutazone tablets. Figure 37 illustrates an in vivo/in vitro correlation of $t_{90\%}$ dissolution values with in vivo data for seven brands of phenylbutazone tablets using the rotating basket method.

7. Filter-Stationary Basket Method (Spin Filter) [112]

Essential features of the spin filter apparatus are a stationary sample basket, a large fluid container, and a rotating filter assembly. The rotating filter,

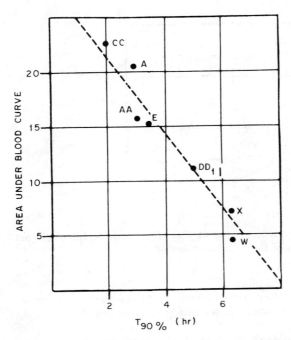

Figure 37. Correlations of $T_{90\%}$ values with in vivo data for seven brands of phenylbutazone tablets. (From Ref. 105; reprinted with permission of the copyright owner.)

employed by Himmelfarb in the cultivation of mammalian cells [133] functions as a liquid agitation device as well as an efficient fluid sampling system.

The rotating filter-stationary basket single-test apparatus was constructed by incorporating necessary modifications into a commercially available microbial cell culture cultivation flask (Flask Model BSC 1000 CA, Virtis Co., Gardiner, N.Y.). Basic features of the apparatus (Fig. 38) are a jacketed dissolution fluid container flask, a stationary sample basket, a rotating filter assembly, and an external variable-speed magnetic stirrer (Magnetic Stirrer Model MS-1, Virtis Co., Gardiner, N.Y.). Dashed lines in Figure 38 represent the optional setup for automated dissolution-rate determinations, in which filtered fluid samples are cycled through a spectrophotometer flow cell by means of 2-mm-ID flexible polyethylene tubing and a peristaltic pump (Model 1210, Harvard Apparatus Co., Millis, Massachusetts). The description of individual parts of the apparatus follows.

Fluid Container Flask and Cover

The jacketed glass flask, suitable for holding up to 1.5 liters of dissolution fluid, has a removable Plexiglas cover secured firmly to the neck of the flask by means of an O-ring and a flexible metal belt. The cover serves as a support

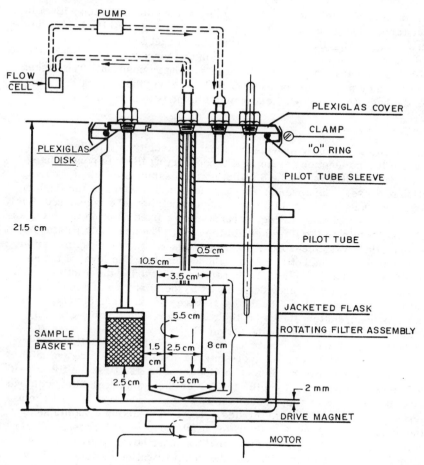

Figure 38. Schematic diagram of the rotating spin filter-stationary basket apparatus. Dashed lines represent the setup for the automated spectrophotometric analysis. (From Ref. 112; reproduced with permission of the copyright owner.)

for the sample basket and the rotating filter assembly. A rabbeted-edge circular opening in the cover, 3 cm in diameter, provides an entrance pathway for the sample basket. There are three other ports in the cover: one in the center for a glass capillary pilot tube, another for a thermometer, and a third for the return of the dissolution fluid from the spectrophotometer flow cell.

Sample Basket

The design features of the stationary sample basket are similar to the basket assembly employed in the official USP-NF Method I apparatus (NF XII), with the exception of using 12-mesh instead of 40-mesh wire cloth screen to facilitate fluid movement through the basket and prevent plugging of the basket screen with solid particles. A rabbeted-edge circular Plexiglas disk is attached to the basket holding rod with a compression fitting, so that when the basket is introduced into the flask through the cover opening, this disk rests in the corresponding rabbeted-edge opening and holds the basket at a preset level in stationary position. The basket level can be varied by moving the position of the disk along the holding rod. In all experiments the basket was held 2.5 cm from the flask bottom (Fig. 38).

Rotating Filter Assembly

The rotating filter assembly provides a variable intensity of mild laminar liquid agitation and it also functions as an in situ nonclogging filter to permit intermittent or continuous filtration of the dissolution fluid samples efficiently during the dissolution process. The assembly is suspended in the center of the flask on the flared end of a glass capillary pilot tube. Since the pilot tube is secured firmly to the cover with a compression fitting, it remains in a fixed position while the assembly can freely rotate on the flared end of the tube. The assembly rotates by means of a controlled, variable-speed, external magnetic stirrer coupling with a magnetic bar embedded in the bottom part of the assembly. The level of the assembly in the flask can be varied simply by raising or lowering the pilot tube. A stainless steel pilot tube sleeve provides support to the pilot tube and prevents subtle vibration of the assembly. The design features of the assembly (Fig. 39) consist of a filter head, bottom flange, cylindrical filter, two flexible gaskets, and a dynamic seal. The filter head and bottom flange are fabricated from 20% glass-filled Teflon with a magnet embedded in the bottom flange. Cylindrical filters of glass fiber, Teflon, ceramic, or sintered stainless steel are available in the 0.2 to 3 μm porosity range. In assembling these parts, first the filter head is suspended on the flared end of the pilot tube, then the cylindrical filter with one flexible gasket on each end is slipped over the filter head, and finally the bottom flange is screwed into the filter head threads. The spring-action dynamic seal slid over the pilot tube positions into the filter head and prevents passage of liquid through the space between the pilot tube and the filter head. Arrows in the cross-sectional diagram of Figure 39 show the liquid filtration system and flow through the assembly. Dissolution fluid upon filtration through the cylindrical filter flows through a hole in the filter head, channels through a helical path around the pilot tube, and then enters the pilot tube capillary. Fluid samples can be withdrawn continuously or intermittently from the upper end of the pilot tube.

In vivo/in vitro correlations have been obtained using the rotating filter-stationary basket apparatus. Figure 40 illustrates the correlation between in vitro dissolution rates ($t_{50\%}$) and total in vivo response obtained with antidiabetic tablets.

8. Multiple-Test Apparatus

An automated multiple-test rotating filter-stationary basket apparatus is capable of monitoring up to six dissolution tests simultaneously. The basic design of this apparatus is similar to the single-test unit, with the exception of using a Plexiglas water bath to thermostat all six units and a six-state controlled variable-speed magnetic stirrer operated by a single motor. The upper panel of the stirrer housing is illuminated by a fluorescent light placed underneath the housing,

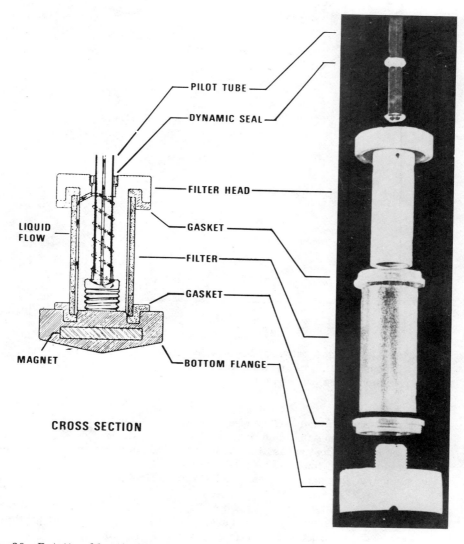

Figure 39. Rotating filter assembly. (From Ref. 112; reproduced with permission of the copyright owner.)

which aids in visual observation of the test environment. Dissolution fluid samples from each flask are continuously cycled by a multichannel pump through one of six flow cells located in the cell compartment of the spectrophotometer. Dissolution rates are monitored by the spectral absorbance recording of the cycling fluid samples at programmed time intervals.

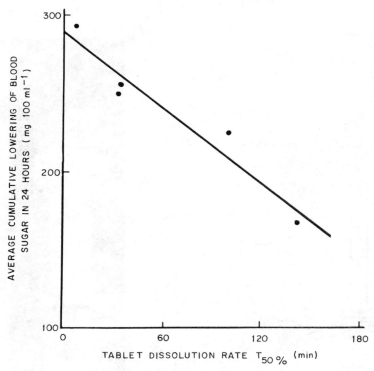

Figure 40. Correlation between the in vitro dissolution rates ($T_{50\%}$) and total in vivo response obtained with antidiabetic tablets. (From Ref. 112; reproduced with permission of the copyright owner.)

Figure 41 shows a comparison of dissolution rates for five antidiabetic tablets obtained by continuous-flow and fixed fluid volume systems. Table 10 shows the correlation between continuous-flow dissolution rates of these antidiabetic tablets and their blood sugar-lowering response in dogs.

In summary, this apparatus has the following advantages:

1. Dissolution rates can be determined by either manual or automated methods.
2. Filtration problems such as clogging of the filter with solid particles is avoided by a dynamic in situ microporous filter element.
3. It permits the determination of dissolution profiles of tablets, capsules, powdered samples, and bulk drug.
4. It permits representative sampling of the bulk dissolution medium because of the relatively large filter area extending over the greater portion of the dissolution fluid.
5. Dissolution-rate determinations can be performed under sink conditions.
6. Mild agitation conditions can be used.
7. Retainment of the microenvironment of the test sample and accurate positioning of the sample have been accomplished. This is a necessary requirement for reliable dissolution studies.
8. Visual observation of the test sample is possible.

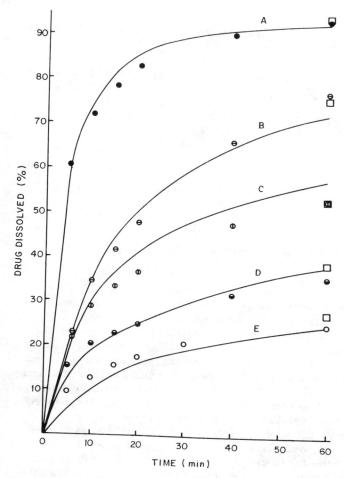

Figure 41. Comparison of dissolution-rate results for tablet samples obtained by continuous-flow and fixed-fluid-volume systems. Lines represent the results obtained by fixed-fluid-volume experiments and points are the values calculated from continuous-flow experiments. (From Ref. 134; reproduced with permission of the copyright owner.)

Some of the disadvantages of the multiple test apparatus are:

1. It is not capable of holding small volumes of fluid in continuous-flow operation. (Shah is modifying the present apparatus.)
2. The cost is approximately $10,000 (Coffman Industries, Inc., Kansas City, Kansas). The basic unit with six stations costs about $5400. (Prices as of 1977.)

9. Sartorius Solubility Simulator

The solubility simulator is used mainly in the development and control of oral pharmaceutical preparations which contain the active ingredient in solid form

Table 10

Correlation Between Continuous-Flow Dissolution Rates of Antidiabetic Tablets and
Their Blood Sugar-Lowering Response in Dogs

Sample	Percent dissolved in 60 min	Total blood sugar-lowering response in 24 hr (mg %)
A	92.3	293
B	76.2	256
C	52.5	250
D	35.3	225
E	24.7	167

Source: From Ref 134; reproduced with permission of the copyright owner.

(tablets, dragees, capsules, powders, suspensions, etc.). Figure 42 shows a
schematic diagram and a photograph of the solubility simulator. It consists of
two main systems: the solution chamber, which simulates the gastrointestinal
tract, and a fraction collector, which represents the biophase. The thermostated
(37° C) solution chambers, in which the solid drugs or drug preparations pass into
solution, contain a fixed amount of inert filling material in addition to the artificial
gastric or intestinal juice. Rotation of the chambers causes a peristaltic movement of the filling material. This both mixes the contents and simulates the mechanical forces in the gastrointestinal tract. The absorption of dissolved drug is
simulated as follows. A sampling pump transports solution (artificial gastric or
intestinal juice) discontinuously from the solution chambers, through filtration
systems, into the fraction collector tubes. An equal volume of buffer flows simultaneously into the chambers to replace the sample volume removed. The sampling interval is set on a time-control dial, which automatically puts the fraction
collector in motion. When the length of the experiment reaches the average time
of stay of a drug in the stomach, the contents of the chamber (artificial gastric
juice) are brought to the pH of the natural intestinal juice. A simple calculation
from the analytically determined drug concentration in the individual samples in
the fraction collector gives the time dependence of the gastrointestinal dissolution
(solubility characteristic) or the resulting rate of absorption (absorption characteristic) for the drug under test.

10. Sartorius Absorption Simulator

The absorption simulator consists of a magnetic stirrer peristaltic pump, thermostat, two containers for the artificial gastric or intestinal juice, and a diffusion
chamber with an artificial lipid barrier. The lipid barrier consists of an inert membrane, the pores of which are filled with a liquid phase. Two different barriers may
be utilized: an artificial stomach-wall barrier and an artificial intestinal-wall barrier. Both are largely impermeable to hydrogen and hydroxyl ions. Thus, the pH

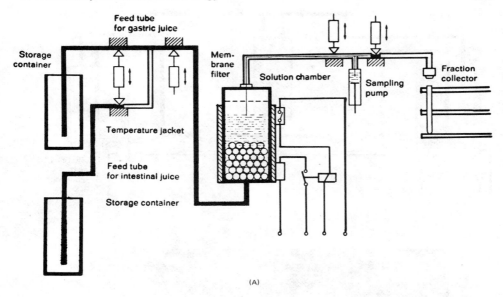

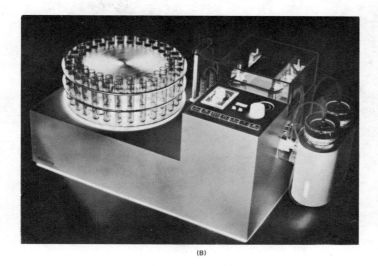

Figure 42. (A) Schematic diagram of the Sartorius solubility simulator, (B) Photograph. (Courtesy of Knut H. Vogel, Sartorius Filter Inc., San Francisco, Calif.)

gradient between the aqueous phases can be held constant over long periods of time. Figure 43 shows a schematic diagram and a photograph of this instrument.

Application of the solubility and absorption simulator has been reported by Stricker [135, 136], who found close agreement between the absorption characteristics measured with the absorption simulator and analogous in vivo studies in

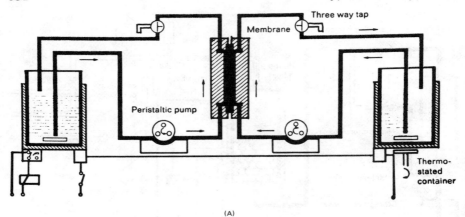

(A)

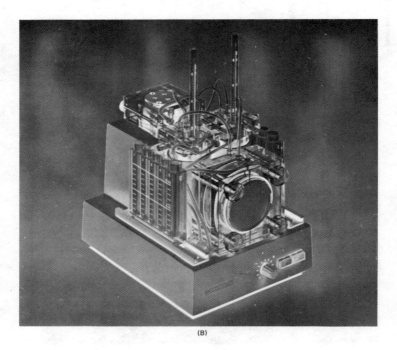

(B)

Figure 43. (A) Schematic diagram of the Sartorius absorption simulator, (B) Photograph. (Courtesy of Knut H. Vogel, Sartorius Filter Ind., San Francisco, Calif.)

humans. Table 11 shows the results obtained with acetylsalicylic acid. The absorption-rate constant for acetylsalicylic acid from the stomach was calculated from blood level measurements following oral administration of dissolved acetylsalicylic acid to a substantial number of test subjects. The value of the diffusion-

Table 11

Absorption-Rate Constant (k_1) for Acetylsalicylic Acid in the Human Stomach[a]

| | $k_1 \times 10^2$ (min^{-1}) | | |
| | In vivo | | |
Test person	Individual values	Mean	In vitro
A.R.	5.5		
H.F.	5.3		
E.S.	5.7		
J.G.	7.6	5.8	5.3 ± 0.5
K.M.	5.3		
I.D.	4.3		
F.H.	7.6		
C.D.	5.0		

[a]In vitro condition: phase I = simulated gastric juice of pH 1.1. In vivo condition: pH of the orally administered solution was 1.2.

Source: From Ref. 135; reproduced with the permission of copyright owner.

rate constant in vitro obtained from the absorption simulator is almost identical with the in vivo average.

Braybrooks et al. [137] examined the effect of mucin on the bioavailability of tetracycline from the gastrointestinal tract using the absorption simulator. Nozaki et al. [138] studied the absorption rate of aspirin and phenylbutazone at various pH levels using this apparatus. The gastric absorption of phenylbutazone decreased in proportion to elevation of pH in the solution. However, the aspirin absorption rate was only rarely increased by changes in pH. Toveraud [139] investigated the permeability of phenobarbital with and without the addition of polyethylene glycol (PEG) 6000 by use of the absorption simulator. Results showed that the rate of permeation was not changed by the addition of PEG 6000, in agreement with findings of Singh et al. [140] and Solvang and Finholt [141].

11. Comments on the USP Policy Statement on Dissolution Requirements

At the 1976 American Pharmaceutical Association meeting in New Orleans, members of the Academy Committee on Dissolution Methodology discussed the "USP Policy Statement on Dissolution Methodology" adopted January 17, 1976, by the USP Executive Committee on Revision.

The following are the comments and suggestions of the Dissolution Methodology Committee:

1. The committee generally favors the USP policy to establish a dissolution test requirement for each USP and NF tablet and capsule. It is felt, however, that the requirement should also include drug suspensions as well as orally administered powders.

2. Two aspects of the following statement are considered inappropriate: "Where dissolution information is totally lacking or is difficult to obtain, limits

may be established to require that the major portion of the drug present in the dosage form shall dissolve in the medium within a reasonable time period (e.g., 80%
dissolution in 30 minutes)." First it is not quite clear how one can establish a dissolution limit for the cases where it is difficult to obtain dissolution information.
Secondly, 80% dissolution in 30 minutes as an example of reasonable dissolution
time period may not be very practical. It would probably encourage the use of
unrealistic test conditions like intense solvent agitation, fluid composition, etc.,
simply to comply with the suggested limits, which could lead to meaningless dissolution tests. Therefore, it is suggested that the above statement may be revised to clarify these points and avoid setting any arbitrary dissolution standards
such as 80% dissolution in 30 minutes.

    3. For dosage forms containing drugs of low aqueous solubility, the policy
statement recommends the use of aqueous-organic solvent systems for testing dissolution rather than the use of extremely large volume of completely aqueous media. Technical problems encountered in using extremely large volume of completely aqueous media (e.g., mixing, representative sampling, multiple testing,
etc.) can be readily recognized. However, the use of aqueous-organic solvent
systems would introduce artifacts in the dissolution data because of the influence
of solvent effects upon disintegration and dissolution processes. An alternative
to using large volumes or organic-aqueous solvents is to use continuous flow-di-
lution systems, whereby a portion of the aqueous dissolution media is replaced
with the fresh media, thus maintaining sink conditions. Successful use of such
systems have been reported in many publications.

    At the present time there is no unique dissolution method that will apply to all
drug dosage forms. The goal should not only be the development of new dissolution methodology and improvements of the present methodology, but the establishment of more discriminating requirements for correlating in vivo/in vitro data.

D. Dissolution Media

Agitation, composition, pH, ionic strength, viscosity, surface tension, and temperature of the dissolution medium have been exhaustively studied. All of these
factors must be considered in order to successfully correlate in vitro data with
the situation in vivo.

    The relative intensity of agitation is extremely important in dissolution-rate
testing. Stirring speeds must be in the correct range to obtain data that will correlate with in vivo results. At a high agitation rate, diffusion control is dimin-
ished and there is a tendency for the dissolution rate to be controlled either by
the rate of release or by solvation of the molecules from the crystalline matrix
[156]. Diffusion control is operative when the rate-determining step is the transport of the solute from the interfacial boundary to the bulk of the surrounding solution. Since diffusion constants are inversely proportional to viscosity, the
passage of solute molecules through the interfacial boundary will decrease as
viscosity is increased.

    Using compressed disks of methyl prednisolone, Hamlin et al. [157] first
showed that agitation intensity was of great importance. More dramatically,
however, Levy and Hayes [123] and Campagna et al. [126] have shown that agitation intensity is of critical concern. An extremely slow stirring technique was

used to correlate the in vitro results with established in vivo differences. Faster
stirring rates distinguished the effects of excipient upon stirring rate which were
not evident with slower stirring [158].

The presence of surface-active agents in the dissolution medium promotes wetting of the solute particles and enhances the dissolution rate, even if the concentration of surfactant is below the critical micelle concentration [156]. This is
extremely important for particles of irregular shape with pores and crevices.
Owing to occlusion by air, the total surface area of these particles may be in-
completely exposed to the solvent. Surface-active agents are discussed in Section III.O.

When neutral ionic compounds or organic additives that are unreactive are
added to the dissolution medium, the dissolution rate of a drug in the combined
medium that is produced may depend significantly on the drug's solubility in the
mixed solvent. Such a dependence was observed for the dissolution rate of benzoic acid in sodium chloride, sodium sulfate, and dextrose solutions [121].

E. Tablet Hardness

A decrease in effective surface area of the active ingredients as a result of granulation and compaction of drug particles can seriously affect the dissolution of
drug from a tablet, unless the process of compaction is easily reversible when
the tablet comes into contact with the dissolution medium.

In pharmacy manufacture, hardness is a measure of resistance of a solid dosage form to mechanical deforming. The assessment of the hardness of tablets
is a very useful quality control check in tablet manufacture, and various techniques have been used, including fracture resistance [159], bending strength,
tensile strength [160], and crushing strength [161].

Huber and Christenson [162] investigated the influence of tablet hardness and
density variation on in vitro dissolution of a dye from controlled-release tablets
made with different types and viscosity grades of hydrophilic polymers. Differences in density and porosity could influence the dissolution rate of drug from the
tablet by affecting the initial rate of penetration of water at the tablet surface and
subsequent disintegration and dissolution. However, these authors reported that
for tablets made of varying hardness, markedly different release characteristics were not observed.

Tablet hardness studies [163] with phenobarbital tablets containing lactose
and silicon dioxide and/or arabinoglactan as binder showed a slight increase in
hardness when the tablets were aged for 16 days at 55° C; however, there was no
decrease in dissolution rate.

Stern [164] investigated the effect of five conventional film-coating materials
on tablet hardness. The author pointed out that the term "tablet hardness" is
widely used in a nonspecific or generic manner as an all-inclusive description
of several important tablet parameters, including bending or attrition resistance
and impact or crushing strength, the later being the most widely used to assess
tablet integrity. Stern demonstrated that placebos showed linear increases in
hardness as coatings were applied. However, the coating process itself did not
alter core hardness, since tablets from which the film could be stripped showed
original values.

F. Adjuvants

In addition to the compressional force used to manufacture a tablet, the chemical components in the formula have also been shown to prolong disintegration times, which subsequently affect the drug dissolution rate and the bioavailability.

Inert fillers have been found to potentiate the chemical degradation of active ingredients and to cause the disintegration time and the dissolution rate of compressed tablets to change with storage. In addition, adjuvants can influence the therapeutic effectiveness of the medicament in a tablet by modifying its absorption characteristics, and can cause changes in tablet color and affect other physical properties such as friability [165].

Alam and Parrott [166] have shown that hydrochlorthiazide tablets granulated with acacia and stored at various temperatures (room temperature to 80° C) increased in hardness with time. The disintegration and dissolution times were also increased. These times were essentially unchanged with tablets granulated with starch and polyvinylpyrrolidone (PVP).

Kornblum and Hirschorn [167] evaluated excipient dilution and compression force effects on the dissolution rate and demonstrated the importance of the excipient/drug ratio to optimize the dissolution rate. The dissolution rate of a quinazolinone compound has been found to increase as the excipient/drug ratio increased. The dissolution data from tablets of 200, 400, and 600 mg, each containing 50 mg of drug, are seen in Figure 44. Changes in compression force were more significant with small tablets, indicating a less pronounced effect as the dilution factor increased. The data supported the conclusion that a larger tablet than necessary for technical reasons could lead to an optimum dissolution rate. The authors also found an increase in the half-lives for dissolution as the compression force increased. The results are seen in Table 12.

By microscopic examination of disintegrated tablets, Johnsgard and Wahlgren [168] found that the greater the ratio of excipients to drug, the less was the tendency for aggregates of the active substance to form. In vitro studies with tablets prepared by wet granulation showed that much aggregation caused a marked decrease in the rate of dissolution of slightly soluble drugs but not of highly soluble substances.

Hydrophilic fillers, such as starch, have been shown to enhance the dissolution of drugs, particularly when the starch was granulated with the drug. Marlowe and Shangraw [149] prepared sodium salicylate tablets by wet granulation techniques using either lactose or a mixture of lactose and cornstarch as filler and found that the presence of starch dramatically increased the dissolution rate. Shotten and Leonard [169] reported that dividing the disintegrant between the interior of the granules and the extragranular void pores can accelerate disintegration into fine particles.

A lubricant is a fine material that functions to enhance flowability of the granulation and decrease die wall friction. Many efficient tablet lubricants are hydrophobic and may retard disintegration and drug dissolution. Owing to the high pressure involved, lubricants are needed to minimize friction, but, if possible, the lubricant effect should be restricted to the die wall because interparticulate lubrication inhibits bonding. The type of lubricant, its concentration, and the method of incorporation must be optimized during formulation development. The efficiency of mixing magnesium stearate with the tablet granulation can influence

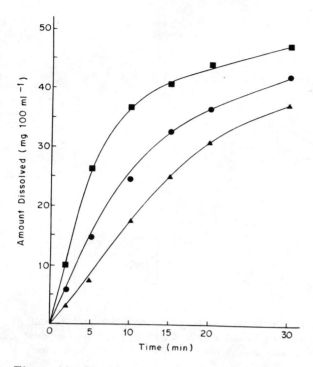

Figure 44. Dissolution of quinazolinone compound in 100 ml of aqueous solution at pH 1.2 from compressed tablets at 24,000 psi. ▲, 200 mg; ●, 400 mg; ■, 600 mg. (From Ref. 167; reproduced with permission of the copyright owner.)

Table 12

Half-Lives (min) of Quinazolinone Compound in 100 ml[a]

Tablet weight half-life pressure applied (psi)	200-mg $t_{50\%}$	400-mg $t_{50\%}$	600-mg $t_{50\%}$
12,000	6.8	4.2	2.5
18,000	9.4	6.4	3.4
24,000	14.8	9.4	4.8

[a]Aqueous solution at pH 1.2 for tablets of 200, 400, and 600 mg at various compression forces.

Source: From Ref. 167; reproduced with permission of the copyright owner.

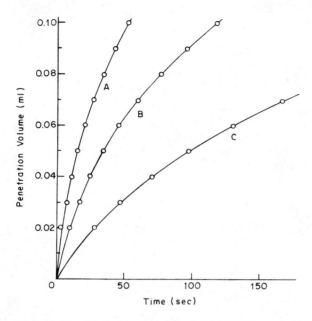

Figure 45. Water penetration into tablets containing lubricant added in different ways. Key: A, 1% magnesium stearate tumbler-mixed with magnesium carbonate powder; B, 1% shear-mixed with powder; C, 0.5% wet-mixed during granulation. (From Ref. 170.)

the lubricant effect and drug release from the granules. The method of incorporating the lubricant [170] can influence penetration into the tablet by the solvent medium, as seen in Figure 45.

Finholt [171] states that the effect of lubricant on the dissolution rates of drugs from tablets will depend upon the properties of the granules and lubricant and upon the amount of lubricant used. If the granule particles are hydrophilic and fast-disintegrating, a surface-active agent would have little effect. However, when the granules are less hydrophilic and slow to disintegrate, a surface-active lubricant such as magnesium lauryl sulfate may enhance dissolution.

The in vitro dissolution of digoxin tablets was shown by Khalil [172] to be suppressed by a commercial antacid containing aluminum hydroxide and magnesium trisilicate. The significance of this finding was later questioned by Loo et al. [173], who found that with mongrel dogs, the antacids had no significant influence on the blood levels of digoxin.

G. Salts and pH Effects

The equilibrium solubility and dissolution rate of a drug are important properties governing the effective concentration that a drug, particularly a relatively insoluble one, achieves at the absorption site in the gastrointestinal tract. The factors that govern solubility of drugs are temperature, particle size, crystalline state, complexation, and variations in pH and salt concentration.

Dissolution is the sum total of various factors involved in the transference of a solute molecule from the solid to the solution phase [174]. Attempts to increase solubility can often be achieved by judicious selection of a suitable excipient or by using a more soluble derivative of the drug.

The dissolution rate of drugs may be increased by adjusting the pH of the microenvironment surrounding the drug particle. The resulting increase in solubility in the diffusion layer in these cases is nearly always due to salt formation following an acid-base reaction.

The solution of a relatively insoluble organic acid in water can be represented by the equilibrium equations

$$[HA] \text{ (solid phase)} \xrightarrow{K_s} [HA] \text{ (solution phase)} \xrightarrow{K_a} [H^+] + [A^-] \tag{34}$$

The equilibrium constant K_s of the first reaction above corresponds to the concentration of the undissociated acid in equilibrium with the solid phase. The equilibrium constant K_a of the second reaction is merely the dissociation constant of the acid,

$$K_a = \frac{[H^+][A^-]}{[HA]} \tag{35}$$

Since the total concentration of the compound in solution c_s would be the sum of the ionized and nonionized form, one can write

$$c_s = [HA] + [A^-] = [HA] + K_a \frac{[HA]}{[H^+]} \tag{36}$$

But since $K_s = [HA]$,

$$c_s = K_s + K_s \frac{K_a}{[H^+]} = K_s \left(1 + \frac{K_a}{[H^+]} \right) \tag{37}$$

When $[H^+] \ll K_a$, $K_a/[H^+]$ is much larger than K_s, and

$$c_s = \frac{K_s K_a}{[H^+]} \tag{38}$$

Expressed in logarithmic form, Equation (38) becomes

$$\log c_s = \log K_s + \log K_a - \log [H^+] \tag{39}$$

or

$$\log c_s = \log K_s + pH - pK_a \tag{40}$$

The solubility c_s of a weak acid actually represents the concentration of the drug in the diffusion layer and [from Eq. (40)] would increase with an increase in pH.

Equivalently, the dissolution of a relatively insoluble organic base can be written as

$$\log c_s = pK_w - pH - pK_b + \log K_s \tag{41}$$

where K_w is the dissociation constant of water and K_b the dissociation constant of the base.

In effect, the solution rate of a weak acid (or base) is not dependent directly on its intrinsic solubility in the medium, but on the solubility that exists in the diffusion layer. The pH of this thin layer for an acidic drug may be increased by including in the formulation agents such as sodium citrate, sodium bicarbonate, and magnesium carbonate. The dissolution rate and the absorption rate of aspirin are increased in buffered tablets as compared to plain aspirin [175]. The pH of the stomach content is significantly altered in the presence of the buffering agent and when the microenvironmental pH is raised sufficiently high to increase the rates of dissolution and absorption.

Techniques for forming sodium, potassium, and other water-soluble salts, such as hydrochloride, has long been used to improve the bioavailability of poorly soluble drugs. Generally, the salt will show higher dissolution rates than the corresponding nonionic drugs at the same pH, even though the final equilibrium solubility of the drug and its salt are alike [176]. Higuchi et al. [176] have shown that under physiological conditions of pH favoring conversion of the salt to a nonelectrolyte, the salt dissolves rapidly and the nonelectrolyte formed then precipitates as fine particles having desirable characteristics for proper redissolution and bioabsorption.

Anderson and Sneddon [177] found this explanation not to be applicable when comparing the dissolution rates in 0.1 N aqueous hydrochloric acid solutions of phenobarbital and sodium phenobarbital tablets produced by the same manufacturer, as displayed in Figure 46. Dissolution of the parent acid compound in both water and acid was very similar. The sodium phenobarbital tablets dissolve rapidly in water; however, dissolution was greatly retarded in acidic media, which, like gastric acid, had a pH of about 1.5. Although 0.1 N hydrochloric acid with or without pepsin is often used as simulated gastric juice for in vitro experiments, Finholt and Solvang [178] discovered that inclusion of a low concentration of a surface-active agent such as polysorbate 80 in the dissolution medium reproduced more closely the conditions in the stomach. The results from the investigation of Anderson and Sneddon found in Table 13 demonstrate that the surfactant had little effect on the formulations tested.

The results of this study [177] are in conflict with an earlier study by Nelson [20], who demonstrated that compressed pellets of phenobarbital dissolved much more slowly than similar pellets of sodium phenobarbital and that this held for acidic, neutral, and alkaline conditions (see Table 14).

The tremendous differences seen in Table 12 for the acid and the salt compound suggest that the tablet formulations and physical properties of the dosage forms (Fig. 46) may exert more influence on drug release than that exerted by the nature of the active ingredient.

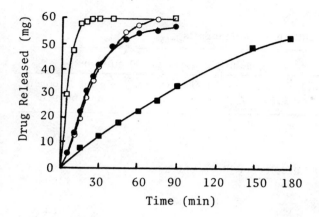

Figure 46. Release of barbiturate from sodium phenobarbital and phenobarbital tablets in water and acid, as a function of time. □, Sodium phenobarbital in water; ○, phenobarbital in water; ■, sodium phenobarbital in 0.1 N HCl, ●, phenobarbital in 0.1 N HCl. (From Ref. 177.)

Table 13

Times for Dissolution (as $T_{50\%}$ Values) of Barbiturate Tablets in Various Media at 37° C

Tablet	Medium	$T_{50\%}$ (min)	Average $T_{50\%}$
Phenobarbital (60 mg)	Water	18, 22, 24	21
	0.1 N hydrochloric acid	19, 20	20
	0.1 N hydrochloric acid with 0.01% polysorbate 80	12, 12	12
	0.1 N hydrochloric acid with 0.05% polysorbate 80	10	10
Phenobarbital sodium (60 mg)	Water	4, 5, 6	5
	0.1 N hydrochloric acid	80, 86	83
	0.1 N hydrochloric acid with 0.01% polysorbate 80	82	82
	0.1 N hydrochloric acid with 0.05% polysorbate 80	75, 84	80

Source: From Ref. 177.

Table 14

Dissolution Rate of Weak Acids and Their Sodium Salts

Compound	pK$_a$	Dissolution rate (mg/100 min/cm^2)		
		0.1 N HCl, pH 1.5	0.1 M phosphate, pH 6.8	0.1 M borate, pH 9.0
Benzoic acid	4.2	2.1	14	28
Sodium salt		980	1770	1600
Phenobarbital	7.4	0.24	1.2	22
Sodium salt		~200	820	1430
Salicylic acid	3.0	1.7	27	53
Sodium salt		1870	2500	2420
Sulfathiazole	7.3	<0.1	~0.5	8.5
Sodium salt		550	810	1300

Source: From Ref. 20; reproduced with permission of the copyright owner.

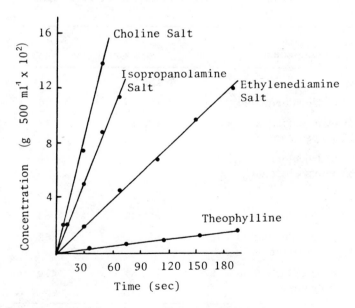

Figure 47. Solution rate of theophylline and salts in 0.1 N hydrochloric acid. (From Ref. 122; reproduced with permission of the copyright owner.)

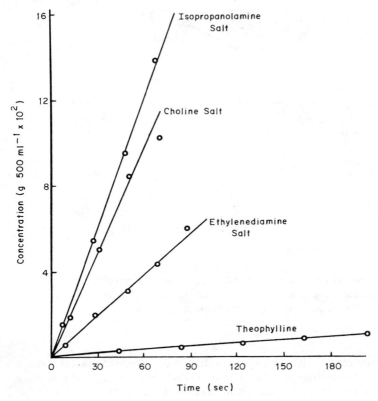

Figure 48. Solution rate of theophylline and salts in 0.1 M phosphate buffer. (From Ref. 122; reproduced with permission of the copyright owner.)

Vivino [179] compared the blood levels of theophylline following the administration of theophylline isopropanolamine and theophylline ethylenediamine to humans. He found that the isopropanolamine salt gave a more rapid rise in blood levels and higher and more prolonged blood levels. In an earlier study, Gagliani et al. [180] showed that choline theophyllinate also gave earlier and higher levels of theophylline in the blood than did theophylline ethylenediamine. These results may be related to the dissolution rates, which appear in Figures 47 and 48. The choline and isopropanolamine salts dissolve between two and three times as fast as the ethylenediamine salt, depending on the media used [122].

Later work by Nelson [181] correlated the excretion rates of tetracycline and its various salts with the dissolution rates as seen in Figure 49.

Correlations between dissolution rates and blood levels in humans have been made with penicillin V and its salts [182]. The rates of solution at pH 2 and 8 occur in the order: potassium salt > calcium salt > free acid > benzathine salt. Studies in human subjects showed that blood levels followed the same sequence, indicating a strong correlation and dependence on the solution rates of the salts.

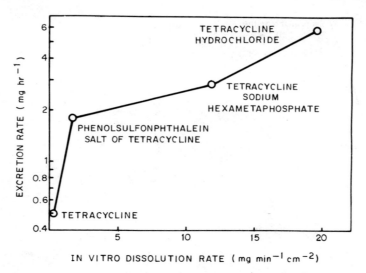

Figure 49. Correlation between excretion rate at 1 hr and in vitro dissolution rate when various tetracyclines are taken in the form of pellets. (From Ref. 181; reproduced with permission of the copyright owner.)

Salt formation does not result in all cases in faster dissolution rates of weak electrolytes in media of various pH. The conversion of a weak acid on the surface of a tablet may form a film that is insoluble in acid media, and this film can prevent penetration of the liquid into the tablet, inhibiting disintegration and dissolution. The precipitation of insoluble alginic acid and carboxymethylcellulose from water-soluble salts of these gums may have a similar effect. Studies with aluminum acetylsalicylate [142, 183], warfarin sodium [184], and benzphetamine pamoate [185] showed that administration of the salt slowed dissolution and subsequent absorption of the drug compared to the nonionized form. This decrease appeared to be a result of precipitation of an insoluble particle or film on the tablet surface.

The formation of salts and esters of drugs has helped to stabilize the active moiety against degradation in the acidic medium of the stomach. Blood levels with erythromycin estolate, an ester, were demonstrated to be several times higher than those obtained with erythromycin base or the stearate salt [186-188]. These differences were found in both fasting and nonfasting subjects, suggesting that food exerted little influence on absorption of erythromycin estolate. This phenomenon is probably due to the high acid stability of the estolate derivative compared to the base and stearate salt. Unfortunately, erythromycin estolate is highly bound to proteins in the blood, and the concentration that is free for antibacterial action in the body is essentially no greater than erythromycin from the salt or base. Furthermore, the estolate is known to cause reversible hepatotoxicity in a small number of cases and must be used with some caution.

The bioavailability of aminosalicylic acid and its sodium, calcium, and potassium salts in tablet form has been examined by Wan et al. [189]. In tests

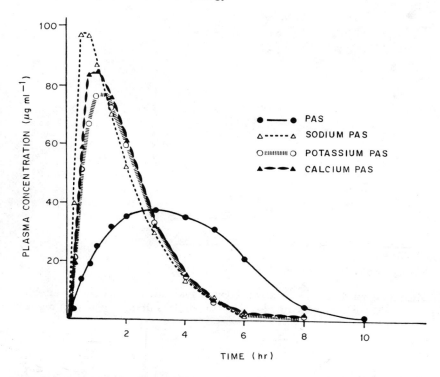

Figure 50. Mean plasma concentrations of unchanged drug from 12 subjects following administration of four different preparations of aminosalicylic acid (PAS). Data were corrected to 70-kg body weight. (From Ref. 189; reproduced with permission of the copyright owner.)

on 12 volunteers, doses of 4 g of the free acid, and 2.8 g and 2.6 g of the sodium, potassium, and calcium salts, were given orally. The absorption from the salts was complete and rapid, but only 77% of the free acid was absorbed, the dissolution rate of this relatively insoluble substance being the rate-limiting factor. The salts gave a greater area under the plasma concentration curve than did the unmetabolized drug, although the absolute amount of free acid absorbed was higher. The authors attribute this phenomenon to the limited capacity of humans to acetylate the drug, especially during the first pass in the gastrointestinal and liver tissues (see Fig. 50).

Berge et al. [190] recently reviewed pharmaceutical salts and discussed the physiochemical properties, bioavailability, and toxicological considerations that must be considered in selecting the most useful salt form of a drug.

H. Particle Size

As stated earlier, drugs administered orally in a solid dosage form must first dissolve in gastrointestinal fluids before they are absorbed. Since dissolution

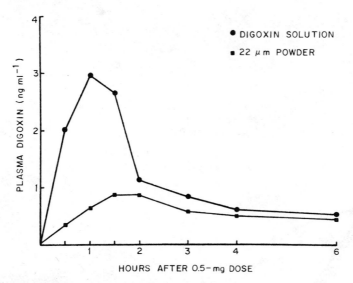

Figure 51. Mean plasma digoxin levels recorded in four healthy volunteers after 0.5-mg doses of (1) digoxin powder of 22-μm mean particle diameter and (2) digoxin in solution. (From Ref. 193.)

rate is directly proportional to surface area [see Eq. (13)], a decrease in size of the primary particles of the drug will create a greater surface area in contact with the dissolution medium, resulting in a faster rate of solution. This becomes important where the absorption is rate-limited by the dissolution process. Particle size is generally important for poorly or slowly soluble drugs. The dissolution of drugs from granules prepared by wet and dry granulating techniques was discussed earlier in the chapter.

The classic works of Bedford and coworkers [191, 192], which showed how griseofulvin blood levels were markedly affected by particle size, are often quoted. Extensive studies on the influence of particle size on the bioavailability of digoxin was recently reported by Shaw and Carless [193] (see Figs. 51 and 52) and by Jounela et al. [194].

Although the reduction in particle size remains an accepted method for increasing dissolution rates, it must not be assumed that finer particles will always exhibit faster dissolution rates than coarser drug particles. Aggregation may reduce the effective surface area in contact with the dissolution medium. During tablet compression, the particle shape [195] and particle size [196] may change.

Solvang and Finholt [141] illustrate the complexities of particle size effect in solid dosage forms. They showed that phenacetin was released faster from granules than from tablets, whereas the reverse was true for prednisone and phenobarbital. These results could be due to a wetting phenomenon, yet other factors besides particle size appear to exert an influence on drug dissolution. Kornblum and Hirschorn [197] compared the dissolution rates of powders and tablets of a quinazolinone drug that had been spray-dried and air-attrited. The drug that was

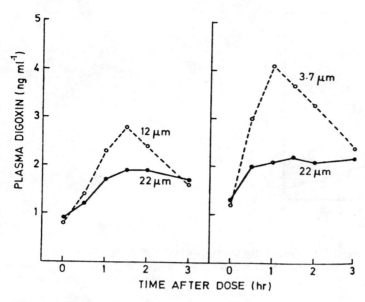

Figure 52. Mean plasma digoxin levels recorded in fasting patients on maintenance dixogin therapy before (●) and after (○) 0.5 mg of digoxin powder of mean particle size 22 μm (four patients) and 12 μm and 3.7 μm (four patients). (From Ref. 193.)

micronized by air attrition had the smaller particle size but formed aggregates in solution; thus, faster dissolution rates were observed for the spray-dried material. The reverse was true when the drug was incorporated into tablets containing microcrystalline cellulose and lactose as filters. The addition of hydrophilic diluents to the hydrophobic drug imparted hydrophilic properties to the tablets, and particle aggregates experienced with the attrited powder did not form.

In addition to compaction during manufacture, other factors, such as adsorption of air on the particle surface, static surface charge, hydrophobicity imparted by adsorption of tablet lubricants, and improper choice of tablet excipients, may cause fine particles to dissolve more slowly than larger particles. In those instances where particle size is important, care must be exercised during moist granulating to prevent crystal growth or condensation into aggregates. These effects must therefore be identified and treated appropriately in the course of good formulation practices.

A reduction in particle size is not desirable in all cases. For example, a particle size reduction of nitrofurantoin will increase dissolution rate (see Fig. 53) and blood levels; however, smaller size particles will also increase gastrointestinal irritation, which explains why a macrocrystalline rather than an amorphous form of nitrofurantoin appears in the marketed product.

Monkhouse and Lach [199] have increased the dissolution rates of various poorly soluble drugs by adsorbing the drug onto an adsorbent and increasing the surface area of the drug in contact with dissolution media. This was accomplished by equilibrating the drug in an organic solvent with an insoluble excipient having an

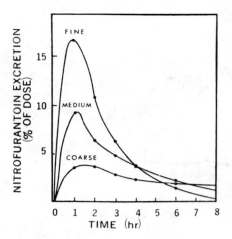

Figure 53. Effect of crystal size of orally administered nitrofurantoin on urinary recovery rate in the rat. Coarse, 50-80 mesh (300-800 μm); medium, 80-200 mesh (180-75 μm); fine, 200 mesh to micronized (75-10 μm or less). (From Ref. 198; reproduced with permission of the copyright owner.)

extensive surface (e.g., fumed silicon dioxide), and evaporating the mixture to dryness. The dissolution data for indomethacin are seen in Figure 54. An increased rate of release from the miniscular drug delivery system, as Monkhouse and Lach called their dosage form, was observed with all drugs studies.

I. Prodrug Approach

A prodrug results from a chemical modification of a biologically active substance to form a new compound, which upon in vivo enzymatic attack will liberate the parent compound [200]. This definition has been extended by Kupchan and Isenberg [201] to include nonenzymatic as well as enzymatic release. Higuchi [202] has outlined the various mechanisms that can be employed to release the agent from the inactive form in the body. These include simple dissolution, dilution, pH changes, action of endogenous esterases, dealkylation, decarboxylation, deamination, oxidation, and reduction.

Stella [203] reported the following applications for prodrugs. They:

1. Facilitate passage through lipid membranes for drugs with poor lipid solubility
2. Eliminate problems associated with drug odor and taste
3. Prolong drug activity in the body by decreasing the absorption rate of the drug
4. Increase water solubility of the drug to allow for direct i.v. injection
5. Simulate natural body transport and storage to lower the toxicity of i.m. injections
6. Increase the stability of compounds that undergo rapid degradation
7. Increase the bioavailability of drugs.

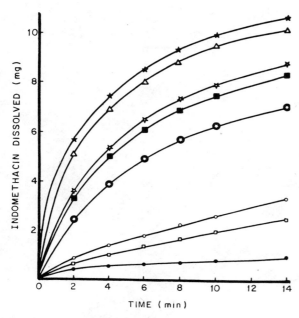

Figure 54. Dissolution profiles of miniscular indomethacin in water at 240 rpm.
★, 20% fumed silicon dioxide EHS; △, 10% fumed silicon dioxide EHS; ✶, 20% fumed silicon dioxide M7; ■, 10% fumed silicon dioxide M7; ◉, 20% silicic acid; ○, 5% fumed silicon dioxide EHS; □, 10% silicic acid; ●, indomethacin powder only. (From Ref. 199; reproduced with permission of the copyright owner.)

The alteration in physical properties and/or modification of the chemistry of active drug substances can in certain instances lead to easier pharmaceutical processing. Candidates with desired melting point, solubility, dissolution, stability, and permeability can be synthesized to allow the dosage-form developer to select, more or less at will, the optimum characteristics desired for the purpose [202].

A wide variety of prodrug chemical linkages are known to be enzymatically hydrolyzed [204]. In many cases, the host tissue in which hydrolysis occurs is also known. Thus, prodrugs administered orally are dependent on enzymes present in the gastrointestinal tract, blood, and liver to regenerate the parent drug. Parenterally administered prodrugs are hydrolyzed by enzymes localized in the circulation and in the liver; whereas site-activated prodrugs are hydrolyzed by enzymes found in specific tissues.

The bioavailability of ampicillin has been improved by the preparation of prodrugs. Pivampicillin was synthesized by Daehne et al. [205] as a prodrug of ampicillin, and as shown in Figure 55 it produced higher blood levels of ampicillin after oral dosing than did ampicillin itself. Pivampicillin is a much more lipophilic derivative of ampicillin; in solution ampicillin exists as a very non-lipophilic ion.

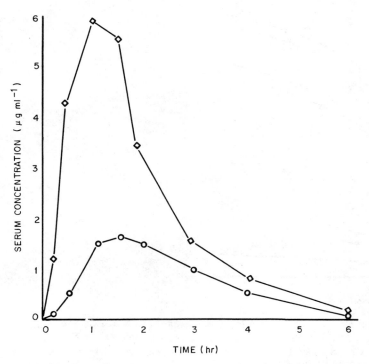

Figure 55. Mean serum levels of ampicillin in normal volunteers following oral administration of 250 mg of ampicillin (○) and 358 mg of pivampicillin HCl (≈250 mg of ampicillin) (◇) on an empty stomach. [Reprinted with permission from Daehne, W. V., Fredericksen, E., Gundersen, E., Lund, F., Morch, P., Peterson, H. J., Roholt, K., Tybring, L., and Godtfredsen, W. O., J. Med. Chem., 13:607 (1970). Copyright by the American Chemical Society.]

   Hetacillin is also a prodrug of ampicillin and may be considered as a condensation product of acetone and ampicillin. Schwartz and Hayton [206] have shown concentrated solutions of hetacillin to be more stable. Prodrugs of carbenicillin [207], lincomycin, and clindamycin [208] have also been made.
   Erythromycin 2'-N-alkylsuccinamate and 2'-N-alkylglutaramate prodrugs afford tasteless derivatives and display blood levels equivalent to or greater than those of erythromycin base. The erythromycin 2'alkylthiosuccinate and thioglutarate prodrugs were reported to be virtually tasteless and extremely stable in a suspension formulation [209].

J. Molecular Dispersion Principles

The dispersion of a drug within a water-soluble carrier effectively causes a reduction in particle size of the dispersed drug. Enhancement of rate of dissolution by this method and thus a possible absorption rate increase has generated considerable interest [210-226].

The unique approach of solid dispersions to reduce the particle size of drugs and increase rates of dissolution and absorption was first demonstrated in 1961 by Sekiguchi and Obi [210]. They prepared a eutectic mixture of the drug sulfathiazole, and the carrier urea, followed by rapid solidifcation. The crushed dispersions were expected to release drug faster in aqueous fluids because of the fine dispersion of the sulfathiazole in the matrix and the rapid dissolution of the urea.

Among the several carriers employed by workers to prepare solid dispersions, the most successful include polyethylene glycol 4000 and 6000, urea, dextrose, citric acid, succinic acid, and PVP.

In addition to the fusion or melt method used by Sekiguchi and Obi, another commonly used technique for the preparation of solid dispersion is the solvent method. A physical mixture of drug and carrier is dissolved in a common solvent, and upon evaporation of the solvent, the dissolved substances are coprecipitated from solution. The obvious advantage to the solvent method is its usefulness for drugs that thermally decompose at relatively low temperatures.

Several factors, including the cooling rate of the melt, choice of solvent, and evaporation rate of the solvent, may contribute to solid dispersions of varying physical characteristics and drug dissolution rates. Recently, McGinity et al. [221] prepared melt and coprecipitates of sulfabenzamide using six carrier systems; a comparison of the dissolution rates indicated that the method of preparation influenced the rate of solution of the sulfabenzamide, as seen in Table 15.

Although the technology of solid dispersion has advanced during the past 15 years, most pharmaceutical studies are restricted to powdered dispersions rather than tablets. The formulation of tablets from solid dispersions provides a real challenge to the formulator. Storage at elevated temperatures for long periods of time may induce changes in crystal shape and size and other physical alterations in the dispersed drug, which in turn may influence bioavailability.

Several authors have correlated in vitro dissolution data with pharmacological response and have demonstrated a significant increase in drug activity from the solid dispersion system [222-224]. Svoboda et al. [222] compared the LD_{50} of the experimental antitumor agent acronycine with an acronycin-PVP coprecipitate and demonstrated a significant decrease in LD_{50} for the coprecipitate over the pure drug.

Stupak and Bates [225] reported that the dissolution rate of reserpine from PVP coprecipitates was significantly faster than from a PVP physical mix with micronized reserpine, as seen in Figure 56. Stoll et al. [223, 224] also showed that PVP coprecipitates of reserpine gave a superior pharmacological response over the pure drug.

K. Polymorphism (and Crystal Form)

Many organic medicinal compounds are capable of existing in two or more crystalline forms with different arrangements of the molecules in the crystal lattice, and these are referred to as polymorphs. Two polymorphs of a given compound may be as different in structure and properties as the crystals of different compounds. The X-ray diffraction patterns, densities, melting points, solubilities, crystal shape, and electrical properties vary with the polymorphic form. However, in the liquid or vapor state, no difference in properties is discernible.

Table 15

Time (min) for 25, 50 and 75% of Sulfabenzamide from Solid Dispersions to Pass into Aqueous Solution

| Carrier | Ratio of drug: carrier | | t_{25} | t_{50} | t_{75} |
	Coprecipitate	Melt			
Dextrose	1:0.5		2.05	9.50	>16.00
	1:1		1.00	2.24	5.95
	1:3		0.60	1.30	2.95
		1:3	0.06	0.10	0.14
Mannitol	1:1		2.25	11.00	>16.00
	1:3		0.83	2.83	10.30
		1:1	4.35	>16.00	>16.00
		1:3	1.10	4.30	>16.00
Urea	1:05		3.20	9.65	>16.00
	1:1		1.38	2.70	9.25
	1:3		0.70	1.25	3.10
		1:3	0.18	0.28	0.45
Polyethylene glycol	1:1		3.60	15.40	>16.00
(PEG) 6000	1:3		1.32	4.40	14.40
	1:6		0.98	2.45	5.55
		1:1	4.35	>16.00	>16.00
		1:3	2.05	7.50	>16.00
		1:6	1.20	3.00	6.40
Citric acid	1:1		2.70	9.90	>16.00
	1:3		1.20	1.58	7.40
	1:6		0.62	1.30	3.55
Succinic acid	1:1		6.00	>16.00	>16.00
	1:3		2.70	10.40	>16.00
	1:10		1.35	3.90	14.50
Control[a]			14.15	>16.00	>16.00

[a]Pure drug, in the absence of carrier.
Source: From Ref. 221.

At room temperature and pressure, one polymorph may be thermodynamically more stable than the other forms in the solid state, as explained by Carstensen [101]. The metastable polymorph possesses a higher solubility and dissolution rate than does the stable form, and this phenomenon may be used to advantage in biopharmaceutics. The appropriate selection and preparation of the most suitable polymorph can often significantly increase the absorption and medicinal value of drugs, particularly those with low solubilities. With poorly soluble drugs it is

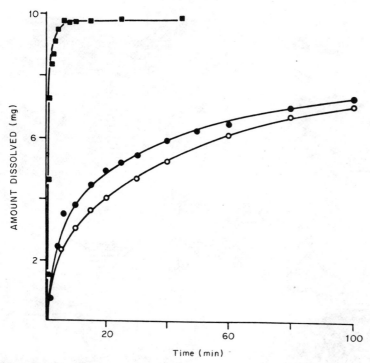

Figure 56. Dissolution rate of reserpine. ○, Reserpine crystals (6-30 μm); ●, 1:5 physical mixture with polyvinylpyrrolidone; ■, 1:5 coprecipitate with polyvinylpyrrolidone. (From Ref. 225; reproduced with permission of the copyright owner.)

possible to increase the solubility simply by modifying their crystalline nature [226, 227]. However, metastable crystalline forms may not be stable and may revert on standing to the stable polymorph; such stability problems must be taken into consideration. When incorporated into the final tablet dosage form it is, of course, necessary to ensure against transformation to a more stable and less soluble crystalline state.

The polymorphism of succinylsulfathiazole has been examined by several investigators [228-233]. Literature reports on this drug suggest a degree of uncertainty concerning the number of crystal forms and the lack of reproducibility in preparation and characterization. Recent studies on this drug by Moustafa et al. [231] showed that physical instability was exhibited by some aqueous suspensions of succinylsulfathiazole. Some of the problems encountered were crystal growth, formation of cementlike precipitates, and difficult resuspendability. These workers isolated six crystal forms and one amorphous form of succinylsulfathiazole. Suspension of all forms in water resulted in a transformation to the more stable form II. The transformation of form I to form II in aqueous suspension is seen in Figure 57.

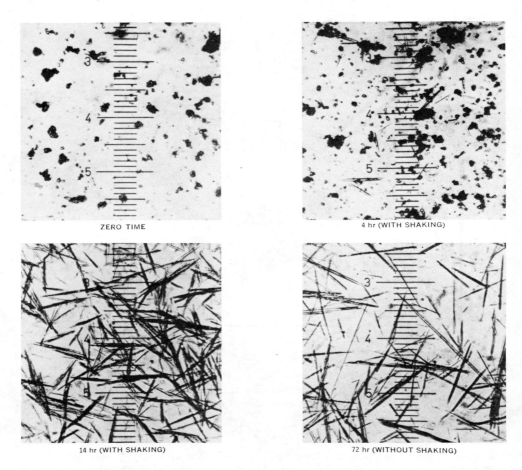

ZERO TIME   4 hr (WITH SHAKING)

14 hr (WITH SHAKING)   72 hr (WITHOUT SHAKING)

Figure 57. Photomicrographs representing various stages in the crystal growth accompanying the transformation of succinylsulfathiazole Form I to Form II in aqueous suspension (1 small micrometer division = 100 μm). (From Ref. 231; reproduced with permission of the copyright owner.)

The formation of polymorphs of a potential tricyclic antidepressant drug was demonstrated by Gibbs et al. [234] to dramatically improve the bioavailability of the drug, as seen in Figure 58. Formulation 1 contained untreated drug and excipient. Drug in formulation 2 was micronized, resulting in a twofold increase in the area under the curve. Drug in formulation 3 was present as a 1:1 (w/w) lyophilized combination of active moiety and poloxamer 407 (Pluronic F-127). The X-ray diffraction, differential thermograms, and infrared analyses confirmed the formation of a more rapidly soluble polymorph in the lyophilized sample. The dissolution profiles of the three formulas appear in Figure 59.

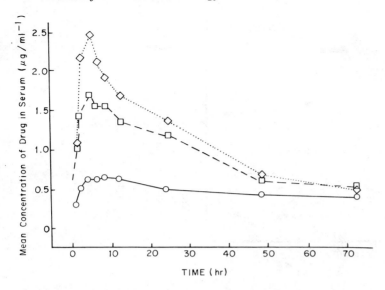

Figure 58. Mean concentrations of unchanged drug in the serum of six healthy male volunteers after oral administration of 200-mg doses of three different capsule formulations of an experimental tricyclic antidepressant drug in a three-way crossover design study. o, Drug plus excipients (AUC = 43.6 μg ml^{-1} hr^{-1}; □, micronized drug plus excipients (AUC = 68.2 μg ml^{-1} hr^{-1}; ◇, lyophilized drug-poloxamer 407 combination plus excipients (AUC = 81.2 μg ml^{-1} hr^{-1}. (From Ref. 234; reproduced with permission of the copyright owner.)

    Theoretical considerations predict that amorphous solids will, in general, be better absorbed than will crystalline ones. These considerations are based on the relative energies involved in the dissolution phenomena. An amorphous solid lacks strong cohesive bonds between the molecules. The molecules are randomly arranged, and less energy is required to separate the molecules of the amorphous material and dissolve the solid in contrast to a crystalline material. Techniques commonly used in preparing drugs in the amorphous state generally reduce the particle size of the drug and result in a faster rate of dissolution than occurs with the crystalline form. Since the amorphous state is predictably unstable, there is a strong tendency to transform to the crystalline state. Macek [235] reported that amorphous forms of the sodium and potassium salts of penicillin G obtained by evaporation from solution are less stable chemically than are their crystalline counterparts. Crystalline potassium penicillin can withstand dry heat for several hours without significant decomposition. Under similar conditions, the amorphous forms lose considerable activity. The amorphous form of novobiocin is 10 times more soluble but less stable than the crystalline form of the drug. Sokoloski [236] utilized methylcellulose to block this transformation from amorphous back to crystalline.

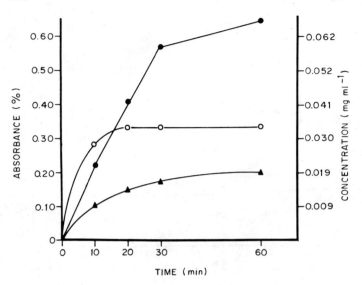

Figure 59. Dissolution profiles in 0.1 N hydrochloric acid (absorbance and concentration versus time) for three capsule formulations of an experimental tricyclic antidepressant drug. ▲, Drug plus excipients; o, micronized drug plus excipients; ●, lyophilized drug-poloxamer 407 combination plus excipients. (From Ref. 234; reproduced with permission of the copyright owner.)

L. Solvates and Hydrates

As a corollary to the importance of polymorphic forms on drug availability, hydrates and solvates of poorly soluble drugs should be considered. Solvates are different from polymorphs; they are the crystalline forms of drugs that associate with solvent molecules. When water is the solvent, the solvate formed is called a hydrate.

A comparative study [229] on the dissolution behavior of hydrated and non-solvated forms of cholesterol, theophylline, caffeine, glutathimide, and succinyl-sulfathiazole, showed that the anhydrous forms dissolved more rapidly in water and in all cases yielded drug concentrations in solution substantially higher than the hydrated states. Conversely, Shefter and Higuchi [229] showed that the solvated forms of fluorocortisone with n-pentanol or ethyl acetate and of succinyl-sulfathiazole with n-pentanol dissolved much more rapidly than did nonsolvated forms of the drugs.

Ballard and Biles [237] studied the in vitro absorption rates of hydrocortisone tert-butyl acetate and prednisolone tert-butyl acetate and their solvates, by a pellet-implantation technique. Their results indicated that drug solvates may exhibit dimorphism (two polymorphic forms) and each form may exhibit different in vivo absorption rates.

Lin and Lachman [238] employed photomicrographic and dissolution methods to study the in situ crystalline transformation of a new antihypertensive drug.

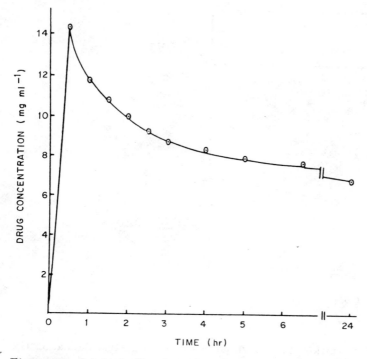

Figure 60. Intrinsic dissolution profile of a new antihypertensive drug in 0.1 N hydrochloric acid at 500 rpm. (From Ref. 238; reproduced with permission of the copyright owner.)

The intrinsic dissolution profile of this drug, as seen in Figure 60, shows an apparent rapid dissolution and attainment of a peak concentration of drug in solution. Following this peak, there is a pronounced decline of drug in solution with time, which was attributed to the formation of a less soluble species, such as a hydrate of the drug.

M. Complexation

The formation of molecular complexes can either increase or decrease the apparent solubility of many pharmaceuticals. Higuchi and Lach [239] reported the use of xanthine to increase the solubility of drugs. The delayed onset of action of drugs in tablets containing agents for the relief of asthma was due to the formation of an insoluble complex. The dissolution of theophylline from various generic tablets is seen in Figure 61. In Figure 62 the bioavailability of theophylline complexed with penobarbital is compared with blood levels of theophylline alone and a physical mix of the two drugs. The complexation of theophylline to the barbiturate resulted in a significant decrease in theophylline blood levels after 0.5- and 1-hr periods.

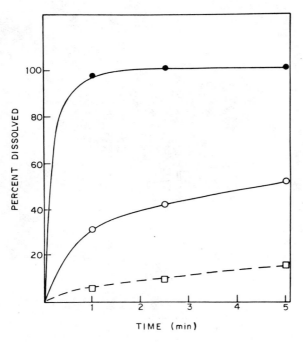

Figure 61. Dissolution profiles of theophylline in simulated gastric fluid at 37° C from theophylline, ephedrine hydrochloride, and phenobarbital tablets. ●, Brand name; ○, generic B; □, generic A. (From Ref. 240.)

In studies with the benzocaine-caffeine complex, Higuchi et al. [241] observed that the fastest rate of dissolution for either compound occurred when the molar ratio was 1:1. Zoglio et al. [242] later showed that caffeine forms soluble complexes with the ergot alkaloids.

Higuchi and Ikeda [243] prepared a rapidly dissolving form of digoxin by complexing the drug with hydroquinone. The dissolution profiles appear in Figure 63. It was suggested that the formation of a complex may overcome the processing problems associated with digoxin solid dosage forms because the complex completely dissociates when dissolved.

N-Methylglucamine, a basic compound with a pK_a of 9.3 and aqueous solubility of 1 g ml^{-1}, has been used successfully employed as a complexing agent to enhance the absorption of Coumermycin A_1 [244]. When the drug was admixed with four parts of the complexing agent and administered to humans, the blood levels of the drug increased significantly, as seen in Figure 64. The in vitro everted intestinal sac preparation was used with this drug, plus two parts of the N-methylglucamine, and compared with the diffusion of the drug alone. The data in Figure 65 suggest that the permeability of drug from solutions was enhanced by the addition of the complexing agent. Overall, it appears that the complexing agent altered both the dissolution and permeability characteristics of Coumermycin A_1, to allow for a more prolonged absorption of an otherwise negligibly absorbed drug.

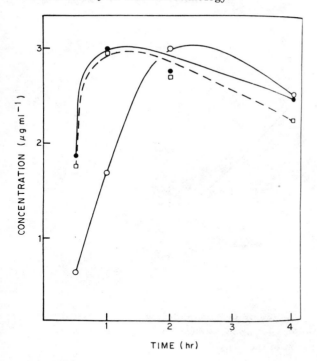

Figure 62. Theophylline serum levels, subject JWB, following a single 100-mg oral dose of theophylline. (1) Physically mixed with phenobarbital, (2) complexed with phenobarbital. ●, Free; ○, complex; □, physical mixture. (From Ref. 240.)

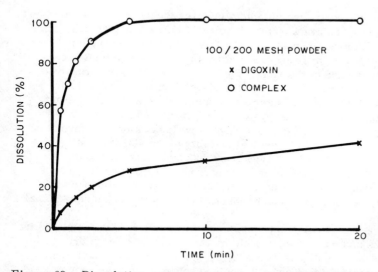

Figure 63. Dissolution-rate profiles obtained for the hydroquinone-digoxin complex and for digoxin itself under comparable conditions. (From Ref. 243; reproduced with permission of the copyright owner.)

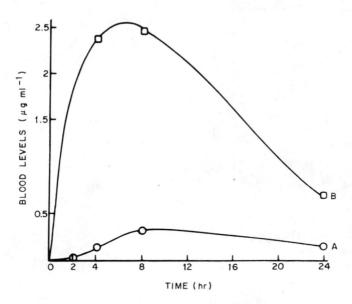

Figure 64. Mean coumermycin blood levels in humans following a single oral dose. A, alone; B, in combination with four parts of N-methylglucamine. (From Ref. 244; reprinted with permission of the copyright owner.)

N. Drug-Excipient Interactions

It is well known that the preparation of tablets involves the use of so-called "inert" ingredients. Excipient or adjuvant materials are added as binding agents, lubricants, disintegrants, diluent, or coating materials and are necessary for the preparation of a good-quality drug product. Since these ingredients often constitute a considerable portion of the tablet, the possibility exists for drug-excipient interactions to influence drug stability, dissolution rate, and drug absorption; but a physical or chemical interaction between the drug and adjuvant may result in the modification of the physical state, particle size, and/or surface area of the drug available to the absorption site. In addition, the formation of a surface complex or changes in chemical stability of the active constituent may result in toxic manifestations. Drugs bound by physical forces to excipients in the solid state generally separate rapidly from the excipient in aqueous solution. However, drugs bound via chemisorption are strongly attached to the excipient, which may result in incomplete absorption through the gastrointestinal membrane.

Several literature reports have appeared over the past decade describing drug-excipient interactions and the influence such interactions may have on drug bioavailability. An intensive review on this subject was conducted by Monkhouse and Lach [96], who stressed that drug products resulting from a generic or trade name manufacturer should be equally efficacious if proper care is taken

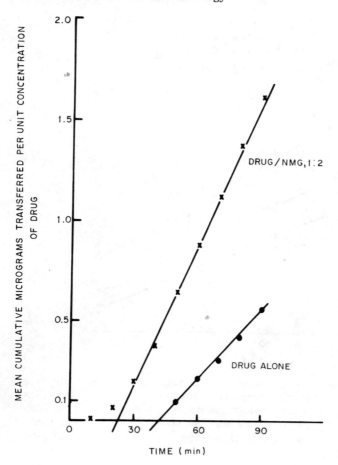

Figure 65. Everted intestinal sac data of a drug exhibiting poor in vitro permeability characteristics with and without the addition of 2 parts N-methylglucamine. (From Ref. 244; reprinted with permission of the copyright owner.)

during the formulation and manufacture of the dosage form to ensure optimum absorption. Space does not allow discussion of the paper by Monkhouse and Lach; however, important excipient studies referred to by them and published in the past few years should be mentioned. The interaction of dicumarol with several excipients was extensively studied by Akers and coworkers [245, 246]. Dicumarol administered with talc, Veegum, aluminum hydroxide, and starch resulted in lower plasma levels of the drug in dogs when compared to the drug alone (see Figs. 66 to 68). Significantly higher plasma levels (up to 180% of control values) were observed when dicumarol was administered with magnesium oxide or hydroxide, and this was thought to be due to the formation of a magnesium

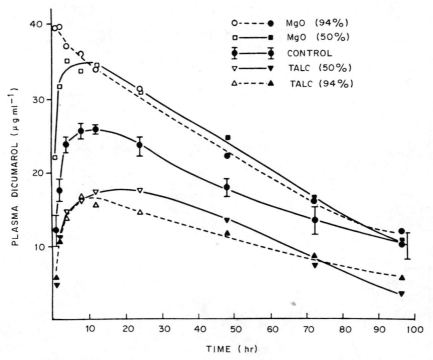

Figure 66. Plasma concentration of dicumarol after single oral doses of the drug given alone (control) or with various excipient materials. The values shown are the mean of four animals. Open data points indicate significant differences from control. Variations about the mean values was not statistically different from that of the control values shown with SEM. (From Ref. 245; reproduced with permission of the copyright owner.)

chelate. The chelate was later isolated and characterized by Spivey [247]. Studies in vivo with dogs confirmed that the dicumarol from the magnesium chelate was more bioavailable than was the dicumarol itself. This effect is very interesting since, to the contrary, chelation has been reported to lower blood levels of drugs (e.g., tetracycline complexes with calcium and iron). Dissolution studies with three commercial dicumarol tablets (see Fig. 69) and in vivo evaluation of these tablets in dogs [246] verified that drug excipient interactions with this drug can be of serious proportions.

In other studies with colloidal magnesium aluminum silicate, cationic drugs were found to bind strongly to the clay [248]. Urinary recovery studies with amphetamine sulfate [249], however, indicated that although absorption was delayed, bioavailability from the amphetamine-clay adsorbate was not significantly different from that with the pure drug.

Sorby [250] studied the influence of attapulgite and activated charcoal on the absorption of promazine and found that charcoal decreased both the rate and extent

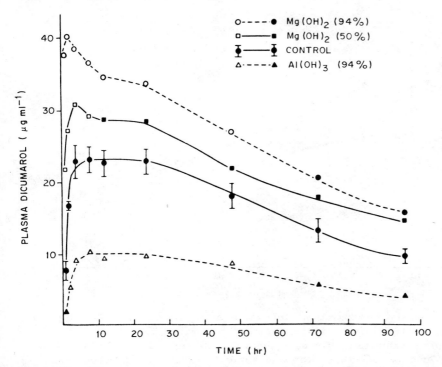

Figure 67. Plasma concentration of dicumarol after single oral doses of the drug given alone (control) or with various excipient materials. The values shown are the mean of four animals. Open data points indicate significant differences from control. Variations about the mean values was not statistically different from that of the control values shown with SEM. (From Ref. 245; reproduced with permission of the copyright owner.)

of absorption. Although attapulgite decreased the initial rate of drug absorption, there was no significant effect on total availability, since the drug was weakly bound to the clay. Later studies by Tsuchiya and Levy [251] suggested that it was possible to make reasonable predictions concerning the relative antidotal effectiveness of activated charcoal in humans on the basis of appropriate in vitro adsorption studies.

O. Surface-Active Agents

The improved oral absorption of drugs when administered with surface-active agents has been attributed to the improved solubility and dissolution rates due to solubilization and/or wetting effects of the surfactants. However, in evaluating the effect of surface-active agents on the absorption rate of a drug, it is essential to establish whether this effect is mediated by an alteration of the absorbing membrane, an interaction with the drug, or by a modification of the

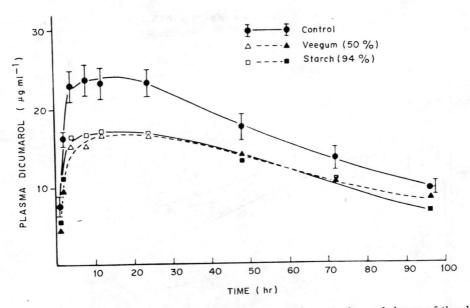

Figure 68. Plasma concentration of dicumarol after single oral doses of the drug given alone (control) or with various excipient materials. The values shown are the mean of four animals. Open data points indicate significant differences from control. Variations about the mean values was not statistically different from that of the control values shown with SEM. (From Ref. 245; reproduced with permission of the copyright owner.)

physical properties of the dosage form. According to Nogami et al. [68, 252, 253], the rate-determining step in tablet disintegration is the penetration of media through the pores in the tablet. An equation was derived [42] which was found applicable to tablets:

$$L^2 = \frac{r\gamma \cos \theta}{2\eta} t = kt \qquad (42)$$

where L is the length penetrated at time t, k the coefficient of penetration, r the average radius of the void space, θ the contact angle, and γ and η the surface tension and viscosity, respectively.

Equation (42) indicates that a surfactant has two effects on penetration of a liquid into the tablet. The addition of a surfactant lowers the surface tension and decreases the contact angle. Thus, the overall coefficient of penetration of a liquid into the tablet rises in the presence of surfactants, and increased penetration generally enhances disintegration. Ganderton [254] examined the effect of including a surfactant such as sodium lauryl sulfate on the breakup and dissolution of phenindione tablets and showed that the surfactant greatly assisted these effects over a wide range of pressures.

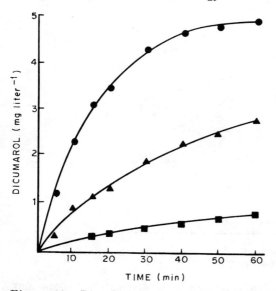

Figure 69. Dissolution rate of dicumarol from three commercial tablets. ▲, Product A; ●, product B; ■, product C. (From Ref. 246; reproduced with permission of the copyright owner.)

The surfactants dioctyl sodium sulfosuccinate and poloxamer 188, which are used internally as fecal softeners, have been shown to improve the dissolution rates and absorption characteristics of various sulfonamides [255-257].

The presence of a surface-active agent in the dissolution medium has also been investigated. At levels of surfactant below the critical micelle concentration (CMC), the principal effect involved would be a wetting phenomenon rather than solubilization, according to Finholt and Solvang [178]. These workers used phenacetin as the model hydrophobic drug and studied the dissolution rate of phenacetin in 0.1 N aqueous hydrochloric acid containing different amounts of polysorbate 80. The data in Figure 70 show the times for 100 mg of drug to dissolve as a function of the surface tension. Other investigators [258, 259] have shown improved dissolution rates at levels of surfactant below the CMC. Recently, Lim and Chen [260] reported that at pH 2.4 and 37° C, the apparent solubility of aspirin increased 17% in solutions of cetylpyridinium chloride above its CMC (0.2%). However, at concentrations below the CMC, dissolution rate and apparent solubility of aspirin decreased (see Fig. 71). Chiou et al. [261] enhanced the dissolution rates of sulfathiazole, prednisone, and chloramphenicol by recrystallization of the drugs in aqueous polysorbate 80 solutions.

Parrott and others [262, 263] have studied the effects of high concentrations of surfactants on the dissolution of benzoic acid. Using concentrations of surfactant exceeding the critical micelle concentration, the dissolution rate rose to a peak and then declined with increase in surfactant concentration, as seen in Figure 72. The total solubility of benzoic acid increased linearly as the concentration of the surfactant increased.

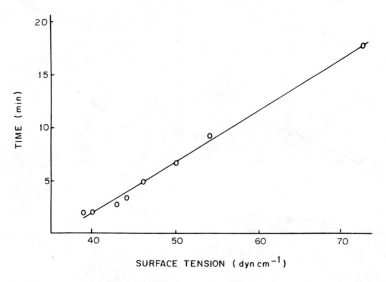

Figure 70. Relationship between the surface tension of the dissolution medium and the time necessary for dissolution of 100 mg of phenacetin (0.21-0.31 mm). Dissolution media: 0.1 N HCl containing different amounts of polysorbate 80. (From Ref. 178; reproduced with permission of the copyright owner.)

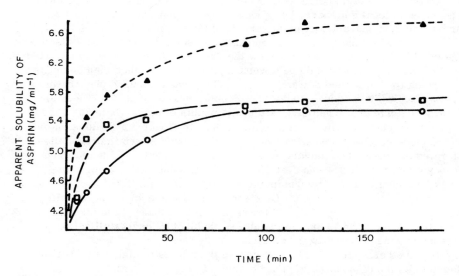

Figure 71. Effect of cetylpyridinium chloride on the apparent solubility of aspirin as a function of time at 37°C in pH 2.4 buffer. ▲, Above CMC, ○, below CMC; □, buffer control. (From Ref. 260; reproduced with permission of the copyright owner.)

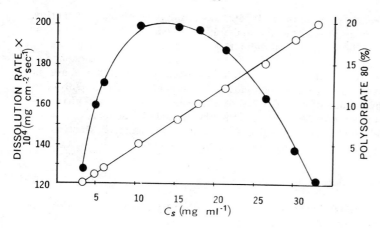

Figure 72. Relationship of total solubility C_S of benzoic acid at 25° C to dissolution rate and concentration of polysorbate 80. •, Rate; o, concentration. (From Ref. 263; reproduced with permission of the copyright owner.)

Elworthy and Lipscomb [264] substantiated these results by reporting that at high concentrations of surfactant, the viscosities of dissolution media were enhanced markedly, slowing the dissolution rate of griseofulvin.

IV. Pharmacokinetic Models and Methods

A basic understanding of pharmacokinetics—the quantitative description of the time course of drugs and metabolites in the body—is essential to the intelligent use of biopharmaceutics in tablet development. So far we have attempted to show that dosage formulation variables affect bioavailability and as a consequence alter clinical efficacy of medicinal agents in a significant way.

In the research laboratories and manufacturing plants of modern drug companies it is not enough to know that complex forces are at play. The scientific foundations of physical pharmacy, biopharmaceutics and pharmacokinetics, have advanced to a point where the pharmaceutical scientist is expected to apply current knowledge to the design of a tablet, suppository, suspension, or microcapsule with release properties and stability characteristics that result in maximum efficacy, safety, and therapeutic control.

These demands on the drug scientist require that he or she have at least an acquaintance with the quantitative aspects of pharmacokinetics and biopharmaceutics.

In order to follow the processes of absorption, distribution, metabolism, and elimination of drugs in the body and to relate these events to pharmacological action and therapeutic response, it is convenient to use models, that is, to represent the body as a system of compartments with the drug entering and leaving the compartments according to a postulated kinetic scheme. Modeling employs techniques of statistics, kinetics, and the devising of mathematical constructs in order to cast the observed data, such as blood levels and cumulative urinary excretion, into an organized sequence of steps which make up the model. The model is a hypothetical scheme, and the simplest mathematical construct that corresponds with the observed facts should be used. If it serves to explain the observed phenomena and allows predictions of results not yet obtained, it should be considered adequate even though it proves to be an oversimplification of the real situation. Only when results obtained from the use of a model fail to correspond to observed pharmacokinetic data should more elaborate compartmental models be sought.

Some of the models that have been used with success in pharmacokinetics and biopharmaceutics are described in the following paragraphs.

A. One-Compartment Model: Single Dosing

The one-compartment model, represented by the following scheme, considers the body as a homogeneous unit with an input and an output rate process.

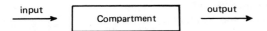

This model does not suggest that the concentration of drug in the blood plasma is equal to the concentration of drug in all tissues or fluids at any one time. The model implies, however, that whatever occurs regarding the drug concentration in the blood plasma is mirrored by changes in other tissues and fluids. Hence, if one could follow the time course of drug concentration in tissues and blood plasma, all levels should decline in a parallel fashion. This is illustrated in Figure 73A and B, where Figure 73B is a semilogarithmic plot of the data in Figure 73A. The ratio of the concentration of drug in blood plasma to the concentration of drug in the tissue at any given point in time is constant.

A convenience in utilizing the one-compartment model is that the output of drug from the body is frequently a first-order process. This means that the elimination of drug from the body is proportional to the amount of drug in the body at that time. The proportionality constant K is the apparent elimination-rate constant, drug elimination taking place by several physiological processes. The apparent first-order elimination-rate constant K is the sum of the individual rate constants for different elimination processes:

$$K = k_e + k_b + k_m + k_s + \cdots \tag{43}$$

where k_e and k_b are apparent first-order elimination-rate constants for renal and biliary excretion, respectively, and k_m and k_s are apparent first-order constants for metabolic and salivary processes.

Let us now turn our attention to the analysis of a one-compartment model after single-dose intravenous administration.

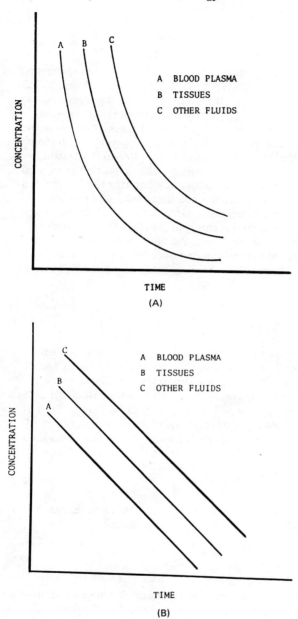

Figure 73.   (A) Time course of drug in body fluids and tissues (B) a semilog-arithmic plot of the data in (A).

1. Intravenous Injection

Plasma Levels

After intravenous injection of a single dose, the drug is distributed throughout the body by means of the vascular network. When the drug is injected rapidly into the bloodstream, it initially mixes with a small volume of blood, forming a bolus or mass of the administered dose. However, as it passes through the various capillary beds, filtration and diffusion effects cause some of the molecules to diffuse into the surrounding tissues. The rate of uptake of a compound into tissues is controlled by several factors, including the rate of blood flow to the tissue, permeability of the compound across tissue membranes, the mass of tissue, and partition characteristics of the compound between plasma and tissues. Partitioning, in turn, is affected by the pH of the medium, complexation, and plasma protein binding. In addition to distribution processes, drugs are metabolized or excreted unchanged in urine, bile, saliva, and other body fluids. In each of these systems the intact drug may undergo recycling into the body rather than direct elimination. If the drug is distributed and eliminated according to a one-compartment model, the rate of loss of drug from the body is given by the first-order expression,

$$\frac{dA}{dt} = -KA \tag{44}$$

where A is the amount of drug at time t after injection, dA/dt the change of the amount of drug dA in the single compartment representing the body with respect to the infinitesimal duration of time, dt and K, as illustrated in Equation (43), is the overall elimination-rate constant. The negative sign in Equation (43) indicates that the amount of drug in the body is decreasing with time.

Equation (44) is a first-order linear differential equation, and integration of this equation according to elementary principles of calculus or by use of Laplace transforms [265-267] results in

$$A = A_0 e^{-Kt} \tag{45}$$

The initial condition for the integration is that $A = A_0$ = initial intravenous (i.v.) dose. Conversion of Equation (45) to Briggsian logarithms leads to

$$\log A = \log A_0 - \frac{Kt}{2.303} \tag{46}$$

It should be understood that owing to the process of distribution, the body cannot be truly considered a homogenous unit, the drug concentration in blood plasma differing from drug concentration in tissues. However, the ratio of blood plasma drug concentration to tissue drug concentration will be constant at any point in time, and a constant relationship exists between the drug concentration C in the plasma and the amount A of drug in the body:

$$A = V_d D \tag{47}$$

where V_d is a proportionality constant termed "apparent volume of distribution"; the units of V_d are volume units. If A is expressed as milligrams of drug per kilogram of body weight and plasma concentration as mg liter^{-1}, V_d has the units liter kg^{-1}. No physiological meaning should be attached to this constant; rather it should be considered simply as a proportionality term which allows one to relate amount A in the body to concentration C.

Equation (5) enables the conversion of Equation (46) to be expressed in concentration terms:

$$\log C = \log C_0 - \frac{Kt}{2.303} \tag{48}$$

Equation (48) yields a straight line and extrapolation to time zero gives C_0, the plasma concentration at initial injection. The value of the apparent first-order elimination-rate constant K can be obtained from the slope of the line. C_0 may be used to calculate the value of the apparent distribution V_d using the relationship

$$V_d = \frac{A_0}{C_0} \tag{49}$$

where A_0 is the i.v. dose.

The graphical representation of Equation (48) is illustrated in Figure 74.

The biological or elimination half-life $t_{1/2}$ is defined as the time required for the drug concentration at any point on the straight line to decrease to one-half of its original value. The half-life can be obtained either graphically as illustrated in Figure 74 or by use of the following relationship:

$$t_{1/2} = \frac{0.693}{K} \tag{50}$$

The best values for K, $t_{1/2}$, and C_0 are obtained by least-squares regression analysis of the data.

Example 1: Sample Calculation of Pharmacokinetic Parameters Using Plasma Concentration-Time Data Following I.V. Administration of a Drug That is Represented by a One-Compartment Model

A subject received an i.v. dose of 100 mg of a drug, and plasma concentrations of drug were determined as a function of time. The results are illustrated in Table 16. Calculate (a) the overall elimination-rate constant K, (b) the volume of distribution V_d, (c) the elimination half-life $t_{1/2}$, and (d) C_0. Assume that the drug is eliminated by an apparent first-order process.

Solution:

Step 1. To solve this problem, start by using Equation (48), which shows that a plot of the logarithm of the drug plasma concentration versus time is linear. The result of plotting the data is illustrated in Figure 75.

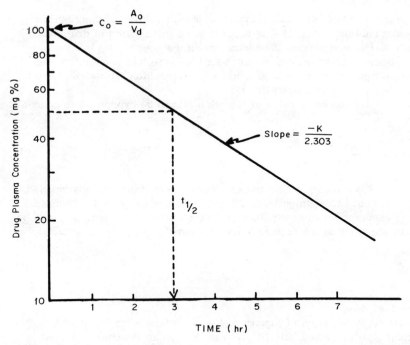

Figure 74. Semilogarithmic plot of the concentration of drug in the blood plasma as a function of time after single intravenous administration.

Table 16

Plasma Concentration of a Drug After
Intravenous Administration of 100 mg

Time (hr)	Plasma concentration (μg ml^{-1})
1	60.65
2	36.79
3	22.31
4	13.53
5	8.21
6	4.98
7	3.02

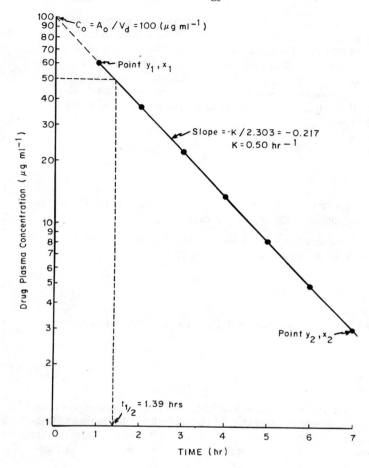

Figure 75. Semilogarithmic plot of the concentration of drug in the blood plasma following intravenous administration of a drug represented by a one-compartment model.

Step 2. Calculate the slope of the line. An equation for obtaining slope is

$$S = \frac{\log y_1 - \log y_2}{x_1 - x_2}$$

Using the points $y_1 = 60.65$, $x_1 = 1$ hr and $y_2 = 3.02$, $x_2 = 7$ hr from Figure 75 we get

$$S = \frac{1.78 - 0.48}{1 - 7} = -0.217$$

The slope of a line is more accurately obtained by use of a pocket calculator that uses linear regression by least squares. The Texas Instrument SR-56 or the Commodore SR 4190R allows one to obtain the slope, intercept, and correlation coefficient for two variables that are related linearly. The Hewlett-Packard 25 or HP 67 are programmable calculators and are easily programmed to solve problems in linear and nonlinear regression analysis.

The slope is equal to -0.217. According to Equation (48), the slope is equal to $-K/2.303$. Thus.

$$-K = \text{slope} \times 2.303$$

$$K = -(0.217 \times 2.303) = 0.5$$

Step 3. Extrapolate the line to time zero to obtain C_0. In this particular example, C_0 is equal to 100 $\mu g/ml^{-1}$ (see Fig. 75.)

Step 4. Knowledge of C_0 and the intravenous dose enables one to calculate the volume of distribution V_d by means of Equation (49).

$$V_d = \frac{100,000}{100} = 1000 \text{ ml} = 1 \text{ liter}$$

Step 5. Calculation of the elimination half-life is accomplished using Equation (50). Thus,

$$t_{1/2} = \frac{0.693}{0.500} = 1.39 \text{ hr}$$

Another method to calculate the half-life is graphical representation of the data. At time t = 0, the drug plasma concentration is 100 $\mu g/ml^{-1}$. Using the definition of half-life at drug plasma concentration of 50 $\mu g/ml^{-1}$, or one-half the original value, the half-life is read from the horizontal axis as roughly 1.4 hr (see Fig. 75).

Urinary Excretion

K, $t_{1/2}$, and C_0 can also be obtained using urinary excretion data, since the amount of unchanged drug in the urine is proportional to the amount of drug in the body. The excretion rate dA_u/dt can be expressed in terms of first-order kinetics as

$$\frac{dA_u}{dt} = k_e A \qquad (51)$$

It is important to recognize that k_e is the apparent first-order elimination-rate constant for unchanged drug. The overall elimination constant K does not appear in this equation, since it is the summation of k_e together with other elimination-rate constants.

Substitution of Equation (45) into Equation (51) leads to

$$\frac{dA_u}{dt} = k_e A_0 e^{-Kt} \qquad (52)$$

dA_u/dt can be approximated by $\Delta A_u/\Delta t$; therefore,

$$\frac{\Delta A_u}{\Delta t} = k_e A_0 e^{-Kt} \tag{53}$$

Taking the logarithm of this equation results in

$$\log \frac{\Delta A_u}{\Delta t} = \log k_e A_0 - \frac{Kt}{2.303} \tag{54}$$

Equation (54) is a straight line when the excretion rate of unchanged drug in the urine $\Delta A_u/\Delta t$, in mg/hr^{-1}, is plotted versus time; it provides a technique called the "elimination-rate method." The slope of the line is $-K/2.303$. Thus, the overall elimination rate constant K can be obtained from this relationship, and the elimination half-life is calculated using Equation (50).

It is important to consider that dA_u/dt is not an instantaneous rate but rather an average rate $\Delta A_u/\Delta t$ obtained over the finite time period Δt. Consequently, when constructing the graph, average excretion rates should be plotted versus the midpoint of a short urine-collection-time interval. At the midpoint of each Δt, the average excretion rate will approximate the instantaneous excretion rate.

Other methods exist to analyze urinary excretion data. Swintosky [268] introduced a technique that can be used when drug elimination continues over long periods of time. This method is also employed when the rate of excretion of drug and metabolite are maximum.

Sigma-Minus Method

Another useful analysis of urinary excretion data can be obtained through the sigma-minus method, a procedure introduced by Martin [269]. This method requires accurate assessment of the total amount of drug or metabolite excreted in the urine. The method becomes impractical when drug elimination is slow or when the data relate to multiple-dose therapy. The sigma-minus method is not applicable when drug elimination is a zero-order process. However, this approach overcomes the problem of fluctuations in the rate of drug elimination which one obtains when using the excretion-rate plot based on Equation (54). Figure 76 illustrates that fluctuations in the rate of drug elimination are reflected to a much greater extent in the excretion-rate method than in the sigma-minus method.

The following mathematical treatment leads to the equation utilized in the sigma-minus method. Integration of Equation (52), assuming that $A_u = 0$ at $t = 0$, yields

$$A_u = \frac{k_e A_0}{K} (1 - e^{-Kt}) \tag{55}$$

where A_u is the cumulative amount of unchanged drug excreted to time t. At time $t = \infty$, Equation (55) reduces to

$$A_u^\infty = \frac{k_e A_0}{K} \tag{56}$$

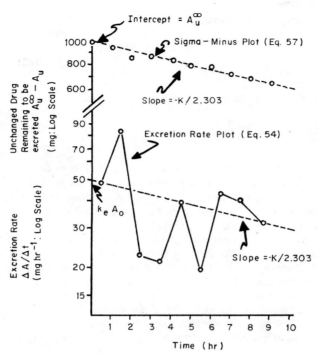

Figure 76. Log sigma-minus plot and corresponding log rate plot relating to data for the excretion of drug in urine. The dashed lines represents a theoretical decline corresponding to $K = 0.05$ hr^{-1}. Fluctuations in the rate of drug elimination are reflected to a much greater extent in the rate plot. (From Ref. 269.)

where A_u^∞ is the total amount of unchanged drug eliminated in the urine. Substitution of A_u^∞ for $k_e A_0/K$ in Equation (55) gives

$$\log (A_u^\infty - A_u) = \log A_u^\infty - \frac{Kt}{2.303} \tag{57}$$

Equation (58) is a straight line with a slope of $-K/2.303$; consequently, K can be determined using urinary excretion data. If the drug is eliminated unchanged in the urine and is not eliminated by other routes, k_e becomes equal to K and from Equation (56) is can be seen that A_u^∞ becomes A_0, which is the initial i.v. dose.

Several practical applications of these methods have been reported in the literature [270-272].

Example 2. Sample Calculation of Pharmacokinetic Parameters Following Intravenous Bolus Injection of a Drug That Is Represented by a One-Compartment Model Using Urinary Excretion Data.

A 100-mg dose of a drug was administered i.v. to a subject and the cumulative amount of drug in the urine was obtained as a function of time. The

Table 17

Cumulative Amount Excreted Unchanged After Intravenous Administration of 100 mg
of a Drug

Time, t (hr)	Cumulative amount A_u (mg)	$t_{midpoint}$	Δt	ΔA_u	$\dfrac{\Delta A_u}{\Delta t}$	$A_u^\infty - A_u$
0	0					28.85
0.5	8.45	0.25	0.5	8.45	16.90	20.40
1.0	14.43	0.75	0.5	5.98	11.96	14.42
1.5	18.65	1.25	0.5	4.22	8.44	10.20
2.0	21.64	1.75	0.5	2.99	5.98	7.21
2.5	23.76	2.25	0.5	2.12	4.24	5.09
3.0	25.25	2.75	0.5	1.49	2.98	3.60
3.5	26.31	3.25	0.5	1.06	2.12	2.54
4.0	27.06	3.75	0.5	0.75	1.50	1.79
5.0	27.96	4.5	1.0	0.90	0.9	0.89
6.0	28.41	5.5	1.0	0.45	0.45	0.44
7.0	28.63	6.5	1.0	0.22	0.22	0.22
8.0	28.75	7.5	1.0	0.12	0.12	0.10
∞	$A_u^\infty = 28.85$					0.0

results are illustrated in Table 17. Using the sigma-minus method and the excretion-rate method, estimate (1) the half-life of the drug, (2) the overall
elimination-rate constant K, (3) the rate constant for elimination of unchanged
drug, and (4) the cumulative amount of drug excreted unchanged at 4.5 hr.

Solution:

Step 1. Equation (54) shows that a plot of log $\Delta A_u / \Delta t$ versus t will result in a
straight line. The slope is equal to $-K/2.303$ and the intercept $k_e A_0$. The use
of this equation requires that log $\Delta A_u / \Delta t$ be plotted against the midpoint of a
short urine-collection interval (see Table 17). According to Figure 77, the
slope and the intercept of the line are -0.30 and 20.0 mg, respectively. Thus,

$$K = -slope \times 2.303 = -(-0.30 \times 3.303) = 0.691 \text{ hr}^{-1}$$

$$k_e = \frac{intercept}{A_0} = \frac{20}{100} = 0.20 \text{ hr}^{-1}$$

Step 2. Equation (58) shows that a plot of log $(A_u^\infty - A_u)$ versus time will result
in a straight line with a slope equal to $-K/2.303$. According to Figure 77, the
slope is equal to -0.30. Thus,

$$K = -slope \times 2.303 = -(-0.30 \times 2.303) = 0.691 \text{ hr}^{-1}$$

This is the same value obtained in step 1 for K, as would be expected.

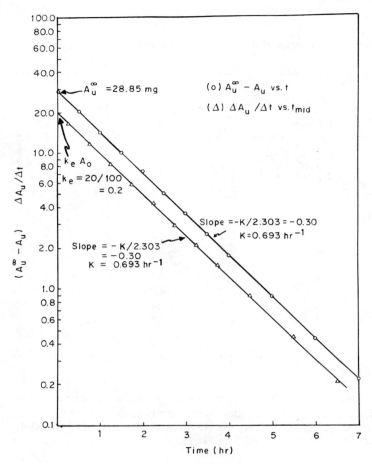

Figure 77. Log sigma-minus plot (o) and corresponding log rate plot (Δ) relating to data for the urinary excretion of a drug following intravenous bolus injection. The drug is represented by a one-compartment model.

Step 3. Another way to calculate k_e is given by Equation (56).

$$k_e = \frac{KA_u^\infty}{A_0} = \frac{0.691 \times 28.85}{100} = 0.20 \text{ hr}^{-1}$$

Step 4. The cumulative amount excreted unchanged up to 4.5 hr can be estimated by means of Equation (55). Thus,

$$A_{u(4.5 \text{ hr})} = \frac{0.20 \times 100}{0.691} (1 - e^{-0.691 \times 4.5}) = 27.61 \text{ mg}$$

2. Oral Absorption

The treatment here follows the excellent description of Gibaldi and Perrier [273]. The reader should also refer to Wagner's explanation of dosage regimen and its calculations; he [274] introduced a number of dose regimen equations. Equation (58) represents the pharmacokinetic model of a drug entering the body by an apparent first-order rate process, as is customarily found for oral, rectal, and intra-muscular administration. The drug, administered as a single dose, is absorbed and eliminated from the body by apparent first-order processes. One-compartment characteristics are observed in this case.

$$G \xrightarrow{k_a} A \xrightarrow{K} U \tag{58}$$

G is the amount of drug at the absorption site, A the amount in the body, and U the amount eliminated unchanged in the urine.

The differential equation describing the change in A is given by

$$\frac{dA}{dt} = k_a G - KA \tag{59}$$

The term k_a is the apparent first-order absorption-rate constant, and K is the apparent first-order overall elimination-rate constant. The rate of loss at the absorption site is given by

$$\frac{dG}{dt} = -k_a G \tag{60}$$

Integration of Equation (60), assuming that G is the dose at t = 0, leads to

$$G = G_0 e^{-k_a t} \tag{61}$$

However, it should be remembered that in most cases only a fraction of the dose is absorbed. Thus,

$$G = F G_0 e^{-k_a t} \tag{62}$$

where F is the fraction of the administered dose G_0 that is absorbed following oral administration. Substituting Equation (62) into Equation (59) and integrating assuming that $A = A_0 = 0$ at t = 0 leads to

$$A = \frac{k_a F G_0}{k_a - K} (e^{-Kt} - e^{-k_a t}) \tag{63}$$

which is expressed in terms of concentration as

$$C = \frac{k_a F G_0}{(k_a - K) V_d} (e^{-Kt} - e^{-k_a t}) \tag{64}$$

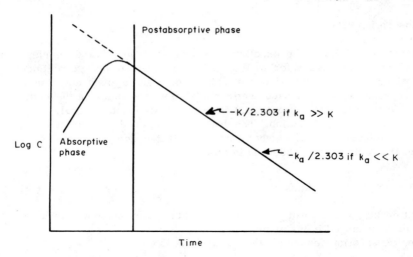

Figure 78. Semilogarithmic plot of drug levels in plasma after oral administration of a single dose of a drug. The slope values are explained in the text.

where V_d is the apparent volume of distribution. It is helpful to consider two situations: the usual case, where absorption is rapid and then subsides to insignificance while elimination continues at a finite rate ($k_a \gg K$); and a second instance in which K is large relative to k_a (that is, $k_a \ll K$), owing to rapid drug elimination or slow release of the drug from its dosage form. In the first case k_a is appreciably greater than K—say, 10 to 100 times as large—then $e^{-k_a t}$ will become quite small as time proceeds, whereas e^{-Kt} remains significant. Equation (64) then reduces to

$$C = \frac{k_a F G_0}{(k_a - K)V_d} e^{-Kt} \tag{65}$$

This case is the one more frequently encountered after oral administration of drugs. Equation (65) describes the concentration of drug in the body after absorption has ceased (i.e., during the postabsorptive period).

The logarithm of Equation (65) is

$$\log C = \log \frac{k_a F G_0}{(k_a - K)V_d} - \frac{Kt}{2.303} \tag{66}$$

Log C may be plotted on the vertical axis of a graph versus time on the horizontal axis to yield a curve as shown in Figure 78. The terminal portion or postabsorptive phase is essentially linear with a slope of $-K/2.303$, following Equation (66). Employing Equation (50), the half-life for elimination can also be calculated.

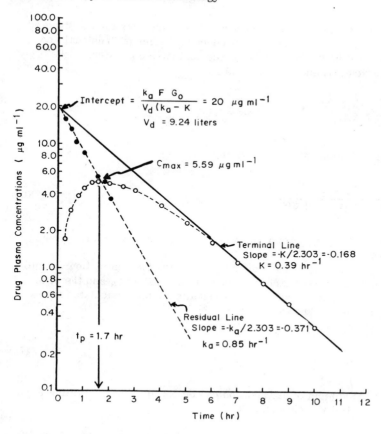

Figure 79. Semilogarithmic plot of the concentration of drug in the blood plasma following single oral administration of a drug represented by a one-compartment model.

In the reverse case where K is significantly greater than k_a, the slope of the line in the terminal phase will now be equal to $-k_a/2.303$. The flip in slope from $-K/2.303$ to $-k_a/2.303$ is called a "flip-flop" model and is usually observed when drugs are rapidly eliminated (K large). An example of this phenomenon is provided by ampicillin kinetics as reported by Doluisio et al. [275]. The value for the rate constant of absorption k_a may be calculated as follows. The "method of residuals" (also called feathering or stripping) is used to obtain a residual line, and the slope of this line for the usual case where $k_a > K$ is $-k_a/2.303$. This is illustrated in Figure 79.

According to Equation (66), the terminal linear portion of the curve with slope $-K/2.303$ may be extrapolated to $t = 0$ to provide an intercept value, I:

$$I = \log \frac{k_a FG_0}{(k_a - K)V_d} \qquad (67)$$

The actual plasma levels of the early portion of the curve are then subtracted from the extrapolated line. This procedure produces a series of "residual" concentrations, Cr, as found in Table 17. These residuals are equivalent to the difference between Equation (64) and Equation (65):

$$Cr = \frac{k_a FG_0}{(k_a - K)V_d} e^{-k_a t} \tag{68}$$

A plot of Cr on a logarithmic scale versus time

$$\log Cr = \log \frac{k_a FG_0}{(k_a - K)V_d} - \frac{k_a t}{2.303} \tag{69}$$

yields a straight line [Eq. (69)] with a slope of $-k_a/2.303$ and an intercept I as given by Equation (67).

By such a method of residuals it is possible to resolve the original curve into its component parameters, particularly the absorption constant k_a and the elimination constant K. The apparent volume of distribution can be calculated from the y intercept if k_a and K are known:

$$V_d = \frac{k_a FG_0}{(k_a - K)I} \tag{70}$$

A better estimate of the volume of distribution can be obtained by integrating Equation (64) from zero to infinity. This leads to

$$\int_0^\infty C \, dt = \frac{FG_0}{V_d K} \tag{71}$$

where the left term of the equation is the area under the plasma concentration–time curve. Rearrangement of Equation (71) gives

$$V_d = \frac{FG_0}{K \int_0^\infty C \, dt} \tag{72}$$

If the total dose administered is absorbed, then F is equal to 1.

Calculating the Time at Peak Concentration t_p

Two quantities are of particular importance in studying the biopharmaceutics of rival products either during the formulation stage or during evaluation of competitive marketed forms of a generic drug. These are the peak or maximum bioconcentration C_{max} attained with a particular dose of the drug, and the time t_p following administration that the blood level reaches its maximum value.

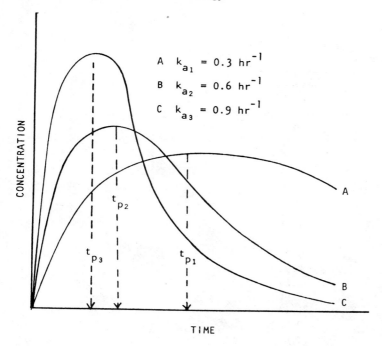

Figure 80. Effect of the absorption rate k_a on the time to peak t_p. As k_a increases, t_p decreases.

Differentiation of Equation (64) with respect to time and assuming that at peak concentration in the plasma concentration-time curve $dc/dt = 0$ results in the expression

$$\frac{k_a}{K} = \frac{e^{-kt_p}}{e^{-k_a t_p}} \tag{73}$$

where t_p is the time to peak.

Further simplification of Equation (73) leads to a solution for the time to peak t_p:

$$t_p = \frac{2.303}{k_a - K} \log \frac{k_a}{K} \tag{74}$$

It will be observed from Equation (74) that as the absorption rate increases, the time to peak decreases. This is illustrated in Figure 80.

Maximum plasma concentration C_{max} is easily estimated by substituting t_p for t in Equation (64), yielding

$$C_{max} = \frac{k_a FG_0}{V_d(k_a - K)} (e^{-Kt_p} - e^{-k_a t_p}) \tag{75}$$

Table 18

Concentration Time Data Obtained Following
Oral Administration of a Drug

Time (hr)	Drug concentration (μg ml^{-1})
0	0
0.25	1.72
0.5	2.97
0.75	3.84
1.0	4.42
1.5	4.95
1.75	5.0
2.0	4.95
2.5	4.65
3.0	4.21
4.0	3.22
5.0	2.34
6.0	1.65
7.0	1.14
8.0	0.78
9.0	0.53
10.0	0.36

Combining Equation (74) and (75) leads to a simple equation for estimating the peak blood level C_{max}:

$$C_{max} = \frac{FG_0}{V_d} e^{-Kt_p} \tag{76}$$

Now that we have presented the equations as derived by Gibaldi and Perrier [273], let us apply them to the oral administration of a drug product.

Example 3: Sample Calculation of Pharmacokinetic Parameters Using Plasma Concentration-Time Data Following Oral Administration of a Drug That Is Represented by a One-Compartment Model.

A subject received a single oral dose of 100 mg in a tablet dosage form, and the drug plasma concentration was obtained as a function of time. The results are illustrated in Table 18. Calculate (a) the absorption-rate constant k_a, (b) the elimination-rate constant K, (c) the volume of distribution V_d, (d) time to peak t_p, and (e) the maximum drug concentration C_{max}. Assume that the fraction of the dose absorbed F is equal to 1.0.

Solution:

Step 1. Plot the values from Table 18 on semilogarithmic paper. Figure 79 provides a graphical representation of the data (open circles).

Table 19

Residual Values: Plasma Concentration-Time Data Following Oral Administration of a Drug

Time (hr)	Drug concentration ($\mu g/ml^{-1}$)	Extrapolated concentration ($\mu g/ml^{-1}$)	Residual concentration ($\mu g/ml^{-1}$)
0.25	1.72	17.5	15.78
0.5	2.97	16.0	13.03
0.75	3.84	14.0	10.16
1.0	4.42	13.0	8.58
1.5	4.95	10.5	5.55
1.75	5.0	10.0	5.0
2.0	4.95	8.6	3.65

Step 2. Extrapolate the terminal linear phase to time zero, where one observes the intercept to be 20.0 $\mu g\ ml^{-1}$.

Step 3. Calculate the slope of the terminal linear phase. According to Equation (66), the slope of the line should be equal to $-K/2.303$. Thus,

$-K$ = slope x 2.303

$\quad = -(0.168 \times 2.303) = 0.39\ hr^{-1}$

Step 4. Using the method of residuals ("feathering"), calculate the residual concentration values. These values are obtained by subtracting the true plasma drug concentration values in the absorptive phase from the corresponding drug concentration values on the extrapolated linear portion of the line. Table 19 illustrates the results.

Step 5. On the same graph, plot the residual values of column 4, Table 19 (see Fig. 79). Calculate the slope of this line using the two-point formula or a desk calculator. The result is -0.371. The slope is equal to $-k_a/2.303$; therefore,

$k_a = -(-0.371 \times 2.303) = 0.85\ hr^{-1}$

Step 6. Equation (66) indicates that the intercept at time zero is equal to $k_aFG_0/(k_a - K)V_d$. This allows us to calculate the volume of distribution. From Figure 79 we see that the intercept I is equal to 20 $\mu g\ ml^{-1}$. Thus,

$$V_d = \frac{k_a FG_0}{(k_a - K)(I)}$$

$$= \frac{0.85 \times 1.0 \times 100}{(0.85 - 0.39)20} = 9.24\ liters$$

A second method to calculate the volume of distribution is given by Equation (72). This requires the estimate of the area under the plasma concentration-time curve from time zero to infinity. In this particular case, the area is approximately equal to 27.75 μg ml^{-1} hr^{-1}. The area under the curve may be calculated using the trapezoidal rule or more elaborate methods, such as Simpson's rule. (A program for using the Simpson rule is provided with the programmable HP-25 hand calculator of Hewlett-Packard, for example.)

$$V_d = \frac{FG_0}{K \int_0^\infty C \, dt} = \frac{1.0 \times 100}{0.39 \times 27.75} = 9.24 \text{ liters}$$

Step 7. Equation (74) allows calculation of time to peak t_p:

$$t_p = \frac{2.303}{0.85 - 0.39} \log \frac{0.85}{0.39} = 1.7 \text{ hr}$$

See Figure 79 for a visual estimation of t_p in comparison with the calculated value, 1.7 hr.

Step 8. Equation (75) provides an expression for calculating maximum plasma concentration on the time curve:

$$C_{max} = \frac{0.85 \times 1 \times 100}{9.24 \, (0.85 - 0.39)} \, (e^{-0.39 \times 1.7} - e^{-0.85 \times 1.7})$$

$$= 5.59 \, \mu g \, ml^{-1}$$

B. One-Compartment Model: Multiple Dosing

The implications and mathematical analysis of multiple-dosing pharmacokinetics on dosage form design have been extensively reviewed by Krüger-Thiemer and others [276-281]. Both Wagner [282, 283] and Gibaldi and Perrier [284] describe multiple dosing in some detail, and readers will profit by familiarizing themselves with these sources and the original literature that is referred to in these books. The treatment of this section on multiple dosing follows the outline of Gibaldi and Perrier [284], and ends with sample calculations that hopefully provide the reader with a better understanding of the somewhat complex equations used to describe multiple dosing. Although the discussion of pharmacokinetics up to this point has centered on the administration of a single dose of drug, the most common therapy involves a practice of multiple dosing with the purpose of reaching and maintaining a desired therapeutic blood concentration over an extended period of time.

In treating an acute headache, a single dose of aspirin may be given. For producing sleep, a single dose of sedative is usually effective. But for mild arthritis, aspirin tablets may be given every 4 hr over a period of days. For effective antibacterial action, antibiotics are ordinarily taken according to a prescribed dosage regimen for perhaps 10 days or longer. In the case of onycomycosis, griseofulvin is recommended to be taken for as long as 6 months to a year, until the infected toe or fingernail shows no more presence of the infecting organism.

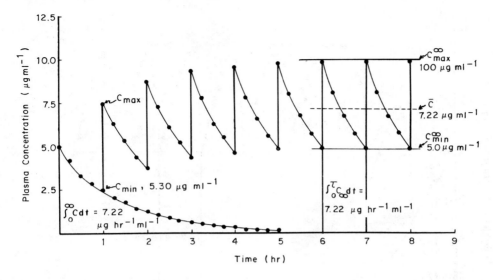

Figure 81. One-compartment model of multiple-dose intravenous administration of equal doses of a drug at a uniform time interval τ.

Figures 75 and 79 show the rise and fall in drug blood level curves for single dosing from time of administration until the concentration of drug in the body can no longer be determined. As previously indicated, the area under the concentration-time curve provides an important means for estimating the relative bioavail-ability of a drug administered in various drug delivery systems.

When a dose of drug is repeated at definite time intervals, the therapeutic regimen is referred to as multiple dosing. Such a sequence of dosing is shown in Figures 81 and 82. It is observed that following the first dose, the blood level of the second dose adds on to the blood level remaining from the first dose. Each new dose elevates the blood level more because it is added to drug concentration remaining from previous doses. The succession of blood level curves have the shape of the single-dose curves. Each curve begins at the time a new dose is ad-ministered, rises to a maximum or peak value C_{max}, and then falls as drug is excreted and each dose is exhausted. In the meantime, at a definite dosing time interval τ, a new dose is administered and another concentration-time curve rises through a peak value and falls to zero.

As observed in Figures 81 and 82, a program of multiple dosing results in both a C_{max} and a C_{min}, and eventually a steady-state plateau is reached where C_{max} and C_{min} no longer change in value with the administration of successive doses. By following the increases in blood level as each new dose is added to the figures, readers can satisfy themselves that the plateau is reached when the first dose is essentially eliminated from the body. Actually, the single-dose value approaches zero asymptotically, and complete elimination is never reached. However, 97% of the plateau value is attained in a period of five half-lives, and 99% is attained after seven half-lives. For a drug with $t_{1/2} = 5$ hr, the plateau is therefore reached in 25 to 35 hr.

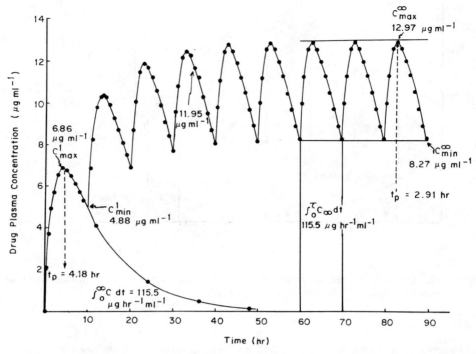

Figure 82. One-compartment model of multiple-dose oral administration of equal doses of a drug at a uniform time interval τ.

1. Multiple Dosing by Intravenous Administration.

Benet introduced a method by which multiple-dose equations can be readily obtained [267]. He has shown that any equation describing the time course of a drug leaving a compartment after a single dose may be changed into a multiple-dose equation by multiplying each exponential term containing t (time) (i.e., $e^{-k_i t}$) by the function

$$\frac{e^{(n-1)k_i \tau} - e^{-k_i \tau}}{1 - e^{k_i \tau}} \tag{77}$$

where τ is the dosing interval, k_i the apparent first-order rate constant in each exponential term, and n is equal to the number of doses.

Based on these considerations, Equation (45) can be converted to the following multiple-dose equation:

$$A \left(\frac{1 - e^{-nK\tau}}{1 - e^{-K\tau}} \right) = A_0 \left(\frac{1 - e^{-nK\tau}}{1 - e^{-K\tau}} \right) e^{-Kt} = A_n \tag{78}$$

which in concentration terms becomes

$$C_n = \frac{A_0}{V_d}\left(\frac{1 - e^{-nK_T}}{1 - e^{-K_T}}\right) e^{-Kt} \tag{79}$$

where t is the time elapsed since dose n was administered. Equation (79) allows the calculation of the drug plasma concentration at any point in time during a dosing interval. It can be seen from this equation that the plasma concentration increases with time and approaches a steady-state level. After multiple dosing for a time equal to seven half-lives, the plasma concentration is within 1% of the steady-state level or plateau level.

To obtain the plasma concentration at steady state, Equation (79) can be used. By setting n to infinity we obtained C_∞, which is the plasma concentration as a function of time at steady state.

$$C_\infty = \frac{A_0}{V_d}\left(\frac{1}{1 - e^{-K_T}}\right) e^{-Kt} \tag{80}$$

Similarly, the minimum plasma concentration C_{min} at steady state can be expressed as

$$C_{min}^\infty = \frac{A_0}{V_d}\left(\frac{1}{1 - e^{-K_T}}\right) e^{-K_T} \tag{81}$$

and the maximum plasma concentration at steady state becomes

$$C_{max}^\infty = \frac{A_0}{V_d}\left(\frac{1}{1 - e^{-K_T}}\right) \tag{82}$$

The "average" concentration of drug at steady state $\overline{C}_\infty$ is frequently referred to in the literature of multiple dosing:

$$\overline{C}_\infty = \frac{\int_0^\tau C_\infty \, dt}{\tau} \tag{83}$$

In Equation (83), $\int_0^\tau C_\infty \, dt$ is the area under the curve at steady state during a dosing interval (see Fig. 81 for a graphical depiction of this area) and is not a true average value of C_{max}^∞ and C_{min}^∞. The area under the curve may be obtained from the Simpson or trapezoidal rule or calculated from the expression

$$\int_0^\tau C_\infty \, dt = \frac{A_0}{V_d K} \tag{84}$$

Substituting Equation (84) into (83) yields

$$\bar{C}_\infty = \frac{A_0}{V_d K} \frac{1}{\tau} \tag{85}$$

Krüger-Thiemer and Bunger [278] have extensively discussed the concept of loading dose when drugs are administered repetitively. If a drug has a long half-life, considerable time may be required before the plateau blood level is reached. This delay may be circumvented by use of a loading dose. The loading dose A_0^* is estimated using the equation

$$A_0^* = A_0 \left(\frac{1}{1 - e^{-K\tau}} \right) \tag{86}$$

where A_0 is the maintenance dose. This equation applies when the drug is administered intravenously and confers one-compartment model characteristics on the body. A practical example of this equation has been illustrated by Krüger-Thiemer et al. [285].

It is interesting to note that if the half-life $(0.693/K)$ of the drug is equal to the dosing interval τ, then Equation (86) becomes

$$A_0^* = 2A_0 \tag{87}$$

which indicates that the loading dose is twice the maintenance dose.

Example 4. Sample Calculation of Pharmacokinetic Parameters Following Multiple Intravenous Administration of a Drug That Is Represented by a One-Compartment Model.

A subject was administered 50 mg of a drug solution intravenously every hour for a period of 9 hr and plasma concentrations of drug were obtained as a function of time. The results are illustrated in Figure 81. Two weeks prior to this treatment the subject received a single intravenous dose of 50 mg of the drug solution. The elimination half-life of the drug, the area under the plasma concentration-time curve, and the volume of distribution were found from the single-dose study to be 1 hr, 7.22 μg hr^{-1} ml^{-1}, and 10 liters, respectively. Assuming that there was no change in renal and metabolic function of the subject, when multiple dosing was conducted, calculate (a) the elimination rate constant K, (b) the plasma concentration of drug 0.5 hr after the second dose, (c) the minimum C_{min}^∞ and maximum C_{max}^∞ concentration of drug at steady state, (d) the average concentration of drug at steady state $\bar{C}$, and (e) the loading dose required to produce an immediate steady-state plasma level of the drug. The area under the plasma concentration-time curve during the 6- to 7-hr dosing interval was found to be 7.22 μg ml^{-1} hr^{-1}. Assume that steady state was achieved after seven doses.

Solution:

Step 1. The elimination-rate constant can be calculated by using Equation (83). Thus,

$$K = \frac{0.693}{t_{1/2}} = \frac{0.693}{1.0} = 0.693 \text{ hr}^{-1}$$

Step 2. The plasma concentration of drug 0.5 hr after the second dose can be calculated using Equation (79). In this case, τ, the dosing interval, is equal to 1 hr. Thus,

$$C = \frac{50}{10} \left(\frac{1 - e^{-2 \times 0.693 \times 1.0}}{1 - e^{-0.693 \times 1.0}} \right) e^{-0.693 \times 0.5}$$

$$= 5.30 \ \mu g \ ml^{-1}$$

Compare with Figure 81 at 1.5 hr.

Step 3. The minimum C_{min} and maximum C_{max} drug plasma concentrations at steady state can be calculated from Equations (81) and (82), respectively. Thus,

$$C^{\infty}_{min} = \frac{50}{10} \left(\frac{1}{1 - e^{-0.693 \times 1.0}} \right) e^{-0.693 \times 1.0} = 5.0 \ \mu g \ ml^{-1}$$

and

$$C^{\infty}_{max} = \frac{50}{10} \left(\frac{1}{1 - e^{-0.693 \quad 1.0}} \right) = 10.0 \ \mu g \ ml^{-1}$$

Compare with Figure 81.

Step 4. The average concentration of drug at steady state $\bar{C}$ can be calculated from Equation (83) or (85). Thus,

$$\bar{C} = \frac{7.22}{1.0} = 7.22 \ \mu g \ ml^{-1}$$

or

$$\bar{C} = \frac{50}{10 \times 0.693 \times 1.0} = 7.22 \ \mu g \ ml^{-1}$$

Compare with Figure 81.

Step 5. Equation (86) allows the calculation of the loading dose. Thus,

$$A^{*}_{0} = 50 \left(\frac{1}{1 - e^{-0.693 \times 1.0}} \right) = 100 \ mg$$

In this particular case, $t_{1/2}$ is equal to τ. Thus, Equation (87) can be employed and the result is

$$A^{*}_{0} = 2 \times 50 = 100 \ mg$$

2. Multiple Dosing with First-Order Absorption (Oral Dosing)

The scheme in Section IV.A.2 may be used to estimate drug plasma levels following multiple oral dosing (usually representing first-order absorption) and assuming a one-compartment model. Applying the method developed by Benet [267], it can be shown that the result of multiplying each exponential term in Equation (64) containing t (time) (that is, $e^{-k_i t}$) by the function given in Equation (80) will yield an equation for calculating multiple oral dosing.

$$C_n = \frac{k_a F G_0}{V_d(k_a - K)} \left[\left(\frac{1 - e^{-nK\tau}}{1 - e^{-K\tau}} \right) e^{-Kt} - \left(\frac{1 - e^{-nk_a\tau}}{1 - e^{-k_a\tau}} \right) e^{-k_a t} \right] \tag{88}$$

Equation (92) is employed to predict the drug plasma concentration at any time during a dosing interval (e.g., the concentration C_3 following the third dose of a drug). The terms of Equation (92) have the same meaning here as in earlier equations in this section.

The terms $e^{-nk_a\tau}$ and $e^{-nK\tau}$ will tend to zero as the number of doses increase. This leads to Equation (93), which describes the drug plasma concentration C_∞ as a function of time at steady state:

$$C_\infty = \frac{k_a F G_0}{V_d(k_a - K)} \left[\left(\frac{1}{1 - e^{-K\tau}} \right) e^{-Kt} - \left(\frac{1}{1 - e^{-k_a\tau}} \right) e^{-k_a t} \right] \tag{89}$$

The average plasma concentration at steady state $\bar{C}_\infty$ is given by an equation analogous to that for intravenous multiple dosing. It can be seen from Equation (90) that $\bar{C}_\infty$ depends on the fraction of the dose absorbed, the magnitude of the dose given, the volume of distribution, the elimination-rate constant, and the dosing interval:

$$\bar{C}_\infty = \frac{F G_0}{V_d K \tau} \tag{90}$$

The area under the plasma concentration-time curve from time zero to infinity following single oral administration is equal to the area under the curve during a dosing interval at steady state. Consequently,

$$\int_0^\infty C \, dt = \int_0^\tau C_\infty \, dt \tag{91}$$

Now, integration of Equation (89) from 0 to τ yields the expression

$$\int_0^\tau C \, dt = \frac{F G_0}{V_d K} \tag{92}$$

Combining Equations (90) and (92), we obtain

$$\bar{C}_\infty = \frac{\int_0^\tau C\, dt}{\tau} \tag{93}$$

Equation (93) allows the calculation of the average plasma concentration of drug at steady state. This equation is useful because it does not require knowledge of the volume of distribution, V_d, or the fraction, F, of the dose absorbed.

3. Time for Maximum Drug Plasma Concentration

Assuming that F remains constant during the multiple-dosing regimen, the time t'_p at which the maximum drug plasma concentration at steady state occurs can be expressed by

$$t'_p = \frac{1}{(k_a - K)} \ln \frac{k_a(1 - e^{-K\tau})}{k(1 - e^{-k_a\tau})} \tag{94}$$

The knowledge of t'_p allows the calculation of the maximum plasma concentration at steady state C_{max}. It is shown by Gibaldi and Perrier [284] that

$$C^\infty_{max} = \frac{FG_0}{V_d}\left(\frac{1}{1 - e^{-K\tau}}\right) e^{-Kt'_p} \tag{95}$$

Similarly, by setting t equal to τ in Equation (89), the following equation for the minimum plasma concentration C_{min} at steady state results:

$$C^\infty_{min} = \frac{k_a FG_0}{V_d(k_a - K)}\left[\left(\frac{1}{1 - e^{-K\tau}}\right) e^{-K\tau} - \left(\frac{1}{1 - e^{-k_a\tau}}\right) e^{-k_a\tau}\right] \tag{96}$$

The maximum drug plasma concentration after the first dose is given by the equation

$$C^1_{max} = \frac{FG_0}{V_d} e^{-Kt_p} \tag{97}$$

where t_p is the time for appearance of maximum plasma concentration of drug after the first dose. The time t_p is given by the expression

$$t_p = \frac{1}{k_a - K} \ln \frac{k_a}{K} \tag{98}$$

Similarly, the minimum plasma drug concentration after the first dose is given by

$$C^1_{min} = \frac{k_a F G_0}{V_d(k_a - K)} (e^{-K\tau} - e^{-k_a\tau}) \tag{99}$$

The loading dose, A^*_0, following first-order input (oral or intramuscular dosing, for example) is calculated using the expression

$$A^*_0 = A_0 \frac{1}{1 - e^{-K\tau}} \tag{100}$$

which is identical to Equation (86) for intravenous administration if the maintenance dose A_0 is administered in the postabsorptive period.

Example 5. Sample Calculation of Pharmacokinetic Parameters Following Multiple Oral Administration of a Drug That Is Represented by a One-Compartment Model.

A subject was administered a tablet dosage form containing 100 mg of a drug every 10 hr for a period of 100 hr. Plasma concentration of drug was obtained as a function of time. The results are illustrated in Figure 82. Two weeks prior to this treatment the subject received a single oral dose of the dosage form and after performing a Wagner-Nelson calculation (see Sec. V.A.1), the absorption-rate constant k_a, the elimination half-life of the drug, the area under the curve from time zero to infinity, and the volume of distribution were found to be 0.5 hr^{-1}, 7.7 hr, 115.5 μg ml^{-1} hr^{-1}, and 10 liters, respectively. Calculate (a) the elimination-rate constant K, (b) the plasma concentration of drug 5 hr after the fourth dose, (c) the minimum C^1_{min}, and maximum C^1_{max} drug plasma concentration after the first dose, (d) the minimum C^∞_{max} drug plasma concentration at steady state, (e) the average drug concentration of steady state, and (f) an estimation of a loading dose assuming that the maintenance dose is equal to 100 mg and is administered in the postabsorptive phase. Assume that the fraction of drug absorbed F is equal to 1.0.

Solution:

Step 1. The elimination-rate constant can be calculated by using Equation (41). Thus,

$$K = \frac{0.693}{t_{1/2}} = \frac{0.693}{7.7} = 0.09 \text{ hr}^{-1}$$

Step 2. The plasma concentration of drug 5 hr after the fourth dose can be calculated using Equation (88). In this case, τ, the dosing interval, is 10 hr. Thus,

$$C = \frac{0.5 \times 1 \times 100}{10(0.5 - 0.09)} \left[\left(\frac{1 - e^{-4 \times 0.09 \times 10}}{1 - e^{-0.09 \times 10}} \right) e^{-0.09 \times 5} \right.$$

$$\left. - \left(\frac{1 - e^{-4 \times 0.5 \times 10}}{1 - e^{-0.5 \times 10}} \right) e^{-0.5 \times 5} \right] = 11.95 \text{ }\mu\text{g ml}^{-1}$$

See Figure 82 for comparison of the result.

Step 3. The minimum concentration of drug C_{min}^1 after the first dose can be calculated using Equation (99). Thus,

$$C_{min}^1 = \frac{0.5 \times 1 \times 100}{10(0.5 - 0.09)} \left(e^{-0.09 \times 10} - e^{-0.5 \times 10} \right)$$

$$= 4.88 \ \mu g \ ml^{-1}$$

The maximum drug plasma concentration C_{max}^1 is given by Equation (97). However, if it is necessary to calculate the time to peak t_p after the first dose, t_p is given by Equation (98). Consequently,

$$t_p = \frac{1}{0.5 - 0.09} \ln \frac{0.5}{0.09} = 4.18 \ hr$$

and

$$C_{max}^1 = \frac{1 \times 100}{10} e^{-0.09 \times 4.18} = 6.86 \ \mu g \ ml^{-1}$$

See Figure 82 for comparison of results.

Step 4. The minimum drug plasma concentration C_{min}^∞ at steady state can be calculated using Equation (95). Thus,

$$C_{min}^\infty = \frac{0.5 \times 1 \times 100}{10(0.5 - 0.09)} \left[\left(\frac{1}{1 - e^{-0.09 \times 10}} \right) e^{-0.09 \times 10} \right.$$

$$\left. - \left(\frac{1}{1 - e^{-0.5 \times 10}} \right) e^{-0.5 \times 10} \right] = 8.27 \ \mu g \ ml^{-1}$$

See Figure 82 for comparison of results.

The maximum drug concentration C_{max}^∞ at steady state can be calculated using Equation (95). However, use of this equation requires knowledge of the time to peak t_p', which is given by Equation (94). Thus,

$$t_p' = \frac{1}{0.5 - 0.09} \ln \frac{0.5(1 - e^{-0.09 \times 10})}{0.09(1 - e^{-0.5 \times 10})} = 2.91 \ hr$$

Consequently,

$$C_{max}^\infty = \frac{1 \times 100}{10} \left(\frac{1}{1 - e^{-0.09 \times 10}} \right) e^{-0.09 \times 2.91} = 12.97 \ \mu g \ ml^{-1}$$

See Figure 82 for comparison of the results.

Step 5. An estimate of a loading dose can be obtained using Equation (100). Thus,

$$A_0^* = 100 \times \frac{1}{1 - e^{-0.09 \times 10}} = 169 \text{ mg}$$

C. Two-Compartment Model: Single Dosing

In the beginning of Section IV it was observed that drugs distribute throughout the body, and this fact prompted investigators to develop a more complex mathematical model, including a central and at least one peripheral compartment. The two-compartment model is sufficiently realistic when viewed on a physiological basis, and it is perhaps mathematically more acceptable than a one-compartment model. However, when calculations using a one-compartment model yield results that correspond satisfactorily with the experimental data, the more complex two-compartment model need not be employed.

1. Intravenous Injection (Single Dose)

The two-compartment model, with bolus intravenous injection and with elimination occurring from the central compartment, can be represented by the scheme

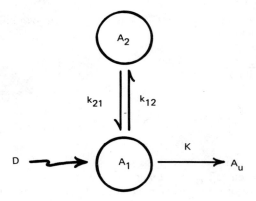

where k_{12} is the first-order rate constant for transfer of drug from compartment 1 to compartment 2, k_{21} the first-order rate constant for transfer of drug from compartment 2 to compartment 1, K the overall first-order rate constant for elimination of drug by all processes from compartment 1, A_1 the amount of drug in compartment 1 at time t, and A_2 the amount of drug in compartment 2 at time t. D is the amount of drug representing the intravenous dose, and A_u is the amount of drug in the urine. The rate of change in amount of drug in compartment 1 can be described by the following differential equation:

$$\frac{dA_1}{dt} = k_{21}A_2 - k_{12}A_1 - KA_1 \tag{101}$$

A second equation may be written to describe the rate of change of the amount of drug in the second compartment:

$$\frac{dA_2}{dt} = k_{12}A_1 - k_{21}A_2 \tag{102}$$

Integration of Equations (101) and (102) leads to

$$A_1 = \frac{D(\alpha - k_{21})}{\alpha - \beta} e^{-\alpha t} + \frac{D(k_{21} - \beta)}{\alpha - \beta} e^{-\beta t} \tag{103}$$

which is referred to as a biexponential equation because of the two terms containing exponents. Equation (103) describes the amount of drug in compartment 1 as a function of time. In this equation, D is the intravenous dose, and thus the amount of drug in compartment 1 at t equals zero; the quantities α and β are hybrid rate constants:

$$\alpha = \frac{1}{2}\left[(k_{12} + k_{21} + K) + \sqrt{(k_{12} + k_{21} + K)^2 - 4k_{21}K}\right] \tag{104}$$

$$\beta = \frac{1}{2}\left[(k_{12} + k_{21} + K) - \sqrt{(k_{12} + k_{21} + K)^2 - 4k_{21}K}\right] \tag{105}$$

and

$$\alpha \cdot \beta = k_{21}K \tag{105}$$

$$\alpha \cdot \beta = k_{12} + k_{21} + K \tag{106}$$

The integrated equation describing the amount of drug A_2 in compartment 2 as a function of time can be described by

$$A_2 = \frac{k_{12}De^{-\beta t}}{\alpha - \beta} - \frac{k_{12}De^{-\alpha t}}{\alpha - \beta} \tag{107}$$

or

$$A_2 = \frac{k_{12}D}{\alpha - \beta}(e^{-\beta t} - e^{-\alpha t})$$

A linear relationship exists between the drug concentration in the plasma C and the amount of drug in compartment 1; that is,

$$A_1 = V_1 C \tag{108}$$

where V_1 is the apparent volume of compartment 1. Equation (108) enables the conversion of Equation (103) from amount to concentration,

$$C = \frac{D(\alpha - k_{21})}{V_1 (\alpha - \beta)} e^{-\alpha t} + \frac{D(k_{21} - \beta)}{V_1 (\alpha - \beta)} e^{-\beta t} \qquad (109)$$

and

$$C = Pe^{-\alpha t} + Qe^{-\beta t} \qquad (110)$$

where the coefficients P and Q of these biexponential equations are defined by the expressions

$$P = \frac{D(\alpha - k_{21})}{(\alpha - \beta)V_1} \qquad (111)$$

and

$$Q = \frac{D(k_{21} - \beta)}{(\alpha - \beta)V_1} \qquad (112)$$

If the logarithm of plasma concentration of drug is plotted against the time t, following Equation (110), a biexponential curve is obtained (see Fig. 83). The curve is referred to as biexponential because it can be factored into two curves by a technique called "feathering" or "stripping." The terminal linear segment of the biexponential curve is extrapolated to time t = 0, and is shown in Figure 83 as a dashed line. The data are feathered or stripped by subtracting each drug concentration value on the extrapolated dashed portion of the biexponential curve from the experimental points above it on the curved part of the biexponential line at that particular time (see Example 6). As observed in Figure 83, the $Pe^{-\alpha t}$ curve will approach zero and $Qe^{-\beta t}$ will retain a finite value. When $e^{-\alpha t}$ has approached closely to zero, this period is referred to as the postdistributive phase. At this point Equation (110) reduces to

$$P = Qe^{-\beta t} \qquad (113)$$

or in logarithmic form,

$$\log P = \log Q - \frac{\beta t}{2.303} \qquad (114)$$

To summarize, one begins the analysis in the case of a two-compartment model by plotting the results on semilogarithmic graph paper, feathering the data so as to obtain two curves, then calculating β using Equation (114), corresponding to the terminal part of the biexponential curve. Q, the coefficient for the β exponential term

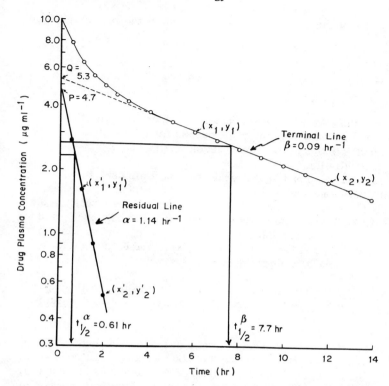

Figure 83. Semilogarithmic plot of the concentration of drug in the blood plasma following single intravenous administration of a drug represented by a two-compartment model.

of Equation (113), is obtained from the extrapolation value [see Eq. (114)], where the dashed line crosses the vertical axis at t = 0. The value of α is obtained from the slope of the linear segment resulting from a plot of the residuals, and the P value is found where this line crosses the vertical axis at zero time.

The half-lives for the α and β phases are obtained in the ordinary manner, employing the equations

$$t^{\alpha}_{1/2} = \frac{0.693}{\alpha}$$

(115)

$$t^{\beta}_{1/2} = \frac{0.693}{\beta}$$

(116)

It should be noted that β is not an elimination-rate constant, but rather depends both on elimination and distribution of the drug according to the expression

$$\beta = fK$$

(117)

where f, the fraction of drug in the central compartment in the postdistributive phase, is

$$f = \frac{k_{21} - \beta}{k_{21} + k_{12} - \beta} \qquad (118)$$

Thus, β is smaller than the elimination-rate constant K, being K multiplied by a fractional quantity f. The quantity K is the rate constant for elimination from the central compartment and β is the elimination constant for the body. The quantity $t^{\beta}_{1/2}$ gives the biological half-life.

If f is unity or near to a value of 1.0, the drug is present almost totally in the central compartment, and a one-compartment model will describe its kinetics. In this case, β simply becomes the elimination-rate constant K. Currently, computer programs are available to fit and feather the data shown in Figure 83, and to give the constants α, β, P, and Q and the half-lives. The computer can also be programmed to calculate and print the values for k_{12}, k_{21}, and K, as well as V_1, the apparent volume of the central compartment.

Example 6. Sample Calculation of Pharmacokinetic Parameters Following Single Intravenous Administration of a Drug Represented by a Two-Compartment Model.

A subject received a single intravenous dose of a drug solution containing 100 mg of drug. The drug plasma concentration was obtained as a function of time. The results are illustrated in Table 20. Calculate (a) the values for α and β, and (b) the half-life for the distributive phase α and the elimination phase β. (c) Write an equation that will give the concentration of drug C as a function of time and calculate the concentration of drug 9.5 hr after administration. Calculate (d) the volume of distribution of the central compartment V_1; (e) the fraction of drug in the central compartment in the postdistributive phase; (f) the values of k_{12}, k_{21}, and K; and (g) the area under the plasma concentration-time curve. Assume that the drug plasma levels are represented by a two-compartment model.

Solution:

Step 1. Plot the data in semilogarithmic graph paper. Figure 83 illustrates the graphical representation of the data (open circles).

Step 2. To calculate the value for the elimination phase β, extrapolate the terminal linear segment of the biexponential to time zero. According to Equation (114), the slope of this line is equal to $-\beta/2.303$. For practical purposes, the points (x_1, y_1) and (x_2, y_2) in the graph will be used to estimate the slope. However, it should be noted that the best way to obtain the slope is by using linear regression analysis.

$$\text{Slope} = \frac{\log y_2 - \log y_1}{x_2 - x_1} = \frac{\log 3.05 - \log 1.77}{6 - 12} = 0.0394$$

Table 20

Concentration Time Data Obtained Following
Intravenous Administration of a Drug

Time (hr)	Drug plasma concentration (μg ml^{-1})
0.5	7.78
1.0	6.40
1.5	5.51
2.0	4.91
2.5	4.89
3.0	4.17
4.0	3.70
5.0	3.35
6.0	3.05
8.0	2.54
10.0	2.12
12.0	1.77
14.0	1.48

Thus,

$$\beta = -(-0.0394 \times 2.303) = 0.09 \text{ hr}^{-1}$$

In order to calculate the value for the distributive phase α, the method of residuals is employed. The residual values are obtained by subtracting from true plasma concentration values in the distributive phase the corresponding drug concentration values on the extrapolated line (dashed line, see Fig. 83). Table 21 illustrates the results. On the same sheet of graph paper, plot the residual values (solid circles, Fig. 83). Calculate the slope of this line using the points (x_1', y_1') and (x_2', y_2').

$$\text{Slope} = \frac{\log y_2' - \log y_1'}{x_2' - x_1'} = \frac{\log 0.51 - \log 1.60}{2 - 1} = -0.497$$

Thus,

$$\alpha = -(\text{slope} \times 2.303) = -(-0.497 \times 2.303) = 1.14 \text{ hr}^{-1}$$

Step 3. To calculate the half-life for the α phase $t_{1/2}^{\alpha}$ and the half-life for the β phase, $t_{1/2}^{\beta}$, Equations (115) and (116) are used. Thus,

$$t_{1/2}^{\alpha} = \frac{0.693}{1.14} = 0.61 \text{ hr}$$

and

$$t_{1/2}^{\beta} = \frac{0.693}{0.09} = 7.70 \text{ hr}$$

Table 21

Residual Values Plasma Concentration-Time Data Following Single Intravenous Administration

Time (hr)	Drug concentration (μg ml^{-1})	Extrapolated concentration (μg ml^{-1})	Residual concentration (μg ml^{-1})
0.5	7.78	5.01	2.77
1.0	6.40	4.80	1.60
1.5	5.51	4.61	0.90
2.0	4.91	4.40	0.51

The half-lives can also be obtained from the graphical representation of the data. The extrapolated line (dashed line, Fig. 83) crosses the y axis at time zero at 5.3 μg ml^{-1} (Q), and the residual line at 4.7 μg ml^{-1} (P). Using the half-life definition, at a drug concentration of 5.3/2, the half-life for the β phase is 7.7 hr, and at a drug concentration 4.7/2, the half-life for the α phase is approximately 0.6 hr.

Step 4. The equation describing the plasma concentration of drug as a function of time is given by

$$C = Pe^{-\alpha t} + Qe^{-\beta t}$$

The values for α and β have been calculated in steps 2 and 3. P and Q are the y intercepts of the residual line and terminal line at t = 0, respectively (see Fig. 83). Thus,

$$C = 4.7e^{-1.14t} + 5.3e^{-0.09t}$$

Therefore, the concentration of drug 9.5 hr postadministration will be

$$C = 4.7e^{-1.14 \times 9.5} + 5.3e^{-0.09 \times 9.5} = 2.25 \ \mu g \ ml^{-1}$$

See Figure 83 for comparison of the calculated result 2.25 μg ml^{-1} with that read from the graph.

Step 5. The value of the central compartment V_1 can be estimated from Equation (110). At time t = 0, Equation (110) reduces to

$$C_0 = P + Q = 4.7 + 5.3 = 10.0$$

and

$$V_1 = \frac{dose}{C_0} = \frac{100,000 \ g \ ml^{-1}}{10 \ g \ ml^{-1}} = 10,000 \ ml \quad or \quad 10 \ liters$$

Step 6. To calculate k_{12}, k_{21}, and K, start by calculating k_{21} from Equation (111) or (112). Thus,

$$k_{21} = \alpha - \frac{P(\alpha - \beta)V_1}{D}$$

$$= 1.14 - \frac{4.7(1.14 - 0.09)10,000}{100,000} = 0.6 \text{ hr}^{-1}$$

or

$$k_{21} = \frac{Q(\alpha - \beta)V_1}{D} + \beta$$

$$= \frac{5.3(1.14 - 0.09)10,000}{100,000} + 0.09 = 0.6 \text{ hr}^{-1}$$

To calculate the elimination-rate constant K, Equation (105) is used. Thus,

$$K = \frac{\alpha \cdot \beta}{k_{21}} = \frac{1.14 \times 0.09}{0.65} = 0.16 \text{ hr}^{-1}$$

And finally, k_{12} can be calculated using Equation (106). Thus,

$$k_{12} = 0.09 + 1.14 - 0.16 - 0.6 = 0.4 \text{ hr}^{-1}$$

Step 7. The fraction of drug in the central compartment in the postdistributive phase can be obtained using Equation (117) or (118):

$$f - \frac{\beta}{K} = \frac{0.09}{0.16} = 0.56$$

or

$$f = \frac{0.6 - 0.09}{0.6 + 0.4 - 0.09} = 0.56$$

In this case f_1 is not unity, and consequently the data cannot be described by a one-compartment model. In addition, it should be remembered that β is smaller than K, and consequently the biological half-life is given by β while the elimination of drug from the central compartment is given by K.

Step 8. The area under the plasma concentration-time curve can be obtained by integrating Equation (110) from time zero to infinity. Thus,

$$\text{area} = \int_0^\infty C \, dt = \frac{P}{\alpha} + \frac{Q}{\beta} = \frac{4.7}{1.14} + \frac{5.3}{0.09} = 63.0 \ \mu\text{g ml}^{-1} \text{ hr}^{-1}$$

2. Urinary Excretion

A drug following the two-compartment model may be subjected to urinary excretion analysis in order to obtain the pharmacokinetic parameters that were described in Section IV.C.1.

According to the following scheme

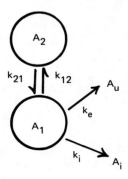

where A_u is the unchanged drug amount eliminated in the urine; A_i the amount of
drug in its various forms eliminated by other excretion pathways, such as salivary
and biliary; and k_e and k_i are the respective first-order elimination-rate constants.
Thus,

$$K = k_e + k_i \tag{119}$$

The rate of excretion of unchanged drug according to the foregoing scheme is given
by

$$\frac{dA_u}{dt} = k_e A_1$$

where A_1, the amount of drug in the central compartment, is given by Equation
(103). Substitution of this equation into Equation (121) leads to

$$\frac{dA_u}{dt} = \frac{k_e D(\alpha - k_{21})}{(\alpha - \beta)} e^{-\alpha t} + \frac{k_e D(k_{21} - \beta)}{(\alpha - \beta)} e^{-\beta t} \tag{121}$$

which can be simplified to

$$\frac{dA_u}{dt} = P'e^{-\alpha t} + Q'e^{-\beta t} \tag{122}$$

where

$$P' = \frac{k_e D(\alpha - k_{21})}{(\alpha - \beta)} \tag{123}$$

and

$$Q' = \frac{k_e D(k_{21} - \beta)}{(\alpha - \beta)} \tag{124}$$

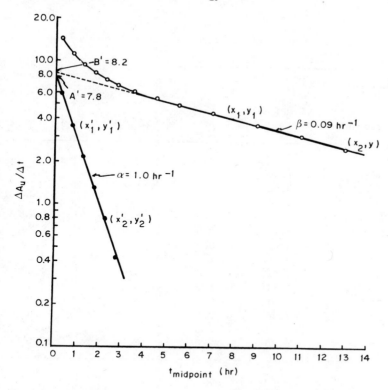

Figure 84. Log rate plot relating to data for the urinary excretion of a drug following intravenous bolus injection. The drug is represented by a two-compartment model.

If the logarithm of the excretion rate dA_u/dt is plotted versus time, a biexponential curve will result. This is illustrated in Figure 84. Using the "method of residuals" or "feathering," the biexponential curve can be broken into two lines. The slope of the terminal line is equal to $-\beta/2.303$ and the slope of the residual line is equal to $-\alpha/2.303$. The respective y intercept at time $t = 0$ are P' and Q'. Gibaldi and Perrier [286] have shown that the elimination-rate constant, k_e, can be calculated using the expression

$$k_e = \frac{P' + Q'}{D} \qquad (125)$$

Similarly,

$$k_{21} = \frac{P'\beta + Q'\alpha}{P' + Q'} \qquad (126)$$

K and K_{12} can be calculated from Equations (105) and (106).

Table 22

Urinary Excretion Data After Intravenous Administration of 100 mg of a Drug Solution

Time (hr)	Cumulative amount of drug excreted unchanged (mg)	ΔA_u	Δt	$\Delta A_u / \Delta t$	$t_{midpoint}$
0	0				
0.5	7.04	7.04	0.5	14.08	0.25
1.0	12.68	5.64	0.5	11.28	0.75
1.5	17.42	4.74	0.5	9.48	1.25
2.0	21.57	4.15	0.5	8.30	1.75
2.5	25.32	3.75	0.5	7.50	2.25
3.0	28.78	3.46	0.5	6.92	2.75
4.0	35.06	6.28	1.0	6.28	3.5
5.0	40.68	5.62	1.0	5.62	4.5
6.0	45.79	5.11	1.0	5.11	5.5
8.0	54.70	8.91	2.0	4.46	7.0
10.0	62.14	7.44	2.0	3.72	9.0
12.0	68.36	6.22	2.0	3.11	11.0
14.0	73.56	5.20	2.0	2.60	13.0

Another approach to calculate the pharmacokinetic parameters from urinary excretion data is the sigma-minus method. This method requires knowledge of the total amount of unchanged drug excreted to time infinity (see Sec. IV.I).

Example 7. Sample Calculation of Pharmacokinetic Parameters Following Intravenous Bolus Injection of a Drug Represented by a Two-Compartment Model Using Urinary Excretion Data.

A subject received an i.v. bolus injection of a solution containing 100 mg of a drug. The cumulative amount of drug in the urine was obtained as a function of time. The results are illustrated in Table 22. Assume that the drug is represented by a two-compartment model. Calculate (1) α, β, P', and Q'; (2) the rate constant k_e for elimination of unchanged drug in the urine; (3) the intercompartmental first-order rate constant k_{21}, the overall elimination rate constant K, and the transfer first-order rate constant k_{12}; and (4) the fraction of unchanged drug excreted in the urine.

Solution:

Step 1. Equation (122) shows that a plot of log $\Delta A_u / \Delta t$ versus t will result in a biexponential curve. The use of this equation requires that log $\Delta A_u / \Delta t$ be plotted against the midpoint of a short urine interval (see Table 22). Figure 84 illustrates the graphical representation of the data (open circles).

Table 23

Residual Values: Urinary Excretion Following Intravenous Dosing

Time (hr)	$\Delta A_u / \Delta t$ (mg hr^{-1})	Extrapolated $\Delta A_u / \Delta t$	Residual value
0.25	14.08	8.1	5.98
0.75	11.28	7.7	3.58
1.25	9.48	7.3	2.18
1.75	8.30	7.0	1.30
2.25	7.50	6.7	0.80
2.75	6.92	6.5	0.42

Step 2. Extrapolate the terminal linear phase to time zero, where one observes the intercept to be 8.2 mg hr^{-1}. Thus,

$$Q' = \text{intercept} = 8.2 \text{ mg hr}^{-1}$$

Step 3. Calculate the slope of the terminal linear phase. The slope of the line is equal to $-\beta/2.303$. Thus,

$$\text{Slope} = \frac{\log y_2 - \log y_1}{x_2 - x_1} = \frac{\log 2.6 - \log 4.46}{13 - 7} = -0.039$$

$$\beta = -(-0.039 \times 2.303) = 0.09 \text{ hr}^{-1}$$

Step 4. Using the method of residuals as previously discussed, calculate the residual amounts. Table 23 illustrates the results.

Step 5. On the same sheet of graph paper, plot the residual values of column 4, Table 23 (see Fig. 84). Calculate the slope of this line, which is equal to $-\alpha/2.303$. It is also observed that the intercept of this line at time zero is 7.8 mg hr^{-1}. Thus,

$$\text{Slope} = \frac{\log y_2' - \log y_1'}{x_2' - x_1'} = \frac{\log 0.8 - \log 3.58}{2.25 - 0.75} = -0.43$$

$$\alpha = -(-0.43 \times 2.303) = 1.0 \text{ hr}^{-1}$$

and

$$P' = \text{intercept} = 7.8 \text{ mg hr}^{-1}$$

Step 6. The first-order elimination-rate constant for unchanged drug in the urine k_e can be calculated using Equation (125). Thus,

$$k_e = \frac{7.8 + 8.2}{100 \text{ mg}} = 0.16 \text{ hr}^{-1}$$

Step 7. The intercompartmental rate constant k_{21} can be calculated from Equation (126). Thus,

$$k_{12} = \alpha + \beta - k_{21} - K = 0.09 + 1.0 - 0.56 - 0.16 = 0.37 \text{ hr}^{-1}$$

Step 8. The fraction of drug excreted unchanged f is given by the ratio of k_e/K. Thus,

$$f = \frac{k_e}{k} = \frac{0.16}{0.16} = 1.0$$

This indicates that 100% of the administered drug was excreted unchanged and that no metabolism took place.

3. Oral Dosing (Two-Compartment Model) with First-Order Absorption

The most practical modality for drug administration is the oral route. A drug is represented by a two-compartment model after oral (assumed to be first-order) absorption is shown in the scheme

where k_a is the first-order absorption-rate constant. The terms k_{12}, k_{21}, K, A_1, and A_u have been previously defined. The amount of drug A_1 as a function of time is given by Equation (127):

$$A_1 = \frac{k_a FG_0 (k_{21} - k_a)}{(\alpha - k_a)(\beta - k_a)} e^{-k_a t} + \frac{k_a FG_0 (k_{21} - \alpha)}{(k_a - \alpha)(\beta - \alpha)} e^{-\alpha t} + \frac{k_a FG_0 (k_{21} - \beta)}{(k_a - \beta)(\alpha - \beta)} e^{-\beta t} \quad (127)$$

where F is the fraction of the dose G_0 absorbed. The quantities α and β have been previously defined. Equation (127) can be converted to concentration terms using the relationship $A_1 = V_c C$. Thus,

$$C = \frac{k_a FG_0 (k_{21} - k_a)}{V_c(\alpha - k_a)(\beta - k_a)} e^{-k_a t} + \frac{k_a FG_0 (k_{21} - \alpha)}{V_c(k_a - \alpha)(\beta - \alpha)} e^{-\alpha t}$$

$$+ \frac{k_a FG_0 (k_{21} - \beta)}{V_c(k_a - \beta)(\alpha - \beta)} e^{-\beta t} \quad (128)$$

where V_c is the volume of the central compartment. Equation (128) can be reduced to

$$C = ne^{-k_a t} + Le^{-\alpha t} + Me^{-\beta t} \quad (129)$$

where

$$N = \frac{k_a F G_0 (k_{21} - k_a)}{V_c (\alpha - k_a)(\beta - k_a)} \tag{130}$$

$$L = \frac{k_a F G_0 (k_{21} - \alpha)}{V_c (k_a - \alpha)(\beta - \alpha)} \tag{131}$$

$$M = \frac{k_a F G_0 (k_{21} - \beta)}{V_c (k_a - \beta)(\alpha - \beta)} \tag{132}$$

The typical kinetic behavior of a drug represented by a two-compartment model indicates that the terms $e^{-k_a t}$ and $e^{-\alpha t}$ in Equation (129) tend to zero as time proceeds. Thus, Equation (129) reduces to

$$C = M e^{-\beta t} \tag{133}$$

or in logarithmic form

$$\log C = \log M - \frac{\beta t}{2.303} \tag{134}$$

According to Equation (129), a plot of the logarithm of the drug plasma concentration C versus time will result in a triexponential curve, and according to Equation (134), the terminal linear segment of the line has a slope equal to $-\beta/2.303$. To obtain α and k_a, the method of residuals is used. In this case two residual lines are obtained. The terminal linear segment of the first residual line has a slope equal to $-\alpha/2.303$, and the second residual line has a slope equal to $-k_a/2.303$. In most instances, it is very difficult to obtain α and k_a from the residual lines and it is advisable that intravenous data be obtained to gain insight into the values of α, β, k_{12}, k_{21}, and K. When α and k_a have values which are close, the triexponential curve will appear more like a biexponential curve, such as the one in Figure 79, obtained following oral administration of a drug that is represented by a one-compartment model. Under normal circumstances the method of Loo and Riegelman (Sec. V.A.2) is employed to calculate the rate constant, k_a. It should be remembered that this method requires i.v. data. An example of Loo-Riegelman calculations is given in Section V.A.2.

Integration of Equation (129) from time zero to infinity will lead to the area under the plasma concentration time curve. This is described by

$$\int_0^\infty C \, dt = \frac{N}{k_a} + \frac{L}{\alpha} + \frac{M}{\beta} \tag{135}$$

The area under the curve is important because it gives an indication of the extent of absorption, as shown in the section of bioabsorption.

The volume of distribution of a drug following oral administration and represented by a one-compartment model is given in Equation (72). Similarly, the volume of distribution for a drug represented by a two-compartment model is given by Equation (136).

$$V_d = \frac{FG_0}{\int_0^\infty C \, dt} \tag{136}$$

D. Two-Compartment Model: Multiple Oral Dosing

For a drug given by first-order input, a class in which most oral dosage regimens fall, the drug plasma concentration as a function of time can be readily obtained by multiplying each exponential term in Equation (129) by the multiple-dosing function developed by Benet [235]. This leads to

$$C_n = N \left(\frac{1 - e^{-nk_a\tau}}{1 - e^{-k_a\tau}} \right) e^{-k_a t} + L \left(\frac{1 - e^{-n\alpha\tau}}{1 - e^{-\alpha\tau}} \right) e^{-\alpha t} + M \left(\frac{1 - e^{-n\beta\tau}}{1 - e^{-\beta\tau}} \right) e^{-\beta t} \tag{137}$$

where N, L, and M have been previously defined. At steady-state levels the terms $e^{-n\alpha\tau}$, $e^{-nk_a\tau}$, and $e^{-n\beta\tau}$ will tend to zero and Equation (137) reduces to

$$C_\infty = N \left(\frac{1}{1 - e^{-k_a\tau}} \right) e^{-k_a t} + L \left(\frac{1}{1 - e^{-\alpha\tau}} \right) e^{-\alpha t} + M \left(\frac{1}{1 - e^{-\beta\tau}} \right) e^{-\beta t} \tag{138}$$

Equation (138) can be used to calculate the drug plasma concentration at any time during a dosing interval at steady state. Integration of Equation (138) from time zero to infinity will give the area under the curve at steady state.

$$\int_0^\infty C_\infty \, dt = \frac{N}{k_a} + \frac{L}{\alpha} + \frac{M}{\beta} \tag{139}$$

It can be observed that Equation (139) is identical to Equation (135) obtained after single oral administration of a drug represented by a two-compartment model. The average drug plasma concentration at steady state is given by Equations (140) and (141).

$$\bar{C}_\infty = \frac{\int_0^\infty C \, dt}{\tau} \tag{140}$$

or

$$\bar{C}_\infty = \frac{\int_0^\infty C_\infty \, dt}{\tau} \tag{141}$$

These equations are the same as Equation (93) for a one-compartment model. Consequently,

$$\bar{C}_\infty = \frac{FG_0}{V_d \beta \tau} \tag{142}$$

Equations (140) to (142) hold as long as elimination of drug occurs only from the central compartment.

The minimum concentration of drug after the first dose can be obtained by setting n equal to unity in Equation (137). Thus,

$$C_{min}^1 = Ne^{-k_a t} + Le^{-\alpha t} + Me^{-\beta t} \tag{143}$$

Similarly, by setting n equal to 1 and t equal to τ in Equation (138), the following equation results for the minimum plasma concentration C_{min}^∞ at steady state.

$$C_{min}^\infty = N \left(\frac{1}{1 - e^{-k_a \tau}} \right) e^{-k_a \tau} + L \left(\frac{1}{1 - e^{-\alpha \tau}} \right) e^{-\alpha \tau} + M \left(\frac{1}{1 - e^{-\beta \tau}} \right) e^{-\beta \tau} \tag{144}$$

The loading dose A_0^* is calculated using the equation

$$A_0^* = A_0 \left(\frac{1}{1 - e^{-\beta \tau}} \right) \tag{145}$$

as long as the maintenance dose A_0 is given in the postabsorptive, postdistributive phase of the loading dose.

Example 8. <u>Sample Calculation of Pharmacokinetic Parameters Following Multiple Oral Administration of a Drug That Is Represented by a Two-Compartment Model</u>.

A subject received a tablet dosage form containing 100 mg of a drug every 4.5 hr for a period of 45 hr, and drug plasma concentrations were determined as a function of time. The graphical representation of the results is illustrated in Figure 85. Two weeks prior to this treatment the subject received a single oral dose of the tablet dosage form. Pharmacokinetic analysis of the drug plasma levels resulting from the single oral dose indicated that the data can be represented by a two-compartment model. The rate constant for absorption k_a was estimated using the method of Loo and Riegelman (see Sec. V.A.2) and was found to be 0.8 hr^{-1}. In addition, k_{12}, k_{21}, K, V_c, α, and β were calculated as 0.4 hr^{-1}, 0.6 hr^{-1}, 0.16 hr^{-1}, 10 liters, 1.14 hr^{-1}, and 0.09 hr^{-1}, respectively. The area under the plasma concentration-time curve after the single oral dose was found to be 58.5 µg ml^{-1} hr^{-1}. Assuming that the renal and metabolic functions of the subject remain the same in the multiple- as in the single-dose regimen, calculate (a) the drug plasma concentration 2 hr after the third dose was given, (b) the average drug plasma concentration at steady state, (c) the drug plasma concentration 0.5 hr after the eighth dose was administered, and (d) a loading dose assuming a maintenance

dose of 100 mg that will be given in the postabsorptive, postdistributive phase
of the preceding dose.

Solution:

Step 1. The drug plasma concentration 2 hr after the third dose can be calculated using Equation (137). However, to use this equation it is necessary to
calculate the coefficients, N, L, and M, given in Equations (130) to (132).
Thus,

$$N = \frac{0.8 \times 1 \times 100(0.6 - 0.8)}{10(1.14 - 0.8)(0.09 - 0.8)} = 6.63 \ \mu g \ ml^{-1}$$

$$L = \frac{0.8 \quad 1 \quad 100(0.6 - 1.14)}{10(0.8 - 1.14)(0.09 - 1.14)} = 12.10 \ \mu g \ ml^{-1}$$

$$M = \frac{0.8 \times 1 \times 100(0.6 - 0.09)}{10(0.8 - 0.09)(1.14 - 0.09)} = 5.47 \ \mu g \ ml^{-1}$$

The drug concentration is given by

$$C = 6.63 \left(\frac{1 - e^{-3 \times 0.8 \times 4.5}}{1 - e^{-0.8 \times 4.5}} \right) e^{-0.8 \times 2}$$

$$- 12.10 \left(\frac{1 - e^{-3 \times 1.14 \times 4.5}}{1 - e^{-1.14 \times 4.5}} \right) e^{-1.14 \times 2}$$

$$+ 5.47 \left(\frac{1 - e^{-3 \times 0.09 \times 4.5}}{1 - e^{-0.09 \times 4.5}} \right) e^{-0.09 \times 2} = 9.65 \ \mu g \ ml^{-1}$$

See Figure 85 for comparison of results for drug plasma concentration 2 hr
after administration of the third dose.

Step 2. The average plasma concentration at steady state $\bar{C}_\infty$ can be calculated
using Equation (141). However, knowledge of the area under the curve during
a dosing interval at steady state is necessary. The area can be obtained using
Equation (139):

$$\int_0^\tau C \ dt = \frac{6.63}{0.8} - \frac{12.10}{1.14} + \frac{5.47}{0.09} + 58.5 \ \mu g \ ml^{-1} \ hr^{-1}$$

Thus, $\bar{C}_\infty$ is given by

$$\bar{C}_\infty = \frac{58.5}{4.5} = 13.0 \ \mu g \ ml^{-1}$$

See Figure 85 for comparison of results.

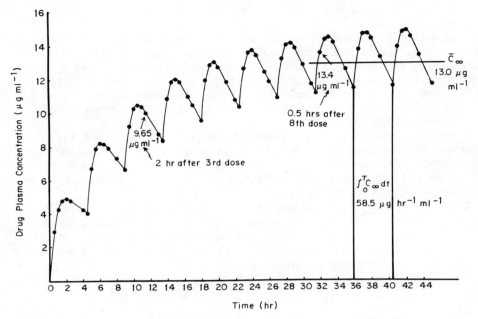

Figure 85. Two-compartment model of multiple-dose oral administration of equal doses of a drug at uniform time interval τ.

Step 3. The drug plasma concentration 0.5 hr after the eighth dose was administered can be calculated using Equation (138). This assumes that we are at steady state. Thus,

$$C = 6.63 \left(\frac{1}{1 - e^{-0.8 \times 4.5}} \right) e^{-0.8 \times 0.5}$$

$$- \ 12.10 \left(\frac{1}{1 - e^{-1.14 \times 4.5}} \right) e^{-1.14 \times 0.5}$$

$$+ \ 5.47 \left(\frac{1}{1 - e^{-0.09 \times 4.5}} \right) e^{-0.09 \times 0.5} = 13.4 \ \mu g \ ml^{-1}$$

Step 4. A loading dose can be calculated using Equation (145). Thus,

$$A_0^* = 100 \left(\frac{1}{1 - e^{-0.09 \times 4.5}} \right) = 300 \ mg$$

V. Kinetics of Bioabsorption

Perhaps the oldest published method for the estimation of the rate of absorption of
a drug into the blood was developed by Dominguez and Pomerene [287]. This technique was based on the assumption that the body is a single compartment or reservoir from which the drug is eliminated by first-order processes. One of the
pitfalls of the method is that estimates of the apparent volume of distribution must
be employed. A number of other procedures using a one-compartment model have
been proposed [288, 289].

Wagner and Nelson [290, 291] published a method for estimating the relative
absorption of drugs using a one-compartment model and collecting either urinary
or blood data. This method has gained wide acceptance because it does not require prior estimate of the volume of distribution and places no limitations on the
order of the absorption-rate constant.

Loo and Riegelman [292] published a second method for calculating the intrinsic absorption of drugs based on a two-compartment model. Let us now examine these two methods, which yield graphs referred to as "percent unabsorbed-
time plots." For a detailed treatment of the subject, the reader should see Gibaldi
and Perrier [293], Wagner [294], and Notari [295].

A. Rate of Absorption: Percent-Unabsorbed-Time Plots

1. One-Compartment Model: Wagner-Nelson Approach

Equation (146) derived by Wagner and Nelson [291] is useful for the determination of the fraction of drug absorbed to time T. We write it in the form

$$\% \text{ absorbed} = \frac{A_T}{A_\infty} \times 100 = \frac{C_T + K \int_0^T C\, dt}{K \int_0^\infty C\, dt} \times 100 \tag{146}$$

The one-compartment scheme on which the Wagner-Nelson method is based can be
depicted as follows:

| DRUG AT ABSORPTION SITE | $\xrightarrow[\substack{\text{1st}\\ \text{order}\\ \text{(ordinarily)}}]{k_a}$ | SINGLE COMPARTMENT $A_T = C_T \times V_c$ | $\xrightarrow[\substack{\text{1st}\\ \text{order}}]{K}$ | CUMULATIVE DRUG IN URINE, A_u |

In this equation A_T is the cumulative amount of drug absorbed from time zero to
time T expressed in convenient units, A is the amount eventually absorbed as expressed in the same units, K is the overall elimination-rate constant given in the
unit of reciprocal time, and C_T is blood, serum, or plasma concentration at time
T. From this equation, fraction-absorbed-time data can be generated based on
plasma concentration of drug and a knowledge of the overall elimination-rate constant.

Example 9. Sample Calculation Illustrating the Wagner-Nelson Method

The following example illustrates the use of Equation (146) for a drug whose kinetics is represented by a one-compartment model. The plasma concentration-time data after oral administration, together with terms required for an analysis of the data by the method of Wagner and Nelson, are found in Table 24. A semilogarithmic plot of percent drug unabsorbed [that is, $100 (1 - A_T/A_\infty]$ versus time is linear, with a slope equal to $-k_a/2.303$. This graphical method yields the absorption-rate constant, 0.50 hr^{-1} (see Fig. 86). In some cases semilogarithmic plots are not linear, and in those cases the rectilinear plot may yield a straight line indicating that absorption is probably occurring by a zero-order process. Examples of more complicated cases have been discussed by Wagner and Nelson [291]. The illustration of Table 24 demonstrates the method of calculating fractional (or percent) absorption of a drug from its oral dosage form. The footnotes of Table 24 describe the steps for carrying out the calculations.

The relative efficiency of absorption of a drug from several tablet formulations can be estimated by this method. Thus, "percent-unabsorbed-time plots" are of use in the design of acceptable dosage forms or in the comparison of the relative bioavailability of marketed generic products. They also provide a means of calculating k_a, the rate of bioabsorption of the drug (see Fig. 86).

Wagner [296] has applied Equation (146) to 12 separate studies with tetracycline combinations from 167 sets of serum tetracycline curves.

Urinary Excretion Data

A method was also developed by Wagner and Nelson [291] in which urinary excretion data were used to obtain the percent of drug absorbed. The following equation is used:

$$\% \text{ absorbed} = \frac{A_T}{A_\infty} \times 100 = \frac{A_u + (1/K)(dA_u/dt)}{A_u^\infty} \times 100 \tag{147}$$

where A_T is the cumulative amount of drug absorbed from time zero to time T given in convenient units; A_∞ the amount eventually absorbed expressed in the same units; K the overall rate constant for elimination from blood, plasma, or serum in units of reciprocal time; dA_u/dt the urinary excretion rate at time T; and A_u the cumulative amount excreted in the same time period.

The value (i.e., the value at $T = \infty$) of the numerator in Equation (147) at times far beyond absorption (i.e., the value at $T \to \infty$) equals the denominator $(A_u)^\infty$, and it is not necessary to determine $(A_u)^\infty$ or to make a complete collection of the urine. There are no assumptions regarding the kinetic order of the absorption process. A semilogarithmic plot of the percent drug unabsorbed versus time will yield a straight line with a slope of $-k_a/2.303$ if absorption occurs by a first-order process. If a rectilinear plot results in a straight line, the absorption of drug may be a zero-order process.

Table 24

Percent Unabsorbed Versus Time Data for a Drug That Is Absorbed by an Apparent First-Order Process and Behaves According to a One-Compartment Model

1	2	3	4	5	6	7
T (hr)	C_T ($\mu g\ ml^{-1}$)	$\int_0^T C\ dt$ ($\mu g\ ml^{-1}\ hr^{-1}$)[a]	$K \int_0^T C\ dt$ ($\mu g\ ml^{-1}$)[b]	$C_T + K \int_0^T C\ dt$ ($\mu g\ ml^{-1}$)[c]	A_T/A_∞ (fraction absorbed)[d]	$100[1 - (A_T/A_\infty)]$ (percent unabsorbed)[e]
0	0	0	0	0	0	100
0.5	2.16	0.54	0.049	2.21	0.212	78.8
1.0	3.75	2.01	0.181	3.93	0.378	62.2
1.5	4.89	4.18	0.376	5.27	0.506	49.4
2.0	5.69	6.82	0.614	6.30	0.606	39.3
3.0	6.59	12.96	1.17	7.76	0.746	25.4
4.0	6.86	19.68	1.77	8.63	0.830	17.0
5.0	6.77	26.50	2.39	9.16	0.880	11.95
6.0	6.50	33.14	2.98	9.48	0.912	8.80
7.0	6.13	39.45	3.55	9.68	0.931	6.89
8.0	5.71	45.37	4.08	9.79	0.942	5.80
12.0	4.11	65.01	5.85	9.96	0.958	4.19
24.0	1.40	98.07	8.83	10.23		
36.0	0.48	109.35	9.84	10.32		
48.0	0.16	113.19	10.19	10.35		
72.0	0.018	115.33	10.38	10.40		
∞	0	115.53	10.40	10.40		

[a]Cumulative areas under the curve are obtained by drawing trapezoids, calculating their areas, and summing the trapezoidal areas to each time T. See the text for use of the trapezoidal method.

[b]K is obtained from a plot of ln C_T versus T (use the data from columns 1 and 2) for times in the 12- to 72-hr range. The value obtained is $K = 0.09\ hr^{-1}$ (graph not shown).

[c]Values are obtained using $K = 0.09\ hr^{-1}$ and the values of columns 2 and 3. For example, for the 2.0-hr time, $C_T + K \int_0^T C\ dt = 5.69 + 0.09(6.82) = 6.30$.

[d]The values are obtained by dividing column 5 values by the column 4 value at $T = \infty$, that is, $K \int_0^\infty C\ dt = 10.40$. For example at time 2.0 hr, $6.30 \div 10.40 = 0.606$. Either column 6 or column 7 may be used as a measure of absorption of a drug from its orally administered dosage form at various times.

[e]A plot of column 7 values on a log scale against time t in hours yields a line with a slope of $-k_a/2.303$, from which k_a, the rate of drug absorption, can be obtained. The value for k_a was found to be $0.5\ hr^{-1}$. See Figure 86.

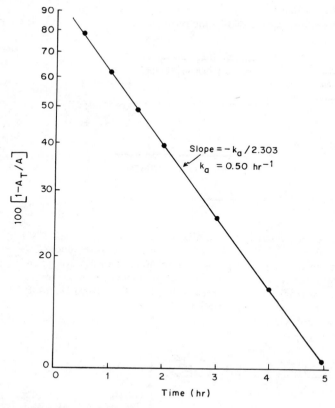

Figure 86. Semilogarithmic plot of percent drug remaining to be absorbed. Data from Table 24.

2. Two-Compartment Model: Loo-Riegelman Approach

Loo and Riegelman [292] pointed out that methods based on the one-compartment model do not result in acceptable estimates of the absorption rates. These methods may yield an incorrect rate constant and occasionally lead to an erroneous assignment of the order of the process. Equation (148), derived by Loo and Riegelman, is useful for the determination of the fraction of drug absorbed to time T. This equation,

$$\% \text{ Absorbed to time } T = \frac{(A_1)_T}{(A_1)^\infty} \times 100 = \frac{(C_1)_T + (C_2)_T + K \int_0^T C_1 \, dt}{K \int_0^\infty C_1 \, dt} \times 100 \qquad (148)$$

is based on the assumption that a drug upon oral or intravenous administration confers upon the body the characteristics of a two-compartment model, which may be represented as

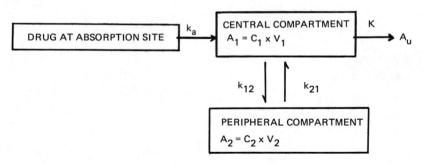

In Equation (148), $(A_1)_T$ is the amount of drug absorbed to time T, $(A_1)_\infty$ the amount of drug absorbed to time ∞, $\int_0^T C\, dt$ the area under the plasma concentration-time curve from time zero to time T, V_1 the volume of the central compartment or compartment 1, $(A_2)_T$ the amount of drug in the peripheral compartment or compartment 2, and K the overall first-order rate constant for elimination of drug by all processes from the central compartment or compartment 1.

Gibaldi and Perrier [293] and Wagner [297] show that the amount of drug in the peripheral compartment $(A_2)_T$ is

$$(A_2)_T = (A_2)_0 e^{-k_{21}t} + \frac{k_{12}(A_1)_0}{k_{21}}(1 - e^{-k_{21}t}) + \frac{k_{12}t^2}{2}\frac{\Delta A_1}{\Delta t} \tag{149}$$

The time interval Δt is the time between two consecutive sampling periods. Division of Equation (149) by V_1 (volume of central compartment) leads to the expression for $(C_2)_T$ required by Equation (148). Thus,

$$(C_2)_T = \frac{(A_2)_T}{V_1} = \frac{(A_2)_0}{V_1}e^{-k_{21}t} + \frac{k_{12}(A_1)_0}{k_{21}V_1}(1 - e^{-k_{21}t}) + \frac{k_{12}t^2}{2}\frac{\Delta A_1}{V_1\,\Delta t} \tag{150}$$

Letting $t = \Delta t$ reduces equation (150) to

$$(C_2)_T = \frac{(A_2)_T}{V_1} = \frac{(A_2)_0}{V_1}e^{-k_{21}\Delta t} + \frac{k_{12}(A_1)_0}{k_{21}V_1}(1 - e^{-k_{21}\Delta t}) + \frac{k_{12}\,\Delta t}{2}\Delta C_1 \tag{151}$$

Criticisms that might be made against this equation are that the drug must be able to be given intravenously, so that an estimate of K and V_1 can be obtained. An estimate of the amount of drug in the peripheral compartment as a function of time after oral administration must also be made on the same subject under carefully replicated conditions. As shown in Equation (151), this is indeed a complex calculation.

Equations (148) and (151) provide the data for calculating percent drug unabsorbed, $100[1 - (A_1)_T/(A_1)_\infty]$, versus time following oral or intramuscular administration. The estimates of K, k_{12}, k_{21}, and V_1 are obtained from intravenous administration of the drug.

Example 10. Sample Calculation Illustrating the Loo–Riegelman Method

The following example will illustrate the use of Equations (148) and (151). Consider a hypothetical drug that confers upon the body the characteristics of a two-compartment model, having a K of 0.16 hr^{-1}, a V_1 of 10 liters, a k_{12} of 0.4 hr^{-1}, and a k_{21} of 0.6 hr^{-1}. The plasma concentration-time data after oral administration is presented in Tables 25 and 26. These tables include the analysis of the data following the method of Loo and Riegelman.

Solution:

Using Equation (151), with $(A_2)_0/V_1$ for time $= 0.25$ hr, one obtains from Table 25, column 10, for the first point,

$$(C_2)_T = 0.0 + 0.0 + \frac{(0.4)(1.69)(0.25)}{2} = 0.085$$

Employing the data of Table 25 and Equation (151), one obtains for the second point at 0.5 hr:

$$(C_2)_T = (0.084)e^{-(0.6)(0.25)} + \frac{(0.4)(0.2577)}{(0.6)}\left[1 - e^{-(0.6)(0.25)}\right]$$

$$+ \frac{(0.4)(1.19)(0.25)}{2} = 0.289$$

See column 10 of Table 25 for comparison.

Column 10 in Table 25 is obtained by adding columns 7, 8, and 9. The percent absorbed to time T of 0.5 hr is then obtained using columns 2, 3, and 4 of Table 26. Thus, for T = 0.5 hr and using Equation (148), one obtains

$$\% \frac{(A_1)_T}{(A_1)_\infty} = \frac{2.88 + 0.289 + 0.25}{10.01} \times 100 = 33\%$$

See column 5 of Table 26 for comparison.

A semilogarithmic plot of percent drug unabsorbed [that is, $100 \times 1 - (A_1)_T/(A_1)_\infty$] (column 6, Table 26) is linear with a slope equal to $-k_a/2.303$. Figure 87 illustrates the semilogarithmic plot of percent drug remaining to be absorbed versus time. From its slope, one obtains a value for k_a of 0.8 hr^{-1}, the rate of absorption of the drug from the gastrointestinal tract or other site (such as intramuscular, rectal, etc.) of administration. Comparative bioavailability of a drug contained in various dosage forms can thus be assessed using percent rate of absorption.

Table 25

Percent–Unabsorbed–Time Data for a Drug That Is Absorbed by an Apparent First-Order Process and Behaves According to a Two–Compartment Model[a]

1	2	3	4	5	6	7	8	9	10
T (hr)	$(C_1)_T$ (μg ml^{-1})	ΔC_1 (μg ml^{-1})	Δt (hr)	$(A_1)_0$ (μg)	$(A_2)_0/V_1$ (μg ml^{-1})	$\dfrac{(A_2)_0}{V_1} e^{-k_{21}\Delta t}$	$\dfrac{k_{12}(A_1)_0}{k_{21}V_1}(1 - e^{-k_{21}\Delta t})$	$\dfrac{k_{21}(\Delta t)}{2}\,\Delta C_1$	$(C_2)_T$
0	0.0								
0.25	1.69	1.69	0.25	0.0	0.0	0.0	0.0	0.085	0.085
0.50	2.88	1.19	0.25	1.69	0.084	0.073	0.157	0.059	0.289
0.75	3.69	0.815	0.25	2.88	0.289	0.248	0.267	0.040	0.557
1.00	4.24	0.542	0.25	3.69	0.557	0.479	0.343	0.027	0.849
1.25	4.58	0.345	0.25	4.24	0.849	0.731	0.393	0.017	1.14
1.50	4.78	0.203	0.25	4.58	1.14	0.983	0.425	0.010	1.42
2.0	4.91	0.129	0.50	4.78	1.42	1.05	0.826	0.013	1.89
2.5	4.83	-0.078	0.50	4.91	1.89	1.40	0.849	-0.008	2.24
3.0	4.66	-0.172	0.50	4.83	2.24	1.66	0.835	-0.017	2.47
3.5	4.54	-0.208	0.50	4.66	2.48	1.84	0.806	-0.021	2.62
4.0	4.24	-0.216	0.50	4.54	2.62	1.94	0.769	-0.022	2.69
5.0	3.83	-0.410	1.00	4.24	2.69	1.48	1.27	-0.082	2.67
6.0	3.47	-0.361	1.00	3.83	2.67	1.46	1.15	-0.072	2.54
7.0	3.15	-0.316	1.00	3.47	2.54	1.40	1.04	-0.063	2.38
8.0	2.87	-0.280	1.00	3.15	2.38	1.30	0.947	-0.056	2.20
10.0	2.39	-0.478	2.00	2.87	2.20	0.661	1.34	-0.191	1.80
12.0	2.00	-0.395	2.00	2.39	1.80	0.544	1.11	-0.158	1.50
14.0	1.67	-0.328	2.00	2.00	1.50	0.452	0.930	-0.131	1.25
16.0	1.39	-0.275	2.00	1.67	1.25	0.377	0.778	-0.110	1.05
20.0	0.98	-0.420	4.00	1.40	1.05	0.095	0.846	-0.336	0.604

^{a}V$_1$ = 10 liters, k_{12} = 0.4 hr^{-1}, k_{21} = 0.6 hr^{-1}, and K = 0.16 hr^{-1}.

Table 26

Percent-Unabsorbed-Time Data for a Drug That Is Absorbed by an Apparent First-Order Process and Behaves According to a Two-Compartment Model[a]

1	2	3	4	5	6
T (hr)	$(C_1)_T$ ($\mu g\ ml^{-1}$)	$k_{el} \int_0^T C\ dt$ ($\mu g\ ml^{-1}$)	$(C_2)_T$ ($\mu g\ ml^{-1}$)	% $(A_1)_T/(A_1)_\infty$ (% absorbed)	$100[1 - (A_1)_T/(A_1)_\infty]$ (% unabsorbed)
0	0.0	0.0	0.0		
0.25	1.69	0.0334	0.085	18.18	81.82
0.50	2.88	0.125	0.289	33.00	66.93
0.75	3.69	0.257	0.557	45.27	54.73
1.00	4.24	0.415	0.849	55.24	44.76
1.25	4.58	0.591	1.14	63.41	36.59
1.50	4.78	0.778	1.42	70.11	29.89
2.0	4.91	1.16	1.89	80.04	19.96
2.5	4.83	1.56	2.24	86.70	13.30
3.0	4.66	1.94	2.47	91.17	8.83
3.5	4.54	2.30	2.62	94.17	5.83
4.0	4.24	2.64	2.69	96.19	3.81
5.0	3.83	3.29	2.67	98.34	1.66
6.0	3.47	3.88	2.54	99.32	0.68
7.0	3.15	4.40	2.38	99.78	0.22
8.0	2.87	4.89	2.20	100.00	0.0
10.0	2.39	5.73	1.80		
12.0	2.00	6.43	1.50		
14.0	1.67	7.02	1.25		
16.0	1.39	7.51	1.05		
20.0	0.98	8.27	0.604		
∞	0.0	10.01			

[a]Continuation of data for Loo-Riegelman method.

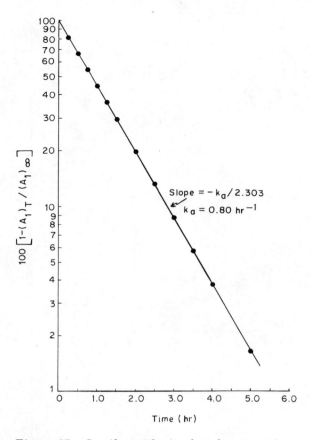

Figure 87. Semilogarithmic plot of percent drug remaining to be absorbed versus time. Data from Tables 25 and 26.

B. Extent of Absorption

1. Assessment of Bioavailability from Plasma Levels

By its definition, bioavailability includes both extent and rate of absorption. The questions to be answered are how fast and how much of an administered drug reaches the systemic circulation. In the preceding section we discussed the Wagner-Nelson and Loo-Riegelman methods to calculate the speed of absorption. Both of these methods are model-dependent. In the following section we discuss methods for estimating absorption extent, which are not model-dependent. It is generally well accepted that the absolute bioavailability of a drug can only be determined by comparison with an intravenous dose, and a widely used method to determine the absorption of a drug is to compare plasma level or urinary excretion following oral administration of a drug (also other routes) with that following intravenous administration of a solution of drug. Absorption extent following intravenous administration of a drug solution is equated to 100% availability.

In many instances intravenous administration is not possible. Examples are drugs that are damaging to the vessels when injected. Suspensions of highly insoluble drugs are not ordinarily administered by the i. v. route. In these cases, the bioavailability of a drug is established by comparing it to a secondary standard (oral solution). Thus, relative bioavailability is determined as opposed to absolute bioavailability, which is obtained when an i. v. dose is used. Lalka and Feldman suggested an approach for approximating the absolute bioavailability without the administration of an intravenous dose; the paper should be seen for details of the method [298].

In order to determine the absolute extent of bioavailability afforded by a drug dosage form, we compare the areas under the plasma concentration–time curve following oral (or other route, excluding i. v.) and intravenous administration of the same dose of drug. This is mathematically expressed as

$$\text{Absolute availability} = \frac{\left(\int_0^\infty C \, dt\right)_{\text{oral}}}{\left(\int_0^\infty C \, dt\right)_{\text{i.v.}}} \tag{152}$$

where $\left(\int_0^\infty C \, dt\right)_{\text{oral}}$ and $\left(\int_0^\infty C \, dt\right)_{\text{i.v.}}$ are the areas under the plasma concentration–time curves after oral and intravenous administration, respectively.

The area under the plasma concentration–time curve can be calculated with the trapezoidal rule:

$$\int_{t_1}^{t_2} C(t) \, dt = \frac{t_2 - t_1}{2} (C_1 + C_2)$$

Using this equation for the time interval 0 to 0.5 hr in Table 24, for example, one obtains for the second point in column 3.

$$\int_0^T C \, dt = \text{area} = \frac{0.5 - 0}{2} (0 + 2.16) = 0.54$$

Some hand calculators, such as the Commodore SR 4190R, are programmed to calculate areas under a curve using the trapezoidal rule.

Following oral administration, the fraction of the dose that is absorbed, or efficiency of absorption F, corrected for intrasubject and intersubject variability in half-life, can be expressed as

$$F = \frac{\left(\int_0^\infty C \, dt\right)_{\text{oral}} (t_{1/2})_{\text{i.v.}}}{\left(\int_0^\infty C \, dt\right)_{\text{i.v.}} (t_{1/2})_{\text{oral}}} \tag{153}$$

Equation (153) is valid regardless of the number of compartments describing the time course of drug in the body. If the half-life for elimination following i.v. injection $(t_{1/2})_{i.v.}$ is identical with the biological half-life following oral administration $(t_{1/2})_{oral}$, then the fraction of dose absorbed by the oral route F of Equation (153) is exactly equal to absolute availability as defined by Equation (152).

As discussed previously, in certain cases intravenous administration of the drug is not possible. In this case the relative bioavailability is given by Equation (154):

$$\text{Relative availability} = \frac{\left(\int_0^\infty C\ dt\right)_{oral}}{\left(\int_0^\infty C\ dt\right)_{oral\ standard}(t_{1/2})_{oral}} \tag{154}$$

in which the standard is administered as an oral solution, suspension, or other form serving as the reference system. The fraction of dose absorbed, when relative availability is being determined, is given by

$$F_{relative} = \frac{\left(\int_0^\infty C\ dt\right)_{oral}(t_{1/2})_{oral\ standard}}{\left(\int_0^\infty C\ dt\right)_{oral\ standard}(t_{1/2})_{oral}} \tag{155}$$

There are a number of cases in which the availability of a drug cannot be obtained after single administration. In these cases the availability of a drug may be determined using steady-state levels of drugs following multiple administration. The following equation is useful to determine a realistic estimate of the relative amount absorbed, under conditions of multiple dosing:

$$F_{rel(mult)} = \frac{\left(\int_0^\infty C(\tau)\ dt\right)_{oral}(t_{1/2})_{oral\ standard}}{\left(\int_0^\infty C(\tau)\ dt\right)_{oral\ standard}(t_{1/2})_{oral}} \tag{156}$$

where $(\int_0^\infty C(\tau)\ dt)_{oral}$ and $(\int_0^\infty C(\tau)\ dt)_{oral\ standard}$ are the area under the plasma concentration-time curve during a dosing interval τ at steady state after oral administration of the test drug dosage form, and the corresponding area for the standard oral dosage form, respectively.

Equation (156) is a valid measure of absorption efficiency regardless of the number of compartments describing the time course of drug in the body. However, it requires that the dosing interval τ be sufficiently large to permit an estimate of half-life from the terminal linear segment. Wagner et al. applied this method for different dosage forms of indoxole [299].

Example 11. <u>Sample Calculation of Relative Bioavailability Employing Extent of Absorption</u>.

A bioavailability study was conducted with the purpose of determining the relative availability (extent of absorption) of a tablet dosage form. A group of subjects received an oral standard preparation (oral solution, treatment A) and a test formulation (tablet, treatment B). On each study day, drug plasma concentration was determined as a function of time. Plasma concentration-times curves were constructed and the elimination half-lives as well as the areas under the curves (AUC) were determined. The following table provides the result:

	Treatment A	Treatment B
Half-life (hr)	12	11
AUC (μg ml^{-1} hr^{-1})	120	113

Calculate the relative bioavailability.

Step 1. Equation (155) allows the calculation of the relative bioavailability. Thus,

$$F_{relative} = \frac{113 \times 12}{120 \times 11} = 1.03$$

It should be noted that $F_{relative}$ can be greater than unity, owing to the ratios of half-lives in Equation (155).

2. Other Techniques for Assessing Bioavailability

Absolute and relative availability of a drug from various dosage forms and routes of administration may also be determined by analysis of unaltered drug in the urine. In cases where the drug is eliminated almost totally by metabolism or where an assay for the metabolite is more adaptable than for the unchanged drug in plasma or urine, an index of comparative bioavailability may be better obtained by comparing areas under the plasma concentration-time curves for metabolites following oral and intravenous administration of the drug at identical dose levels.

3. Assessment of Bioavailability From Pharmacological Response

The use of pharmacological data as an alternative to direct assay data for performing bioavailability and pharmacokinetics analyses of drug has been examined by Smolen and co-workers [300]. Chlorpromazine was used as a model drug for the application of pharmacological data to the study of bioavailability. The work consisted of monitoring changes in pupil size, intraocular pressure, heart rate, body temperature, blood pressure, drug-induced changes in ECG, and spontaneously and visually evoked response EEG. Figure 88 illustrates the time variation of averaged miotic response intensities observed in crossover

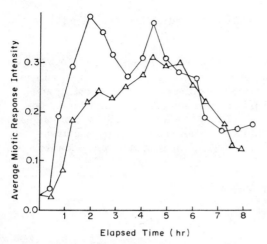

Elapsed Time (hr)

Figure 88. Time variation of average miotic response intensities observed in crossover experiments following oral dosing of nine normal human subjects with 100-mg oral doses of chlorpromazine syrup (O) and tablets (Δ). (From Ref. 300.)

experiments following oral chlorpromazine syrup and tablets. The areas under the pharmacological intensity versus time curves have the same interpretation with regard to reflecting extent of bioavailability as areas under blood level versus time curves [301-304]. The results of these studies present the opportunity to further evaluate bioavailability from pharmacological response. This is a noninvasive method which deals not only with bioavailability but also with therapeutic equivalency.

As a result of some of these studies, the FDA has included in their regulations measurement of an appropriate acute pharmacological effect as a general approach for determining bioavailability [2].

VI. In Vitro, In Situ, and In Vivo Methods to Study Physiologic Factors Affecting Drug Absorption

As mentioned previously, various physiological factors may affect the absorption of drugs from the gastrointestinal tract. The characterization of the absorption behavior of a drug will permit the development and/or improvement of drug dosage forms. In vitro, in situ, and more recently new in vivo techniques have assisted the investigator in examining absorption characteristics of drugs. Apparatus and techniques for studying in vitro dissolution have already been discussed (Sec. III.C). Absorption studies include examination of the region of the gastrointestinal tract for maximum absorption, investigation of the processes by which drugs are absorbed (i.e., passive diffusion and active transport), and elucidation of the physicochemical factors affecting dosage form behavior (i.e., active ingredient/excipient ratio, film versus coated tablets, and solubility parameters).

Table 27

In Vitro, In Situ, and In Vivo Methods to Study Physiological Factors Affecting Drug Absorption

In Vitro	In Situ	In Vivo
Everted sac (Weisman and Wilson [305])	Perfusion technique (Schanker et al. [39])	Direct methods: blood levels, urinary levels
Everted sac modification (Crane and Wilson [306])	Rat gut technique (Doluisio et al. [310])	Indirect methods: pharmacologic response (Irwin et al. [313], De Cato et al. [314], Levy [315])
Circulation technique (Fisher and Parsons [307], Wiseman [308], Darlington and Quastel [319])	Intestinal loop technique (Levine and Pelikan [311])	Short-lived isotope methods (Digenis et al. [316])
Everted ring or slice technique (Crane and Mandelstam [309])	Rat stomach technique (Schanker et al. [312], Doluisio et al. [310])	
Everted sac flow-through technique (Newburger and Stavchansky [318])		

In vitro and in situ methods are simple and reproducible. In vivo animal models usually consist of lower experimental animals, such as rats, hamsters, rabbits, and sometimes dogs and monkeys. These provide clues to drug absorption and action but must be used with caution when comparison is made with clinical studies. In vivo human experimentation provides the most useful information, but the work is expensive, difficult to interpret, and limited by stringent restrictions, such as patient consent, particularly in the case of pediatric and geriatric subjects. In vitro and in situ studies are therefore of value as more direct and economical studies of drug absorption and action.

Table 27 summarizes some of the better known techniques available to the pharmaceutical scientist for the purpose of characterizing drug absorption. These are elaborated on in the following paragraphs.

A. Everted Sac Technique

The everted sac method, devised by Wilson and Wiseman [305], involves isolating a small segment of the intestine of a rat or hamster, inverting the intestine, and filling the sac with drug-buffered solution. Both ends of the segment are tied off and the sac is immersed in an Erlenmeyer flask containing a large volume of a buffer solution. The flask and its contents are oxygenated and agitated at 37° C for a specified period of time and the fluids are assayed for drug content. The major disadvantage of the method is the difficulty in obtaining more than one sample per intestinal segment.

B. Single-Segment Modification of the Everted Sac Method

A modification of the original everted sac technique was introduced by Crane and
Wilson [306] to permit the testing of different solutions with a single intestinal
segment. The major change from the original everted sac technique is the at-
tachment of the intestine to a cannula from which frequent samples can be obtained.
Several investigators have used this method to study active and passive transport
processes [320-322].

C. Circulation Technique

The circulation method involves isolating the entire small intestine of a rat or
hamster [307], or a segment [308, 319] with circulation of oxygenated buffer
through the lumen and serosal side of the intestinal membrane. Absorption rates
are calculated after drug content is determined in the lumen and serosal solutions.

D. Everted Ring or Slice Technique

Crane and Mandelstam [309] devised an everted ring technique, which involves
cutting the entire small intestine or a segment of the intestine into ringlike slices
0.1 to 0.5 cm in length. The slices are oxygenated with Krebs buffer and dried
with filter paper and placed in a flask containing a drug in buffered solution at
37°C. At selected time intervals the slices are assayed for drug content. This
technique has been used by several investigators to examine active and passive
absorption processes [309, 323, 324].

E. Everted Sac Flow-Through Technique

Newburger and Stavchansky [318] modified the Crane and Wilson method. The
major advantage of this technique is that solutions placed inside the everted preparation can be removed by a simple flushing process. Other techniques require a
sampling device to be placed inside the intestine, thereby possibly causing damage
by "raking" the intestinal wall as the sampling device is introduced or removed.
Also, the orifice of the sampling device may become occluded against the intestinal
wall, thus preventing withdrawal of the sample.
        The apparatus is illustrated in Figure 89. It consists of a glass tube permanently
secured inside a plastic jacket through which water is circulated at 37°C. The top of
the tube is closed with a rubber stopper which supports a gas dispersion tube of medium porosity through which oxygen is bubbled. Also supported in the stopper are a
thermometer; a hypodermic needle, which acts as a pressure-relief valve for the
escaping oxygen; a polyethylene tube inserted through the hypodermic needle to allow the outside drug solution to be sampled; and a beaded pipet over which the intestinal segment has been everted and secured with a silk suture. A piece of Tygon
tubing is connected to the top of the pipet to which a three-way plastic valve is attached. The bottom of the glass tube is closed with another rubber stopper which
supports a constricted glass connector. The other end of the everted intestinal
segment is secured with a silk suture to this connector. To the outside of the
glass connector a three-way plastic valve is connected by a piece of Tygon tubing.
One of the other ends of the three-way plastic valve is connected to a glass L by a

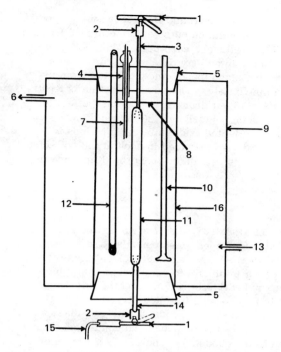

Figure 89. Everted intestinal segment flow through apparatus. 1, three-way valve; 2, Tygon tubing; 3, beaded pipet; 4, hypodermic needle; 5, rubber stopper; 6, water outlet; 7, polyethylene tube; 8, drug solution level; 9, constant-temperature jacket; 10, gas dispersion tube; 11, intestinal segment; 12, thermometer; 13, water inlet; 14, connecting tube; 15, glass L; 16, inside container. (From Ref. 318.)

piece of Tygon tubing. The glass tube must be long enough to accommodate a 10-cm length of intestine which is completely immersed in the drug solution, but to leave an air space above the top of the solution to prevent the bubbling of the solution up through the hypodermic needle with the escaping oxygen. The oxygen flow rate is adjusted to a minimum so that the bubbling of the solution can be observed. Distilled water is circulated through the jacket by connecting hoses from the circulating pump to the inlet and outlet ports of the container. A constant temperature of 37° C is attained before the animal surgery is started. The apparatus is supported on a ring stand during the experiments.

Newburger [318] employed this technique to examine the metabolism of quaternary ammonium compounds in the presence and absence of trichloroacetic acid.

F. Perfusion Technique

The perfusion method of Schanker et al. [39] involves anesthetizing the animal with pentobarbital and then exposing small intestine by a midline abdominal

incision. The intestine is cannulated at the duodenal and ileal ends with polyethylene cannulas having inside diameters of 2.5 mm and outside diameters of 3.5 mm.
The stomach and cecum are closed off by ligatures, care being taken not to oc-
clude major blood vessels. The bile duct may or may not be ligated. The intestine is replaced in the abdomen, the incision closed, and perfusion from pylorus to ileocecal junction is started immediately. The small intestine is first
cleared of particulate matter by perfusion with a drug-free solution (buffer) for
30 min. The solution containing drug is then perfused for 30 min to displace the
previous wash, after which samples are collected at definite time periods from
the ileal outflow. The concentration of drug is measured in each of the collected
samples and the relative rate of absorption is calculated from the difference in
concentration of drug entering and leaving the intestine.

G. Rat Gut Technique

In this method, introduced by Doluisio et al. [310], the small intestine is exposed
by a midline abdominal incision, and two L-shaped glass cannulas are inserted
through small slits at the duodenal and ileal ends. Care is taken to handle the small
intestine gently and to reduce surgery to a minimum to maintain an intact blood supply. The cannulas are secured by ligation with silk suture, and the intestine is returned to the abdominal cavity to aid in maintaining its integrity. Four-centimeter
segments of Tygon tubing are attached to the exposed ends of both cannulae, and a
30-ml hypodermic syringe fitted with a three-way stopcock and containing perfusion fluid warmed to 37° C is attached to the duodenal cannula. As a means of
clearing the gut, perfusion fluid is then passed slowly through it and out the ileal
cannula and discarded until the effluent is clear. The remaining perfusion solution
is carefully expelled from the intestine by means of air pumped in from the syringe,
and 10 ml of drug solution is immediately introduced into the intestine by means of
the syringe. A stopwatch is started, and the ileal cannula is connected to another
30-ml syringe fitted with a three-way stopcock. This arrangement enables the
operator to pump the lumen solution into either the ileal or the duodenal syringe,
remove a 0.1-ml aliquot, and return the remaining solution to the intestine within
10 to 15 sec. To assure uniform drug solution concentrations throughout the gut
segment, aliquots are removed from the two syringes alternately. The apparatus
is shown schematically in Figure 90.
    The Doluisio rat gut technique has been useful in examining the behavior of
weakly acidic and basic drugs. In addition, the effects of membrane storage on
the kinetics of drug absorption have been determined [325].

H. Intestinal Loop Technique

Levine and Pelikan [311] devised an intestinal loop procedure involving the formation of either single or multiple intestinal loops. The single-loop method consists
of anesthetizing the animal under light ether anesthesia, then exposing the intestine
and placing the proximal ligature about 6 in. from the pylorus. The length of the
loop (about 4 in.) is determined in vivo by counting off four mesenteric blood vessels between the proximal and distal ligatures. No major blood vessels are occluded by these ties. After the drug solution is injected quantitatively into the loop
(without puncturing the gut wall between ligatures), the proximal ligature is secured and the incision closed. The rat used in the study reported appeared fully

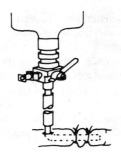

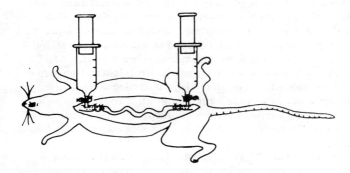

Figure 90. Experimental arrangement for determining rates of absorption of drugs from rat intestinal lumen in situ. (From Ref. 130; reproduced with permission of the copyright owner.)

recovered from the procedure within 5 min. After 3 hr, the animal is again anesthetized with ether and, before the animal is killed, the loop of the gut is removed for chemical analysis and determination of its quantity of unabsorbed drug.

The multiple-loop procedure is similar to that for the single-loop preparation. The proximal ligature of the first loop is placed about 6 in. from the pylorus, four mesenteric blood vessels counted off, and the second ligature placed and secured. The second and third loops, each of which is about 4 in. long, are prepared similarly, leaving about 0.5 in. of intestine between loops. The appropriate solution is injected quantitatively into each loop. At the end of 3 hr, each loop is excised and analyzed separately. The portion of the gut used in the single-loop preparation is always found to be macroscopically free of food. In the multiple-loop preparation, the more distal portions of the gut have to be cleared of visible boluses of food; the boluses are removed by a gentle milking technique.

I. Rat Stomach Technique

There are two widely used rat stomach procedures: a method developed by Schanker et al. [312] and a modification introduced by Doluisio et al. [310]. The

latter allows a determination of the amount of drug absorbed as a function of time.
The rat stomach is exposed, cannulated at the cardiac and duodenal ends, and
washed from the cardiac end with perfusion solution until the effluent is clear.
The perfusion solution is expelled with air, and 5 ml of drug solution is introduced through the cardiac cannula. A stopwatch is started and a 15-cm section
of 0.011-cm-ID polyethylene tubing, connected to a 2-ml syringe and fitted with
a three-way stopcock, is inserted through the duodenal cannula. At specified intervals the stomach contents are sampled by withdrawing about 0.5 ml of the solution into the syringe, removing a 0.1-ml aliquot, and returning the remainder.

J. In Vivo Methods

The methods described above were of the in vitro type. In vivo method have also
been successfully employed to characterize the absorption characteristics of drugs.
Direct methods employ blood or urine data to calculate absorption rates. Indirect
methods use pharmacologic response data for the purpose of examining physiological and physicochemical factors influencing drug absorption. Irwin et al. [313]
and Newburger [314] utilized mydriases to demonstrate gastrointestinal absorption of quaternary ammonium compounds. DeCato [314] used blepharoptic assay
procedures to study the absorption of reserpine. Smolen et al. [300] examined
mydriasis response to determine the bioavailability of chlorpromazine preparations. Levy [315] has reviewed the methods for estimating absorption rates from
pharmacologic response data.

Recently, Digenis et al. [316] used ^{99m}Tc-labeled triethylenetetraminepoly-
styrene resin for measuring gastric emptying in humans. Quantitative dynamic
data were obtained with these radionucleides without physical or physiological influences on the gastrointestinal tract [317]. In addition, excellent scintigraphic
images of the stomach, intestines, and colon were obtained with a low-target-
organ, total-body-radiation dose. Figure 91 illustrates the rate of clearance of
^{99m}Tc-labeled polystyrene beads bearing triethylenetetramine functions from the
stomach of a normal human subject. The authors reported a half-life time of
gastric emptying of 51 min.

VII. Sustained-Release Medication

Sustained-release dosage forms provide a prolonged dosing of drug from the product by supplying an initial amount or loading dose, perhaps one-half of the total
dose released, followed by a gradual and uniform release of the remainder of the
drug over the desired time period.

It is not difficult to write equations that describe the release characteristics
of sustained action tablet and capsule forms. It is another matter to formulate
and manufacture products that faithfully deliver the drug uniformly under variable
conditions of patient physiology and therapy and that reflect the desired plasma
level profiles designed into the dosage form. Cabana and Kumkumian [326] recently outlined the position of the FDA regarding the design of controlled-release
products for use in humans, and requirements for substantiating safety and efficacy and providing proper labeling of these products.

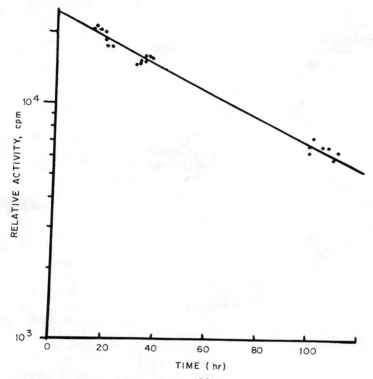

Figure 91. Rate of clearance of ^{99m}Tc-labeled polystyrene beads bearing tri-ethylenetetramine functions from the stomach of a normal human male subject (half-time of gastric emptying = 51 min). (From Ref. 316; reproduced with permission of the copyright owner.)

 The formulation and manufacture of sustained-release products is the subject of another chapter in this series of monographs. It is our intention here only to introduce equations that describe the time course of drug in the body following administration of a sustained-action formulation.

 Sustained-release forms are designed to provide adequate blood levels over a sufficient period of time at the pharmacological site so as to result in clinical advantages.

 Antihistamines, sedative, and tranquilizers are particularly well adapted to sustained action, as the blood levels in these cases are desired to be maintained over prolonged periods of time.

 Time-release preparations have no rational for drugs with a long biologic half-life in the body ($t_{1/2} > 12$ hr). The half-life of some drugs are found in Table 28. Furthermore, highly potent drugs are not candidates for sustained release. It is desirable to be able to alter dosage or withhold the potent drug at will during the regimen, and such control is lost when the patient is under continuous medication with an 8- to 12-hr sustained-dose form.

Table 28

Biological Half-Lives of Drugs

Acetosal	20 min	Xylocaine	75 min
Salicylic acid	4-4 1/2 hr	Pentazocine	2 hr
Phenacetine	45-90 min	Norephedrine	4 hr
Phenazone	10-15 hr	Ephedrine	3-4 hr
Phenylbutazone	3 days	Methylephedrine	4-5 hr
Hydroxyphenylbutazone	3 days	Methoxyphenamine	8-15 hr
Aminophenazone	3 hr	Dexamphetamine	6-7 hr
Paracetamol	95-170 min	(+)-Methamphetamine	12-14 hr
Barbital	4-5 days	(+)-Ethylamphetamine	13-17 hr
Phenobarbital	3-1/2 days	(+)-Isopropylamphetamine	2-3 hr
Butobarbital	30-45 hr	(+)-Dimethylamphetamine	5 1/2-6 hr
Pentobarbital	42 hr	Phentermine	19-24 hr
Thiopental	16 hr	Mephentermine	17-18 hr
Hexobarbital	17 hr	Chlorphentermine	37-38 hr
Gluethimide	10 hr	Pipradrol	22-27 hr
Paraldehyde	7-1/2 hr	Fencamfamin	10-12 hr
Diphnylhydantoin	9 hr	Caffeine	3 1/2-6 hr
Meprobamate	11-14 hr	Lysergide (LSD)	3 hr
Diazepam	27-28 hr	Imipramine	3 1/2 hr
Ethylbiscoumacetate	1-2 hr	Desipramine	30-35 hr
Discoumarol	32 hr	Mepacrine	5 days
Warfarine	30-40 hr	Hexamethonium	1 1/2 hr
Heparine	60-90 min	Tubocurarine	12-15 min
Digitoxine	4-6 days	Succinylcholine	3 1/2 min
Digoxine	40-50 hr	Noscapine	40-50 min

Source: From Ref. 327 and other sources.

Let us suppose that a new potent ephedrine-like tablet, 15 mg when taken four times during the day for its nasal decongestant effect, is found to be therapeutically effective. The daily dose is 4 × 15 = 60 mg. The dosing interval τ is 24 hr, although the drug is administered only during the waking hours of each day: 8 a.m., 12 p.m., 4 p.m., and 8 p.m. The plasma levels fluctuate greatly as each dose is absorbed and eliminated, and it is desired to prepare a sustained release form that would allow administration only once or twice a day. It is expected that this would be more convenient for the patient and provide more uniform blood levels. Let us see how such a product might be formulated. In this example we follow the treatment of Notari [328].

The average steady-state plasma concentration for this drug, following the regimen above, is given by

$$\overline{C} = F \frac{A_0}{V_d K \tau} \tag{157}$$

for drug concentration at steady state following first-order absorption according to a one-compartment model. We obtain the result

$$\overline{C} = 0.86 \frac{60 \text{ mg}}{18,000 \text{ ml} \times 0.231/\text{hr} \times 24 \text{ hr}} = \frac{51.6}{99,792} = 5.171 \times 10^{-4} \text{ mg ml}^{-1}$$

$$= 0.517 \ \mu\text{g ml}^{-1}$$

In this example we have assumed that the fraction of drug absorbed from the gastrointestinal tract into the systemic circulation, F, equals 0.86. The 24-hr dose (four doses × 15 mg) of the ephedrine tablet A_0 is 60 mg. The apparent volume of distribution V_d is 18,000 ml, and K, the elimination-rate constant, is 0.231 hr^{-1}.

To prepare a sustained-release product, we design it so that one 60-mg tablet is taken each 12 hr, or two tablets of 30 mg each are taken over 24 hr. It is assumed that the drug is absorbed orally and eliminated in the urine by first-order processes.

It would be more desirable to have the drug released from its preparation and absorbed from the gastrointestinal tract by zero-order kinetics, providing 60 mg/ 24 hr or a steady release of 2.5 mg of drug each hour. But true zero-order release products are not yet commercially available; we must therefore satisfy ourselves for the present with first-order release from the dosage form.

To overcome the time lag following administration before the drug reaches steady-state concentration in the body, as was noted earlier under intravenous administration, some sustained action products are currently formulated with a loading dose in the outer coating together with the sustained-release mass in the core of the tablet. Care must be taken, however, that this administration form does not lead to an accumulation of drug as each new dose is taken. Accumulation will occur if sufficient time is not allowed for all drug to be cleared from the body between doses. Gibaldi and Perrier [329] discuss this difficulty.

If, however, the sustained-release tablet is given in 30-mg dose twice a day (once each 12 hr), and if its first-order absorption half-life is, for example, 2 hr, then six half-lives transpire before the new dose is taken. This allows a sufficient washout period of the first dose so that only 1.5% of the drug remains in the gastrointestinal tract when the second dose is administered.

In the case of the product we are formulating, the tablet contains 30 mg of drug and for a first-order absorption process has a half-life of 2.0 hr. In the gut it is released over a period of 12 hr before the second dose is given, so that accumulation of drug does not occur in the body.

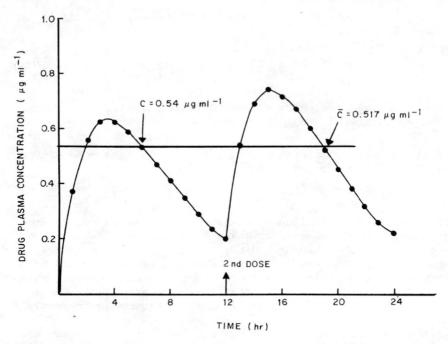

Figure 92. Plasma levels of a hypothetical ephedrine derivative resulting from the oral administration of a sustained-release tablet containing 30 mg of the drug. The drug is released at an apparent first-order rate with a half-life of 2 hr.

The equation used to describe the concentration of drug in the plasma over a 24-hr period is, according to Gibaldi and Perrier [329]:

$$C_n = F \frac{k_a A_0}{V_d(k_a - K)} \left[\left(\frac{1 - e^{-nK\tau}}{1 - e^{-k\tau}} \right) e^{-kt} - \left(\frac{1 - e^{-nk_a\tau}}{1 - e^{-k_a\tau}} \right) e^{-k_a t} \right] \tag{158}$$

where n is the dose number, 1 and 2. For our tablet A = 30 mg, K = 0.231 hr^{-1}, V_d = 18 liters, τ = 12 hr, F is 0.86, and k_a = 0.693/2.0 = 0.347 hr^{-1}. Using this equation, we can evaluate C at 6 hr after the first tablet is administered:

$$C_1 = \frac{(0.86)(0.347)(30)}{18(0.347 - 0.231)} \left[\left(\frac{1 - e^{-(1)(0.231)(12)}}{1 - e^{-(0.231)(12)}} \right) e^{-(0.231)(6)} \right.$$

$$\left. - \left(\frac{1 - e^{-(1)(0.347)(12)}}{1 - e^{-(0.347)(12)}} \right) e^{-(0.347)(6)} \right] = 0.54 \ \mu g \ ml^{-1}$$

Thus, we see in Figure 92 that after 6 hr, the plasma concentration C_6 of the ephedrine derivative has risen to a concentration of 0.54 $\mu g \ ml^{-1}$. Calculating

C_2 with n = 2 in Equation (158) and letting t = 9 gives the computed point on C = 0.38 μg ml^{-1} at a 21-hr running time on the right-hand side of Figure 92. The horizontal line in the figure signifies the "average" steady-state plasma concentration $\bar{C}$ = 0.517 μg ml^{-1}.

It is evident that the two sustained-release tablets do not provide a steady-state blood level approximating $\bar{C}$. Instead, the profile for the two-30-mg tablets actually provides the body with periods of greater than and less than a uniform blood level. Nevertheless, the formulation of this product into sustained-action tablets provides convenience for the patient and relatively continuous blood levels over a 24-hr period, the peaks and valleys of which are probably in the range of therapeutic efficacy. Thus, pharmacokinetic modeling can assist the formulator to make a realistic appraisal of what can be expected at the present stage of technology in designing sustained-release dosage forms.

References

1. Teorell, T., Arch. Int. Pharmacodyn., 57:205 (1937).
2. Bioequivalence Requirements and in Vivo Bioavailability Procedures, Fed. Regist., Jan. 7, 1977.
3. MacDonald, H., Pisano, F., Barger, J., Dornbush, A., and Pelcak, E., Clin. Med., 76:30 (1969).
4. Barr, W. H., Gerbracht, L. M., Letchen, K., Plant, M., and Strahl, N., Clin. Pharmacol. Ther., 13:97 (1972).
5. Glazko, A. J., Kinkel, A. W., Alegmani, W. C., and Holmes, E. L., Clin. Pharmacol. Ther., 9:472 (1968).
6. Wagner, J. G., Christensen, M., Sakmar, E., Blair, D., Yates, P. W., III, and Sedman, A. J., J. Am. Med. Assoc., 224:199 (1973).
7. Lindenbaum, J., N. Engl. J. Med., 285:1344 (1971).
8. Van Pettin, G., Feng, H., Withey, R. J., and Lettau, H. F., J. Clin. Pharmacol., 11:177 (1971).
9. Choiu, W. L., J. Clin. Pharmacol., 12:296 (1972).
10. Blair, D. C., Barnes, R. W., Wildner, E. L., and Murray, W. J., J. Am. Med. Assoc., 215:251 (1971).
11. Brice, G. W., and Hammer, H. F., Drug Inf. Bull., 3:112 (1969).
12. Catz, B., Ginsburg, E., and Salenger, S., N. Engl. J. Med., 266:136 (1962).
13. Sullivan, T. J., Sakmar, E., Albert, K. S., Blair, D. C., and Wagner, J. G, J. Pharm. Sci., 64:1723 (1975).
14. Aguiar, A. J., Wheeler, L. M., Fusari, S., and Zelmer, J. E., J. Pharm. Sci., 57:1844 (1968).
15. Bioavailability Requirement for Prescription Drugs, Fed. Regis., Jan. 3, 1973.
16. Drug Bioequivalence—A report of the Office of Technology Assessment Drug Bioequivalency Study Panel. Superintendent of Documents, U.S. Government Printing Office, Washington, D.C., 1974.
17. Levy, G., Leonards, J. R., and Procknal, J. A., J. Pharm. Sci., 54:1719 (1965).
18. Wagner, J. G., Generic Equivalence and Inequivalence of Oral Products. In: Biopharmaceutics and Relevant Pharmacokinetics, Drug Intelligence Publications, Hamilton, Ill., 1971, pp. 166-179.

19. Barr, W. H., Pharmacology, 8:55 (1972).
20. Nelson, E., J. Am. Pharm. Assoc., Sci. Ed., 47:297 (1958).
21. Levy, G., J. Pharm. Sci., 50:388 (1961).
22. MacDonald, H., Pisano, F., Burger, J., Dornbush, A., and Pelcak, E., Drug Inf. Bull., 3:76 (1969).
23. Bergan, T., Oydvin, B., and Lundo, I., Acta Pharmacol. Toxicol., 33:138 (1973).
24. Bates, T. R., Lambert, D. A., and Johns, W. H., J. Pharm. Sci., 58:1468 (1969).
25. Gibaldi, M., and Weintraub, H., J. Pharm. Sci., 59:725 (1970).
26. Guidelines for Biopharmaceutical Studies in Man. American Pharmaceutical Association, Academy of Pharmaceutical Sciences, Washington, D.C., 1972.
27. Calter, P., Problem Solving with Computers, McGraw-Hill, New York, 1973; J. M. Smith, Scientific Analysis on the Pocket Calculator, Wiley, New York, 1975; R. Hamming, Numerical Methods for Scientists and Engineers, McGraw-Hill, New York, 1973.
28. Wagner, J. G., Pharmacology, 8:102 (1972).
29. Skelly, J. R., Bioavailability Policies and Guidelines. In Industrial Bio-availability and Pharmacokinetics: Guidelines, Regulations and Controls (A. Martin and J. T. Doluisio, eds.), Drug Dynamics Institute, College of Pharmacy, The University of Texas at Austin, Austin, Tex., 1977.
30. Dittert, L. W., and DiSanto, R., J. Am. Pharm. Assoc., NS13(8):421 (1973).
31. Levy, G., and Jusko, W., J. Pharm. Sci., 55:285 (1966).
32. Schanker, L. S., and Tocco, D. J., J. Pharmacol. Exp. Ther., 128:115 (1960).
33. Goldstein, A., Aronow, L., and Kalman, S. M., eds., Principles of Drug Action, 2nd ed., Wiley, New York, 1974, p. 143.
34. Schanker, L. S., and Jeffrey, J. J., Biochem. Pharmacol., 11:961 (1962).
35. Evered, D. F., and Randall, H. G., Biochem. Pharmacol., 11:371 (1962).
36. Higuchi, T., Thermodynamics, Kinetics and Mechanisms of Interface Transport of Organic Ammonium Species, seminar presented at The Upjohn Company, July 12, 1967.
37. Shore, P. A., Brodie, B. B., and Hogben, C. A. M., J. Pharmacol. Exp. Ther., 119:361 (1957).
38. Hogben, C. A. M., Tocco, D. J., Brodie, B. B., and Schanker, L. S., J. Pharmacol. Exp. Ther., 125:275 (1959).
39. Schanker, L. S., Tocco, D. J., Brodie, B. B., and Hogben, C. A. M., J. Pharmacol. Exp. Ther., 123:81 (1958).
40. Brodie, B. B., and Hogben, C. A. M., J. Pharm. Pharmacol., 9:345 (1957).
41. Schanker, L. S., J. Med. Chem., 2:343 (1960).
42. Brodie, B. B., in: Absorption and Distribution of Drugs (T. B. Binns, ed.). William & Wilkins, Baltimore, Md., 1964, p. 42.
43. Suzuki, A., Higuchi, W. I., and Ho, N. F. H., J. Pharm. Sci., 59:644 (1970).
44. Suzuki, A., Higuchi, W. I., and Ho, N. F. H., J. Pharm. Sci., 59:651 (1970).
45. Koizumi, T., Arita, T., and Kakemi, K., Chem. Pharm. Bull., 12:413 (1964).
46. Koizumi, T., Arita, T., and Kakemi, K., Chem. Pharm. Bull., 12:421 (1964).

47. Kakemi, K., Arita, T., and Muranishi, S., Chem. Pharm. Bull., 13:861 (1965).
48. Kakemi, K., Arita, T., Hori, R., and Konishi, R., Chem. Pharm. Bull., 15:1534 (1967).
49. Davenport, H.W., Physiology of the Digestive Tract, 3rd ed. Year Book Medical Publ. is here, Chicago, 1971, Chap. 13.
50. Levy, G., and Jusko, W., J. Pharm. Sci., 54:219 (1965).
51. Okuda, K., Proc. Soc. Expl. Biol. Med., 103:588 (1960).
52. Lish, P. M., Gastroenterology, 41:580 (1961).
53. Necheles, H., and Sporn, G., Am. J. Gastroenterol., 41:580 (1961).
54. Hawkins, G. K., Margolin, S., and Thompson, J. J., Am. J. Gastroenterol., 24:193 (1953).
55. Crone, R. S., and Aroran, G. M., Am. J. Gastroenterol., 32:88 (1957).
56. Weikel, J. H., Jr., and Lish, P. M., Arch. Int. Pharmacodyn, Ther., 119:398 (1959).
57. Consolo, S., and Ledinsky, H., Arch. Int. Pharmacodyn. Ther., 192:265 (1971).
58. Bianchine, J. R., Calimlin, L. R., Morgan, J. P., Dryurene, C. A., and Lasagna, L., Ann. N.Y. Acad. Sci., 179:126 (1971).
59. Beermann, B., Hellstrom, K., and Rosen, A., Circulation, 43:852 (1971).
60. Jaffee, J. M., Colaizzi, J., and Barry, H., J. Pharm. Sci., 60:1646 (1971).
61. Bates, T. R., Sequeira, J. A., and Tembo, A. V., Clin. Pharmacol. Ther., 16:63 (1974).
62. Conklin, J. D., in Bioavailability of Drugs (B. B. Brodie and W. H. Heller, eds.). S. Karger, New York, 1972, p. 178.
63. Klein, J. O., and Finland, M., N. Engl. J. Med., 269:1019 (1963).
64. Wagner, J. G., Can. J. Pharm. Sci., 1:55 (1966).
65. Rosenblatt, J. E., Barrett, J. E., Brodie, J. L., and Kirby, W. M. M., Antimicrob. Agents Chemother., 1:286 (1961).
66. Hirch, H. A., and Finland, M., Am. J. Med. Sci., 237:693 (1959).
67. Crounse, R. G., J. Invest. Dermatol., 37:529 (1961).
68. Nogami, H., Fukuzawa, H., and Nakai, Y., Chem. Pharm. Bull., 11:1389 (1963).
69. Koysooko, R., and Levy, G., J. Pharm. Sci., 63:829 (1974).
70. Koysooko, R., Ellis, E. F., and Levy, G., J. Pharm. Sci., 64:299 (1975).
71. Houston, J. B., and Levy, G., J. Pharm. Sci., 64:1504 (1975).
72. Marks, V., and Kelly, J. F., Lancet, 1:827 (1973).
73. Elias, E., Gibson, G. J., Greenwood, L. F., Hunt, J. N., and Tripp, J. H., J. Physiol., 194:317 (1968).
74. Hunt, J. N., and Knox, M. T., J. Physiol., 201:161 (1969).
75. Wagner, J. G., Am. J. Pharm., 141:5 (1969).
76. Gibaldi, M., and Feldman, S., J. Pharm. Sci., 59:579 (1970).
77. Bates, T., Gibaldi, M., and Kanig, J. L., Nature (Lond.), 210:1331 (1966).
78. Faloon, W. W., Paes, I. C., Woolfolk, D., Nankin, H., Wallace, K., and Haro, E. N., Ann. N.Y. Acad. Sci., 132:879 (1966).
79. Thompson, G. R., Barowman, J., Gutierrez, L., and Dowling, R. H., J. Clin. Invest., 50:319 (1971).
80. Schneierson, S. S., and Amsterdam, D., Nature (Lond.), 182:56 (1958).
81. Glazko, A. J., Dill, W. A., and Wolf, L. M., Fed. Proc., 9:48 (1950).

82. Gibaldi, M., and Schwartz, M. A., Br. J. Pharmacol. Chemother.,
     28:360 (1966).

83. Nelson, E., unpublished data.

84. Levine, R. R., Blair, M. R., and Clark, B. B., J. Pharmacol. Exp.
     Ther., 114:78 (1955).

85. Boston Collaborative Drug Surveillance Program: Clinical Depression of
     the Central Nervous System Due to Diazepam and Chlordiazepoxide in Re-
     lation to Cigarette Smoking and Age, N. Engl. J. Med., 288:277 (1973).

86. Boston Collaborative Drug Surveillance Program: Decreased Clinical Ef-
     ficacy of Propoxyphene in Cigarette Smokers, Clin. Pharmacol. Ther.,
     14:259 (1973).

87. Boston Collaborative Drug Surveillance Program: Drowsiness Due to
     Chlorpromazine in Relation to Cigarette Smoking, Arch. Gen. Psychiatry,
     31:211 (1974).

88. Kerri-Szanto, M., and Pomeroy, J. R., Lancet, 1:947 (1971).

89. Pantuck, E. J., Hsiao, K. C., Maggio, A., Nakamura, K., Kuntzman, R.,
     and Conney, A. H., Clin. Pharmacol. Ther., 14:9 (1974).

90. Beckett, A. H., and Triggs, E. J., Nature (Lond.), 216:587 (1967).

91. Hunt, S. N., Jusko, W. J., and Yurchak, A. M., J. Clin. Pharm. Ther.,
     19:546 (1976).

92. Riegelman, S., Pharmacology, 8:118 (1972).

93. Levy, G., Pharmacology, 8:33 (1972).

94. Heizer, W. D., Smith, T. W., and Goldfinger, S. E., N. Engl. J. Med.,
     285:257 (1971).

95. Beermann, B., Hellstrom, K., and Rosen, A., Acta Med. Scand.,
     193:293 (1973).

96. Monkhouse, D. C., and Lach, J. L., Can. J. Pharm. Sci., 7:29 (1972).

97. Wagner, J. G., Drug Intell. Clin. Pharm., 3:189 (1969); 4:77 (1970).

98. Higuchi, W. I., J. Pharm. Sci., 56:315 (1967).

99. Goyan, J. E., J. Pharm. Sci., 54:645 (1965).

100. Noyes, A. A., and Whitney, W. R., J. Am. Chem. Soc., 19:930 (1897).

101. Carstensen, J. T., Pharmaceutics of Solids and Solid Dosage Forms.
     Wiley, New York, 1977.

102. Higuchi, T., J. Pharm. Sci., 52:1145 (1963).

103. Robinson, J. R., and Eriksen, S. P., J. Pharm. Sci., 55:1254 (1966).

104. Goodhart, F. W., McCoy, R. H., and Ninger, F. C., J. Pharm. Sci.,
     63:1748 (1974).

105. Parnarowski, M., in: Dissolution Technology (L. Leeson and J. T.
     Carstensen, eds.). Industrial Pharmaceutical Technology Section,
     Academy of Pharmaceutical Sciences, Washington, D.C., 1974, p. 58.

106. Lettir, A., Abrégé de pharmacie galénique, Masson et Cie., Paris, 1974,
     p. 109.

107. Hersey, J. A., Manuf. Chem. Aerosol News, 40:32 (1969).

108. Baun, C. D., and Walker, C. G., J. Pharm. Sci., 58:611 (1969).

109. Swarbrick, J., in: Current Concepts in the Pharmaceutical Sciences:
     Biopharmaceutics (J. Swarbrick, ed.). Lea & Febiger, Philadelphia,
     1970, p. 276.

110. Stricker, H., In Vitro Studies on the Dissolution and Absorption Behavior
     of Orally Administered Drugs, and the Connection to Their Bioavailability.
     In: The Quality Control of Medicines (P. B. Deasy and R. F. Timoney,
     eds.), Elsevier, Amsterdam, 1976, Chap. 16.

111. Wagner, G. J., Biopharmaceutics and Relevant Pharmacokinetics. Drug Intelligence Publications, Hamilton, Ill., 1971, p. 110.
112. Shah, A. C., Peot, C. B., and Ochs, J. F., J. Pharm. Sci., 62:671 (1973).
113. Hanson, W., personal communication.
114. Gershberg, S., and Stoll, D. F., J. Am. Pharm. Assoc., Sci. Ed., 35:284 (1946).
115. Huber, H. E., Dale, B. L., and Christenson, L. G., J. Pharm. Sci., 55:974 (1966).
116. Kaplan, L. L., J. Pharm. Sci., 54:457 (1965).
117. Schroeter, C. L., and Hamlin, J. W., J. Pharm. Sci., 51:957 (1962).
118. Schroeter, C. L., and Wagner, J. G., J. Pharm. Sci., 51:957 (1962).
119. Lazarus, J., Pagliery, M., and Lachman, L., J. Pharm. Sci., 53:798 (1964).
120. Simoons, J. R. A., Drukkery Wed. G. Van Soeste N. V. Amst. (1962).
121. Parrott, E. L., Wurster, D. E., and Higuchi, T., J. Am. Pharm. Assoc., Sci. Ed., 44:269 (1955).
122. Nelson, E., J. Am. Pharm. Assoc., Sci. Ed., 46:607 (1957).
123. Levy, G., and Hayes, B., N. Engl. J. Med., 262:1053 (1960).
124. Levy, G., J. Pharm. Sci., 52:1039 (1963).
125. Levy, G., and Procknal, J. A., J. Pharm. Sci., 53:656 (1964).
126. Campagna, F. A., Cureton, G., Mirigian, R. A., and Nelson, E., J. Pharm. Sci., 52:605 (1963).
127. Niebergall, P. J., and Goyan, J. E., J. Pharm. Sci., 52:29 (1963).
128. Gibaldi, M., and Feldman, S., J. Pharm. Sci., 56:1238 (1967).
129. Castello, R. A., Jeelinek, G., Konieczny, J. M., Kwan, K. C., and Toberman, R. O., J. Pharm. Sci., 57:485 (1968).
130. Paikoff, M., and Drumm, G., J. Pharm. Sci., 54:1693 (1965).
131. Poole, J. W., Drug Inf. Bull., 2:8 (1968).
132. Pernarowski, M., Woo, W., and Searl, R. O., J. Pharm. Sci., 57:1419 (1968).
133. Himmelfarb, P., Thayer, S. P., and Martin, E. H., Science, 164:555 (1969).
134. Shah, A. C., and Ochs, F. J., J. Pharm. Sci., 63:110 (1974).
135. Stricker, H., Drugs Made in Ger., 14:93 (1971).
136. Stricker, H., Drugs Made in Ger., 14:80 (1973).
137. Braybrooks, P. M., Barry, W. B., and Abbs, T. B., J. Pharm. Pharmacol., 27:508 (1975).
138. Nozaki, M., Hayashi, M., Shibuya, T., Tsurumi, K., and Fujimura, H., Proceedings of the 5th Symposium on Drug Metabolic Action, Shirvoka, Japan, Nov. 9-10, 1973.
139. Toverud, L. E., Medd. Nor. Farm. Selsk., 36:87 (1974).
140. Singh, P., Guillory, J. K., Sokoloski, T. D., Benet, L. Z., and Bhatia, V. N., J. Pharm. Sci., 55:63 (1966).
141. Solvang, S., and Finholt, P., J. Pharm. Sci., 59:49 (1970).
142. Levy, G., and Sahli, B. A., J. Pharm. Sci., 51:58 (1962).
143. Souder, J. C., and Ellenbogen, W. C., Drug Stand., 26:77 (1958).
144. Vleit, E. B., Drug Stand., 27:97 (1959).
145. Cook, D., Chang, H. S., and Mainville, C. A., Can. J. Pharm. Sci., 1:69 (1966).
146. Cook, D., Can. J. Pharm. Sci., 2:91 (1967).

147. Langenbucher, F., Pharm. Acta Helv., 49:187 (1974).
148. Marshall, K., and Brook, D. B., J. Pharm. Pharmacol., 21:790 (1969).
149. Marlowe, E., and Shangraw, R. F., J. Pharm. Sci., 56:498 (1967).
150. Barzilay, R. B., and Hersey, J. A., J. Pharm. Pharmacol., 20:232S (1968).
151. Northern, R. E., Lach, J. L., and Fincher, J. H., J. Am. Hosp. Pharm., 30:622 (1975).
152. Goldberg, A. H., Gibaldi, M., Kanig, J. L., and Shanker, J., J. Pharm. Sci., 54:1722 (1965).
153. Edmunson, I. C., and Lees, K. A., J. Pharm. Pharmacol., 17:193 (1965).
154. Tingstad, J. E., and Riegelman, S., J. Pharm. Sci., 59:692 (1970).
155. Niebergall, P. J., Patel, M. Y., and Sugita, E. G., J. Pharm. Sci., 56:943 (1967).
156. Wurster, D. E., and Taylor, P. W., J. Pharm. Sci., 54:169 (1965).
157. Hamlin, W. E., Nelson, E., Ballard, B. E., and Wagner, J. G., J. Pharm. Sci., 51:432 (1962).
158. Levy, G., Antkowiak, J. M., Procknal, J. A., and White, D. C., J. Pharm. Sci., 52:1047 (1963).
159. Endicott, C. J., Lowenthall, and Gross, H. M., J. Pharm. Sci., 50:343 (1961).
160. Nelson, E., Drug Stand., 24:1 (1956).
161. McCallam, A., Butcher, J., and Albrecht, R., J. Am. Pharm. Assoc., Sci. Ed., 44:83 (1955).
162. Huber, H. E., and Christenson, G. C., J. Pharm. Sci., 57:164 (1968).
163. Jacob, J. T., and Plein, E. M., J. Pharm. Sci., 57:802 (1968).
164. Stern, P. W., J. Pharm. Sci., 65:1291 (1976).
165. Lachman, L., J. Pharm. Sci., 54:1519 (1965).
166. Alam, A. S., and Parrott, E. L., J. Pharm. Sci., 60:263 (1971).
167. Kornblum, S. S., and Hirschorn, J. O., J. Pharm. Sci., 60:445 (1971).
168. Johnsgard, M., and Wahlgren, S., Medd. Nor. Farm. Selsk., 32:25 (1971).
169. Shotten, E., and Leonard, G. S., J. Pharm. Pharmacol., 24:798 (1972).
170. Ganderton, D., J. Pharm. Pharmacol., 21:9S (1969).
171. Finholt, P., in Dissolution Technology (L. J. Leeson and J. T. Carstensen, eds.). Industrial Pharmaceutical Technology Section, Academy of Pharmaceutical Sciences, Washington, D.C., 1976, p. 119.
172. Khalil, S. A. H., J. Pharm. Pharmacol., 26:961 (1974).
173. Loo, J. C. K., Rowe, M., and McGilveray, I. J., J. Pharm. Sci., 64:1728 (1975).
174. Monkhouse, D. C., Ph.D. thesis, University of Iowa, Iowa City, Iowa, 1970.
175. Levy, G., J. Pharm. Sci., 50:388 (1961).
176. Higuchi, W. I., Parrott, E. L., Wurster, D. E., and Higuchi, T., J. Am. Pharm. Assoc., Sci. Ed., 47:376 (1958).
177. Anderson, R. A., and Sneddon, W., Med. J. Aust., 1:585 (1972).
178. Finholt, P., and Solvang, S., J. Pharm. Sci., 57:1322 (1968).
179. Vivino, E. A., J. Pharm. Sci., 43:234 (1954).
180. Gagliani, J., DeGraff, A. C., and Kupperman, H. S., Int. Rec. Med. Gen. Prac. Clin., 167:251 (1954).
181. Nelson, E., J. Am. Pharm. Assoc., Sci. Ed., 48:96 (1959).

182. Juncher, H., and Raaschov, F., Antibiot. Med. Clin. Ther., 4:497 (1957).
183. Levy, G., and Procknal, J. A., Antibiot. Med. Clin. Ther., 51:294 (1962).
184. O'Reilly, R. A., Nelson, E., and Levy, G., Antibiot. Med. Clin. Ther., 55:435 (1966).
185. Higuchi, W. I., and Hamlin, W. E., Antibiot. Med. Clin. Ther., 52:575 (1963).
186. Griffith, R. S., and Black, H. R., Antibiot. Chemother., 12:398 (1962).
187. Griffith, R. S., and Black, H. R., Am. J. Med. Sci., 247:69 (1964).
188. Bell, S. M., Med. J. Aust., 2:1280 (1971).
189. Wan, S. H., Pentikainen, P. J., and Azarnoff, D. L., J. Pharm. Sci., 63:708 (1974).
190. Berge, S. H., Bighley, L. D., and Monkhouse, D. C., J. Pharm. Sci., 66:1 (1977).
191. Bedford, C., Busfield, D., Child, K. J., MacGregor, I., Sutherland, P., and Tomich, E. G., Arch. Dermatol., 81:735 (1960).
192. Atkinson, R., Bedford, C., Child, K. J., and Tomich, E. G., Nature (Lond.), 193:588 (1962).
193. Shaw, T. R. D., and Carless, J. E., Eur. J. Clin. Pharmacol., 7:269 (1974).
194. Jounela, A. J., Pentikainen, P. J., and Sothmann, A., Eur. J. Clin. Pharmacol., 8:365 (1975).
195. Strickland, W. A., Nelson, E., Busse, L. W., and Higuchi, T., J. Am. Pharm. Assoc., Sci. Ed., 45:51 (1956).
196. Armstrong, A., and Haines-Natt, R. F., J. Pharm. Pharmacol., 22:85 (1970).
197. Kornblum, S. S., and Hirschorn, J. O., J. Pharm. Sci., 59:606 (1970).
198. Paul, H. E., Hayes, K. J., Paul, M. F., and Borgmann, A. R., J. Pharm. Sci., 56:882 (1967).
199. Monkhouse, D. C., and Lach, J. L., J. Pharm. Sci., 61:1430 (1972).
200. Harper, N. J., Prog. Drug Res., 4:221 (1962).
201. Kupchan, S. M., and Isenberg, A. C., J. Med. Chem., 10:960 (1967).
202. Higuchi, T., Acta Pharm. Suec., 13(Suppl.):3 (1976).
203. Stella, V. J., Aust. J. Pharm. Sci., NS2:57 (1973).
204. Sinkula, A. A., Acta Pharm. Suec., 13(Suppl.):4 (1976).
205. Daehne, W. V., Frederiksen, E., Gundersen, E., Lund, F., Morch, P., Peterson, H. J., Roholt, K., Tybring, L., and Godtfredsen, W. O., J. Med. Chem., 13:607 (1970).
206. Schwartz, M. A., and Hayton, W. L., J. Pharm. Sci., 61:906 (1972).
207. Butter, K., English, A. R., Knirsch, A. K., and Korst, J. J., Del. Med. J., 43:366 (1971).
208. Sinkula, A. A., and Lewis, C., J. Pharm. Sci., 62:1757 (1973).
209. Sinkula, A. A., Acta Pharm. Suec., 13(Suppl.):7 (1976).
210. Sekiguchi, K., and Obi, N., Chem. Pharm. Bull., 9:866 (1961).
211. Sekiguchi, K., Obi, N., and Ueda, Y., Chem. Pharm. Bull., 12:134 (1964).
212. Goldberg, A. H., Gibaldi, M., and Kanig, J. L., J. Pharm. Sci., 54:1145 (1965).
213. Goldberg, A. H., Gibaldi, M., and Kanig, J. L., J. Pharm. Sci., 55:482 (1966).
214. Goldberg, A. H., Gibaldi, M., and Kanig, J. L., J. Pharm. Sci., 55:487 (1966).

215.   Goldberg, A. H., Gibaldi, M., Kanig, J. L., and Mayersohn, M.,
       J. Pharm. Sci., 55:581 (1966).
216.   Chiou, W. L., and Riegelman, S., J. Pharm. Sci., 58:1505 (1969).
217.   Chiou, W. L., and Riegelman, S., J. Pharm. Sci., 60:1281 (1971).
218.   Chiou, W. L., and Riegelman, S., J. Pharm. Sci., 60:1569 (1971).
219.   Chiou, W. L., and Niazi, S., J. Pharm. Sci., 60:1333 (1971).
220.   Chiou, W. L., and Smith, L. D., J. Pharm. Sci., 60:125 (1971).
221.   McGinity, J. W., Maness, D. D., and Yakatan, G. J., Drug Dev.
       Commun., 1:369 (1975).
222.   Svoboda, G. H., Sweeney, M. J., and Walkling, W. D., J. Pharm. Sci.,
       60:333 (1971).
223.   Stoll, R. G., Bates, T. R., Nieforth, K. A., and Swarbrick, J.,
       J. Pharm. Sci., 58:1457 (1969).
224.   Stoll, R. G., Bates, T. R., and Swarbrick, J., J. Pharm. Sci., 62:65
       (1973).
225.   Stupak, E. I., and Bates, T. R., J. Pharm. Sci., 61:400 (1972).
226.   Aguiar, A. J., Krc, J., Jr., Kinkel, A. W., and Samyn, J. C.,
       J. Pharm. Sci., 56:847 (1967).
227.   Haleblian, J. K., J. Pharm. Sci., 64:1269 (1975).
228.   Armour Research Foundation of Illinois Institute of Technology, Anal.
       Chem., 21:1293 (1949); through Chem. Abstr., 44:13003 (1950).
229.   Shefter, E., and Higuchi, T., J. Pharm. Sci., 52:781 (1963).
230.   Mesley, R. J., and Houghton, E. E., J. Pharm. Pharmacol., 19:295
       (1967).
231.   Moustafa, M. A., Khalil, S. A., Ebian, A. R., and Motawi, M. M.,
       J. Pharm. Sci., 63:1103 (1974).
232.   Moustafa, M. A., Khalil, S. A., Ebian, A. R., and Motawi, M. M.,
       J. Pharm. Sci., 64:1481 (1975).
233.   Moustafa, M. A., Khalil, S. A., Ebian, A. R., and Motawi, M. M.,
       J. Pharm. Sci., 64:1485 (1975).
234.   Gibbs, I. S., Heald, A., Hacobson, H., Wadke, D., and Weliky, I.,
       J. Pharm. Sci., 65:1380 (1976).
235.   Macek, T. J., Am. J. Pharm., 137:217 (1965).
236.   Sokoloski, T. D., Hosp. Pharm., 3:15 (1968).
237.   Ballard, B. E., and Biles, J. A., Steroids, 4:273 (1964).
238.   Lin, S. L., and Lachman, L., J. Pharm. Sci., 58:377 (1969).
239.   Higuchi, T., and Lach, J. L., J. Am. Pharm. Assoc., Sci. Ed., 43:524
       (1954).
240.   Bettis, J., Hood, J., and Lach, J. L., Am. J. Hosp. Pharm., 30:240
       (1973).
241.   Higuchi, W. I., Nir, N. A., and Desai, S. J., J. Pharm. Sci., 54:1405
       (1965).
242.   Zoglio, M. A., Maulding, H. V., and Windheuser, J. J., J. Pharm. Sci.,
       58:222 (1969).
243.   Higuchi, T., and Ikeda, M., J. Pharm. Sci., 63:809 (1974).
244.   Kaplan, S. A., in Dissolution Technology (L. Leeson and J. T. Carstensen,
       eds.). Industrial Pharmaceutical Technology Section, Academy of Phar-
       maceutical Sciences, Washington, D.C., 1974, pp. 183-185.
245.   Akers, M. J., Lach, J. L., and Fischer, L. J., J. Pharm. Sci., 62:391
       (1973).

246. Akers, M. J., Lach, J. L., and Fischer, L. J., J. Pharm. Sci., 62:1192 (1973).
247. Spivey, R., Ph.D. thesis, University of Iowa, Iowa City, Iowa, 1976.
248. McGinity, J. W., and Lach, J. L., J. Pharm. Sci., 65:896 (1976).
249. McGinity, J. W., and Lach, J. L., J. Pharm. Sci., 66:63 (1977).
250. Sorby, D. L., J. Pharm. Sci., 54:677 (1965).
251. Tsuchiya, T., and Levy, G., J. Pharm. Sci., 61:587 (1972).
252. Nogami, H., Nagai, T., and Uchida, H., Chem. Pharm. Bull., 14:152 (1966).
253. Nogami, H., Hasegawn, J., and Miyamoto, W., Chem. Pharm. Bull., 15:279 (1967).
254. Ganderton, D., Pharm. Acta Helv., 42:152 (1967).
255. Gouda, M. W., Malik, S. N., and Khalil, S. A., Can. J. Pharm. Sci., 10:24 (1975).
256. Khalafallah, N., Gouda, M. W., and Khalil, S. A., J. Pharm. Sci., 64:991 (1975).
257. Reddy, R. K., Khalil, S. A., and Gouda, M. W., J. Pharm. Sci., 65:115 (1976).
258. Levy, G., and Gumtow, R. H., J. Pharm. Sci., 52:1139 (1963).
259. Weintraub, H., and Gibaldi, M., J. Pharm. Sci., 58:1368 (1969).
260. Lim, J. K., and Chen, C. C., J. Pharm. Sci., 63:559 (1974).
261. Chiou, W. L., Chen, S. J., and Athanikar, N., J. Pharm. Sci., 65:1702 (1976).
262. Parrott, E. L., and Sharma, V. K., J. Pharm. Sci., 56:1341 (1967).
263. Braun, R. J., and Parrott, E. L., J. Pharm. Sci., 61:175 (1972).
264. Elworthy, P. H., and Lipscomb, F. J., J. Pharm. Pharmacol., 20:923 (1968).
265. Mayersohn, M., and Gibaldi, M., Am. J. Pharm. Ed., 34:608 (1970).
266. Benet, L. Z., and Turi, J. S., J. Pharm. Sci., 60:1593 (1971).
267. Benet, L. Z., J. Pharm. Sci., 61:536 (1972).
268. Swintosky, J. V., Nature (Lond.), 179:98 (1957).
269. Martin, B. K., Br. J. Pharmacol. Chemother., 29:181 (1967).
270. Wilkinson, G. R., and Beckett, A. H., J. Pharmacol. Exp. Ther., 162:139 (1968).
271. Taylor, J. A., Clin. Pharmacol. Ther., 13:710 (1972).
272. Bray, H. G., Thorpe, W. V., and White, K., Biochem. J., 48:88 (1951).
273. Gibaldi, M., and Perrier, D., Pharmacokinetics. Dekker, New York, 1975, Chap. 1.
274. Wagner, J. G., Fundamentals of Clinical Pharmacokinetics. Drug Intelligence Publications, Hamilton, Ill., 1975, Chap. 3.
275. Doluisio, J. T., LaPiana, C. J., and Dittert, L. W., J. Pharm. Sci., 60:715 (1971).
276. Krüger-Thiemer, E., J. Am. Pharm. Assoc., Sci. Ed., 49:311 (1960).
277. Krüger-Thiemer, E., J. Theor. Biol., 13:212 (1966).
278. Krüger-Thiemer, E., and Bünger, P., Chemotherapia, 10:61 (1965/1966).
279. Krüger-Thiemer, E., and Bünger, P., Chemotherapia, 10:129 (1965/1966).
280. Krüger-Thiemer, E., Bünger, P., Dettli, L., Spring, P., and Wempe, E., Chemotherapia, 10:325 (1965/1966).
281. Krüger-Thiemer, E., J. Theor. Biol., 23:169 (1969).

282. Wagner, J. G., Biopharmaceutics and Relevant Pharmacokinetics. Drug
      Intelligence Publications, Hamilton, Ill., 1971, pp. 272, 292.
283. Wagner, J. G., Fundamentals of Clinical Pharmacokinetics. Drug Intel-
      ligence Publications, Hamilton, Ill., 1975, pp. 144-148.
284. Gibaldi, M., and Perrier, D., Pharmacokinetics. Dekker, New York,
      1975, Chap. 3.
285. Krüger-Thiemer, E., Berlin, H., Brante, G., Bünger, P., Dettli, L.,
      Spring, P., and Wempe, E., Chemotherapia, 14:273 (1969).
286. Gibaldi, M., and Perrier, D., Pharmacokinetics. Dekker, New York,
      1975, p. 63.
287. Dominguez, R., and Pomerene, B., Proc. Soc. Exp. Biol. Med., 60:173
      (1945).
288. Dost, F. H., Der Blutspiegel., Georg. Thieme Verlag, Leipzig, East
      Germany, 1953.
289. Diller, W., Antibiot. Chemother., 12:85 (1964).
290. Wagner, J. G., and Nelson, E., J. Pharm. Sci., 52:610 (1963).
291. Wagner, J. G., and Nelson, E., J. Pharm. Sci., 53:1392 (1964).
292. Loo, J. C. K., and Riegelman, S., J. Pharm. Sci., 57:918 (1968).
293. Gibaldi, M., and Perrier, D., Pharmacokinetics. Dekker, New York,
      1975, pp. 130-145.
294. Wagner, J. G., Fundamentals of Clinical Pharmacokinetics. Drug Intel-
      ligence Publications, Hamilton, Ill., 1975, pp. 174-184, 185-201.
295. Notari, R. E., Biopharmaceutics and Pharmacokinetics. Dekker, New
      York, 1975, pp. 89, 93.
296. Wagner, J. G., J. Clin. Pharmacol., 7:89 (1967).
297. Wagner, J. G., Fundamentals of Clinical Pharmacokinetics. Drug Intel-
      ligence Publications, Hamilton, Ill., 1975, pp. 185-187.
298. Lalka, D., and Feldman, H., J. Pharm. Sci., 63:1812 (1974).
299. Wagner, J. G., Gerard, E. S., and Kaiser, D. G., Clin. Pharmacol.
      Ther., 7:610 (1966).
300. Smolen, V. F., Murdock, H. R., Stoltman, W. P., Clevenger, J. W.,
      Combs, L. W., and Williams, E. J., J. Clin. Pharmacol., 15:734
      (1975).
301. Smolen, V. F., Barile, R. D., and Teophamous, T. G., J. Pharm. Sci.,
      61:467 (1972).
302. Smolen, V. F., Turrie, D. B., and Weigand, W. A., J. Pharm. Sci.,
      61:1941 (1972).
303. Smolen, V. G., J. Pharm. Sci., 60:354 (1971).
304. Smolen, V. F., and Wiegand, W. A., J. Pharmacokinet., Biopharm.,
      1:329 (1973).
305. Wilson, T. H., and Wiseman, G., J. Physiol., 123:116 (1954).
306. Crane, R. K., and Wilson, T. H., J. Appl. Physiol., 12:145 (1958).
307. Fisher, R. B., and Parsons, D. S., J. Physiol. (Lond.), 110:36 (1949).
308. Wiseman, G., in: Methods in Medical Research, Vol. 9 (J. H. Quastel,
      ed.). Year Book Medical Publishers, Chicago, p. 287.
309. Crane, R. K., and Mandelstam, P., Biochim. Biophys. Acta, 45:460
      (1960).
310. Doluisio, T. J., Billups, F. N., Dittert, L. W., Sugita, E. G., and
      Swintosky, V. J., J. Pharm. Sci., 58:1196 (1969).

311. Levine, R. R., and Pelikan, W. E., J. Pharmacol. Exp. Ther., 131:319 (1961).
312. Schanker, L. S., Shone, B. A., Brodie, B. B., and Hogben, M. A., J. Pharmacol. Exp. Ther., 120:528 (1957).
313. Irwin, G. M., Kostenbauder, H. B., Dittert, L. W., Staples, R., Misher, A., and Swintosky, J. V., J. Pharm. Sci., 58:313 (1969).
314. De Cato, L., Malone, M. H., Stoll, R., and Nieforth, D. A., J. Pharm. Sci., 58:273 (1969).
315. Levy, G., Clin. Pharmacol. Ther., 7:362 (1966).
316. Digenis, A. G., Beihn, M. R., Theodorakis, C. M., Shambhu, B. M., J. Pharm. Sci., 66:442 (1977).
317. Harvey, F. R., Brown, J. N., Machie, D. B., Keeling, H. D., and Davies, T. W., Lancet, 1:16 (1970).
318. Newburger, J., Ph.D. thesis, University of Kentucky, Lexington, Ky., 1974; J. Newburger and S. Stavchansky, unpublished data.
319. Darlington, W. A., and Quastel, J. H., Arch. Biochem., 43:194 (1953).
320. Aguiar, A. J., and Fifelski, R. J., J. Pharm. Sci., 55:1387 (1966).
321. Taraszka, M. J., J. Pharm. Sci., 60:946 (1971).
322. Reuning, R., and Levy, G., J. Pharm. Sci., 57:1355 (1968).
323. Agar, W. T., Herd, F. J. R., and Sidhu, G. S., Biochim. Biophys. Acta, 14:80 (1954).
324. Finch, L. R., and Herd, F. J. R., Biochim. Biophys. Acta, 43:278 (1960).
325. Doluisio, J. T., Crouthamel, G. W., Tan, H. G., Swintosky, J. V., and Dittert, L. W., J. Pharm. Sci., 59:72 (1970).
326. Cabana, B. E., and Kumkumian, C. S., A View of Controlled Release Dosage Forms. In: Industrial Bioavailability and Pharmacokinetics (A. Martin and J. T. Doluisio, eds.). Drug Dynamics Institute, The University of Texas at Austin, Austin, Tex., 1977, p. 51.
327. Van Rossum, J. M., Significance of Pharmacokinetics for Drug Design and the Planning of Dosage Regimens. In: Medicinal Chemistry, Vol. 1 (E. J. Ariens, ed.), Academic Press, New York, 1971, p. 470.
328. Notari, R. E., Biopharmaceutics and Pharmacokinetics: An Introduction. Dekker, New York, 1975, p. 163.
329. Gibaldi, M., and Perrier, D., Pharmacokinetics. Dekker, New York, 1975, p. 172.

7

Pharmaceutical Tablet Compression Tooling

George F. Loeffler

Thomas Engineering Incorporated
Hoffman Estates, Illinois

I. Introduction

The compaction tooling involved in the manufacture of the tablet is as critical as the formulation or the tablet press if a quality product is to result. It must meet many requirements to satisfy the needs of dosage uniformity, production efficiency, and aesthetic standards. A basic knowledge of the subject will be of assistance in eliminating unnecessary delays in vendor communication and "starting off on the wrong track" with a proposed novel tablet design. An added plus would be lengthening the service life of the tooling involved.

The intention of this chapter is not to make the pharmacist a tool designer or a line mechanic, but rather to give sufficient background on the subject so that possible production pitfalls (unfortunately inherent in many new products) can be avoided or at least reduced in magnitude.

II. Terminology

To best understand the following material, it is necessary to be familiar with the commonly accepted terminology (see Fig. 1). The tooling depicted is for the most popular single-stroke and rotary machines.

Punch land	Area between the edge of the punch cup and the outside diameter of the punch tip.
head	End of the punch that is controlled by the machine camming.
head flat	Area receiving the force of the compression rolls at the time that the tablet is being formed.
head angles	"Inside" and "outside" are the contact areas with the machine cams.
neck	Clearance provided for the cams.

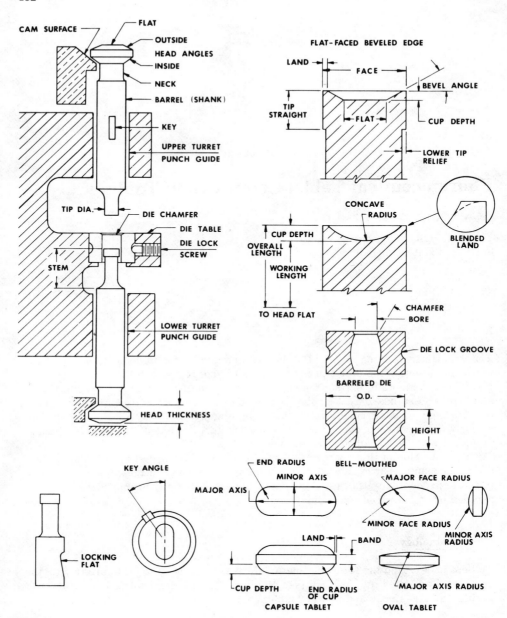

Figure 1. Tooling terminology.

barrel	(Shank) Vertical guiding surface for the tool in the machine.
tip straight	Axial section of the punch, upper or lower, that maintains the exact contour of the punch face.
overall length	Total length of the punch.

working length	Length of the punch from the bottom of the cup to the head flat (critical length).
Bakelite relief	Extra-deep undercut below the lower punch tip straight.
key angle	Relationship of the punch key to the tablet shape.
galling	Roughly worn areas on the metal surfaces.
core rod	Special punch configuration to produce a tablet with a center hole.
"Rockwell"	Hardness of the tool.
fluting	Vertical grooves in the punch barrel.
Die groove	Accepts the press locking screw.
chamfer	Entry angle on the die bore.
taper	Gradual increase in the die bore diameter from the point of compaction to the die chamfer area.
barreled bore	Diameter at the center is larger than at either or both of the ends.
bell-mouthed bore	Converse of the above.
ring	Eroded area in the die bore at the point of compaction.
carbide insert	High-wear lining for the die bore.
Tablet flash	Semicompressed material formed on the perimeter of the tablet due to the punch tip to die bore clearance.
capping	Laminar separation.
picking	Granulation adherance to the punch face.
compaction ratio	Thickness of uncompressed material relative to compacted tablet.
Punch face embossing	
stroke	Width and depth of the engraving cut.
islands	Isolated "mesas" formed by certain letters or numbers, such as a "B" and "8."
striking	(Slug) Formed metal pressing of the punch face design. Used for approval of the punch face design.
overlay	Outline of the tablet face on a glass or plastic film. Used for checking the tablet monogram with the aid of an optical comparitor.

The most common tools employed in the Industry are referred to as BB tools. These are 5 1/4 in. long and have a nominal 3/4-in. barrel diameter with a 1-in. head diameter. The tablet machines that employ these punches usually are available with either of two die sizes: 0.945 in. outside diameter to accept up to a 7/16-in. round or 9/16-in. capsule tablet, and a 1 3/16-in.-OD die, which can make a tablet up to 9/16 in. round or 3/4-in. capsule, all with a maximum depth of fill of 11/16 in.

B tool machines are identical to the above except that the lower punches are only 3 9/16 in. long.

The next most popular machines use D tools. These are also 5 1/4 in. long, but have a 1-in. barrel diameter with a 1 1/4-in. head diameter. The two standard die sizes available are a 1 1/2 in. OD, to accept up to a 1-in. round or capsule tablet, and a 1 3/16-in. OD die, which can make up to a 3/4-in.-major-axis tablet. The maximum depth of fill is 13/16 in.

III. Tablet Design

The tools must mold the granulation or powder to the required shape and face design, while minimizing the possibility of adherence of the product to the punch face.
Consideration must be given to the compaction forces that will be required, potential packaging problems, and possible limitations to the tableting machine output.
Selecting the proper tablet design is very critical to the performance of the tools
in the machine. Round tablets usually run best on the highest-speed rotary machines since they do not normally require keying to maintain orientation of the
upper punch while out of the die. This permits them to rotate, presenting a better
distribution of the lubrication.

Dosage size or marketing requirements, however, may dictate an irregular
shape, such as capsules, ovals, triangles, or squares. Although these shapes
require a little more attention to the mechanical lubrication of the tooling, they
can be operated at the higher machine output speeds more readily if severe "self-
locking" shapes are avoided.

A. Punch-to-Die Binding

One of the more important pitfalls to avoid in the design of the tablet is to introduce the possibility of a self-locking effect between the lower punch tip and the die
bore. This is the result of peculiar radii combinations of the tablet perimeter
that permit a wedging action between the punch tip and the die wall as the punch
rotates through its available clearance.

The rotation is due to the inside head angle of the punch contacting only one
side of the fill cam in the machine. The resultant rotational force or torque on
the punch is increased as the punch is pulled down by the cam, causing an increase
in the tip to bore binding, which in turn causes an increase in the applied torque
etc. The result can be severe enough to twist the lower punch stem, damage the
cam contact areas, or even to the extent of pulling the tips off the smaller tools.

The fill cams are normally double-sided; that is, they have contact lips on both
sides of the inside head angle of the punch for theoretical even pulldown to eliminate the adverse rotational effect. Unfortunately, there are a number of machining
tolerances that are required for the manufacture of the various involved press components that can negate the probability of absolute even pulldown.

The severity of the self-locking effect will be dependent on several factors: (1)
the angle formed between the two tablet face radii and the rotational radius of the
punch (keep the angle as large as possible; Fig. 2); (2) the coefficients of friction
between the punch tip/die bore and between the punch inside head angle/cam lip
(good lubrication is a major factor); (3) the size of the tablet relative to the punch
head diameter (if the tablet is small, it would be better to run it on a machine that
employs BB size tooling rather than the larger "D" tooling); (4) the degree of misalignment of the cam with the punch flight; (5) the concentricity of the punch head
with its barrel; and (6) the slope of the weight cam.

To be on the safe side, it would be best to avoid any shape that approaches
this hazardous condition (see Fig. 2). If in doubt on a selected shape, it would
be advisable to submit the tablet proposal to the tooling manufacturer for his advice. The involved forces can be calculated to a degree and a reasonable prog-
nosis can be given.

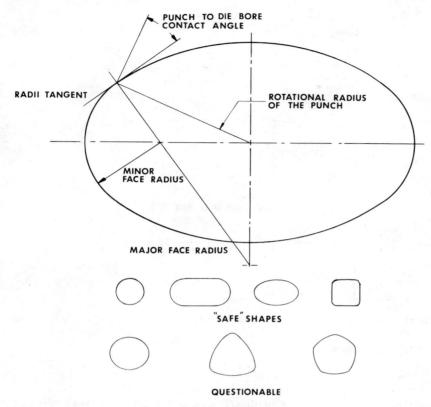

Figure 2. Punch tip "self-locking" shapes.

B. Punch Cup Contour

Next in importance is the proper selection of the punch cup contour. If heavy compaction forces are anticipated, the sturdier shapes should be selected if possible. For example, shallow or standard concave cups are preferable to the flat-face beveled edge, deep, and modified ball shapes.

The pressure required to compress the tablet (which can range up to 150,000 lb/in.^{2}) has a lateral-force component that tends to bend the punch cup edge outward each time a tablet is made (Fig. 3). This continued flexing can cause premature failure if excessive. The degree of this flexing pressure is a function of the angle between the cup and the tip straight for a given compaction force. The more acute the angle, the greater the relative bending force.

There are several ways to strengthen the selected cup shape if the problem is anticipated; (1) increase the width of the land to permit more metal in this more fragile area (this can be "blended" to reduce the visual effect and aid in coating if involved; see Fig. 1); (2) alter the steel and heat-treating specifications for greater ductility; (3) increase the radius between the flat and the bevel on

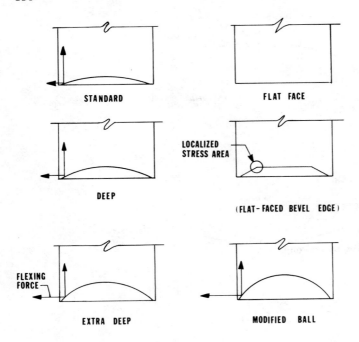

Figure 3. Punch tip shapes.

flat-faced beveled-edge tooling to better distribute the stresses; and (4) specify that the tooling be kept at minimum cup depth to reduce the area that the bending force can act on. Deep punch cup contours should be avoided if the granulation has a tendency to cap because of air entrapment.

C. Engraving

The third major concern in the design of the tablet is the engraving. It must avoid any tendency of the granulation to adhere to the punch face (pick) and must have the mechanical strength to withstand the tumbling action involved in dedusting, film coating, and packaging. Above all, it must be legible on the tablet.

Often, the company involved has an excellent trademark or monogram which they would like to reproduce on their new products. This design as it appears on their stationery or in their advertising might be an inch in height with considerable fine detail. In reducing this logo to fit on a small tablet, most of the fine lines must be sacrificed. Sometimes this detail is so important that the reduced design becomes a meaningless blob.

Broad, simple block letters and numbers should be selected whenever possible (Fig. 4). Script letters and fine lines which may present a beautiful appearance on a letterhead can cause problems with all of the foregoing requirements. "Fine lines" on the punch also will not withstand as much wear because of granulation abrasion and therefore will reduce the usable life of the tool. The design should

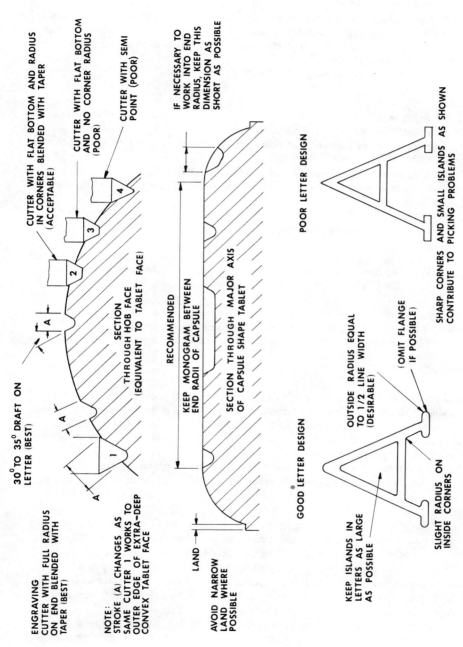

Figure 4. Tablet engraving.

be recessed in the tablet face, as raised letters will not withstand tumbling action. Square corners and small "islands" in the engraving are apt to cause picking. Where islands are necessary, as in "B" and "8," the tendency for the granulation to stick in these areas can be reduced by reducing their height and/or making them as large as possible (e.g., make them equal in size, dropping the cross bar in the "A" or opening the "4," as shown). The height in the island area can also be reduced (or eliminated).

Some design rules of thumb are as follows:

1. Stroke width = 1/5 letter height.
2. Stroke depth = 1/2 stroke width.
3. Space between letters = stroke width.
4. Space between letter and edge of bevel on flat-faced beveled-edge tablets = stroke width (minimum).
5. Monogram should not exceed 75% of face width of tablet.
6. Avoid sharp outside corners if possible. Use 1/2 of the stroke width for outside radii.
7. 30° draft angle on uncoated tablets; 35° draft angle for film-coated tablets.
8. Place deepest embossing on the upper punch face (aids in tablet take-off from the machine).
9. When designing a new logo intended for a range of tablet sizes, work with the smallest tablet on which it will be employed. Significant detail may have to be sacrificed if proportioning down is required.

Following these suggestions does not guarantee success, but it will increase the probability of a good legible debossing, while decreasing the chances of "picking" or tool breakage due to the weakening effect of the grooving.

D. Keying Angle

All tablets, other than rounds, require a device on the upper punch to keep it aligned when the punch tip is out of the die bore to permit proper reentry. This device is customarily a projection or key on the barrel. This key rides in a vertical groove in the turret bore, thereby providing vertical travel freedom but preventing rotation of the punch.

The turret keyway is normally located in the line of travel of the compressing station, so the angle between the punch key and the major axis of the tablet will determine where the tablet take-off blade will strike the periphery of the tablet.

It is usually best to have the largest flat (or if no flat is available, such as on an oval tablet, the largest radius) make the initial contact with the take-off blade. This becomes more critical when friable tablets are compacted at the higher machine speeds and where heavy lower punch embossing is present.

The conventional angle between the punch key and the major axis of the tablet is 35°; that is, when facing the upper punch cup with the key at 12 o'clock, the major tablet axis would be at approximately 1 o'clock.

Although the conventional manufacturing angle is 35°, many presses do not have their take-off blade mounted at this angle. So if a take-off problem is anticipated, it would be best to measure the required angle on the press to be employed and transmit this information with the tooling order.

IV. Specifications and Information Required by the Vendor

One major problem that a vendor has is that of communication. The time spent in clarifying the requirements on a new project unfortunately often exceeds the actual manufacturing time for the tooling. To initiate and preserve a position of confidence with the customer, a vendor must know what the customer wants and needs. This, coupled with the "state of the art" in manufacturing, can produce the best tooling for the particular application in the shortest period of time.

A good drawing of the tablet with accurate dimensioning and compatible tolerances will greatly reduce the overall time involved in completing a set of tools. Any information available on the proposed product, such as abrasiveness, required compaction pressure, excessive ejection pressures, tendency to cap or laminate, and previous tooling problems, is very helpful in the design of the new tooling. Adverse effects, if present, can often be alleviated or eliminated entirely in the design of the new tooling so that problems in production can be minimized.

Very often with older products, a good drawing is not available. The vendor can copy an existing punch or tablet and will prepare a proper drawing. However, its accuracy will be dependent on the condition of the sample furnished and where it fell within the original manufacturing tolerance. This may result in slight appearance deviations in the tablets produced from the new tooling. Reputable tooling manufacturers will supply a drawing as part of their services.

Additional information that is required with the request for a quotation or an order is: (1) the tablet press to be employed (if the press has been modified to accept other than standard tooling, this should be noted); (2) "standard" or "premium" steel (this may be questioned by a vendor if it is felt that it is not compatible with other information received); and (3) the quantity of tools needed and whether overruns will be accepted.

Overruns are a necessary evil with a manufacturer. Because of the number of close-tolerance machining operations involved in producing a tool, a number of tools may be discarded during the course of their manufacturing cycle. This "shrinkage" can account for up to 10% of the order. As a consequence, it is customary to start out with approximately 10% more tools than the customer requested.

Since the loss is not always as severe, the quantity of completed tools may exceed that called for on the order. These overruns are priced at the full set rate. Accepting these tools has an advantage to the supplier in keeping overall costs down (and therefore, ultimately, the customer's) and to the user as spares to replace the inevitable handling accident.

A. Steel and Hardness Section

Several types of tool steel are normally used in the fabrication of compression tooling. Since each has its advantages and disadvantages relative to a particular compressing application, the proper selection becomes critical to a successful overall operation.

The steel characteristics to be looked for in descending order of importance are:

1. Toughness to withstand the cyclic compacting forces
2. Wear resistance
3. Cost

The latter is not necessarily the initial cost but rather the cost per tablet produced.

OVAL TABLET

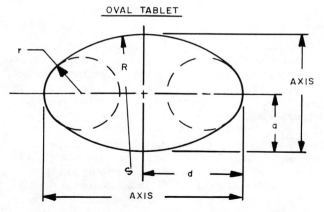

a = HALF THE LENGTH OF SHORT AXIS (in)
d = HALF THE LENGTH OF LONG AXIS (in)
R = RADIUS OF LONG SIDE (in)
r = RADIUS OF SMALL END (in)

$$R = \frac{a^2 + d^2 - 2rd}{2(a-r)}$$

$$d = r + (r^2 - 2Rr + 2Ra - a^2)^{1/2}$$

$$a = R - (R^2 - 2Rr + 2dr - d^2)^{1/2}$$

$$r = \frac{a^2 - 2aR + d^2}{2(d-R)}$$

FLAT FACED BEVEL EDGED CUP

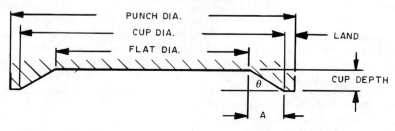

$$\text{CUP DEPTH} = A \, \text{TAN} \, \theta$$

$$A = \frac{\text{CUP DEPTH}}{\text{TAN} \, \theta}$$

Figure 5. Tablet calculations.

ENGRAVING CUT RADIUS

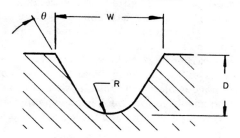

GIVEN: W, D, AND θ FIND: R $\Phi = 45° - \frac{\theta}{2}$

$$R = \frac{\frac{W}{2} - (D\ TAN\ \theta)}{TAN(45° - \frac{\theta}{2})}$$ OR $$\frac{\frac{W}{2} - (D\ TAN\ \theta)}{TAN\ \Phi}$$

$$D = \frac{\frac{W}{2} - R\ TAN(45° - \frac{B}{2})}{TAN\ \theta}$$

$$W = 2(R\ TAN\ \Phi + TAN\ \theta)$$

MONO RADIUS CUP

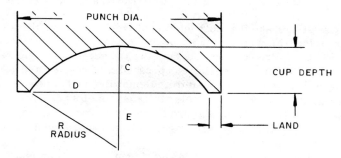

$$R = \frac{D^2 + C^2}{2C}$$ OR $$R = \frac{(2D)^2 + 4C^2}{8C}$$ $$R^2 = D^2 + E^2$$

$$E = R - C$$

$$E = \sqrt{R^2 - D^2}$$ OR $$E = \frac{D^2 - C^2}{2C}$$

$$D = \sqrt{R^2 - E^2}$$

$$C = R - E$$

$$R = \sqrt{E^2 + D^2}$$

The industry-accepted terminology groups the steels used into a standard or premium category. The former is usually an S5-classified, shock-resistant silicone steel which has good ductility and toughness after hardening. Occasionally, when a very fragile cup shape is involved, the vendor may recommend a 3% nickel steel, which has greater ductility but is less resistant to abrasion than the S5.

The premium steels are usually high carbon/high chrome alloys classified as D2 or D3. These steels have a much greater resistance to wear but have considerably less ductility and therefore are more subject to breakage when fragile cup shapes are involved. They should not be specified for deep punch cups or flat-faced beveled-edge tools unless relatively light compaction forces are anticipated.

The steel numbers S5, D2, and so on, are formulae designations by the American Institute of Steel Industries (AISI). They are adhered to by the various tool steel manufacturers to a close degree; however, slight variation can exist.

Unfortunately, there is no single steel available that combines the quality of high wear resistance with high ductility and toughness. The selection of the best steel for the job must be based on experience and the accumulated history of the product being tableted.

Figure 6 is an empirically derived chart depicting the relation of wear to "breakage" resistance for the more common steels employed. The S7 steel shown is an intermediate premium grade, employed where the punch cup geometry and required compaction pressure would not tolerate the more fragile D2 steel. The relationship shown can be altered to some degree by variations in the heat treatment.

In order for the vendor to make the most intelligent steel selection, the following information must be available: (1) the shape of the punch tip (tablet face), (2) the compressing force required to form the tablet to the acceptable weight and thickness, (3) whether the material being compressed is abrasive, and (4) if the compressed material is corrosive in nature. Generally, with a new product, where sufficient background is not available, the steel and its hardness should be selected for the best ductility. Failure due to premature wear is certainly to be preferred over failure by cup breakage, with its associated possibility of metal contamination of the product.

Stainless steel tools are recommended when resistance to corrosion is a major consideration. The absolute need should be well evaluated before specifying because of the negative aspects involved:

1. Higher initial cost and less wear resistance then premium steel tools
2. Relatively poor ductility compared with standard steel punches (refer to Fig. 6)

Often, a corrosive product can be successfully tableted without recourse to stainless steel by maintaining proper room humidity levels and by not allowing the material to remain on the press overnight.

The stainless steel that is normally employed in the manufacture of the majority of pharmaceutical and chemical equipment can be divided into two basic categories: austenitic and martensitic.

The former encompasses the Series 300 steels, which contain nickel-stabilized austenite. This is the type most widely used in tanks, sinks, sterile equipment, and so on. These steels will not accept heat treatment to achieve the proper qualities required for punches and dies.

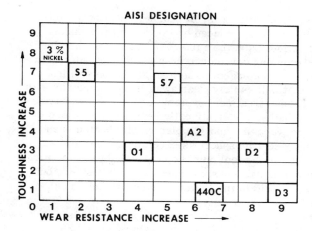

Figure 6. Tool steel wear/toughness chart.

The martensitic or Series 400 steels, containing little or no nickel, can be properly heat-treated by quenching and tempering. The 440C grade is the type that meets the requirements of concern here. It has very little corrosion resistance in the unhardened state and must be heat-treated to produce a hardness of at least 56 Rc to achieve a good degree of resistance to chemical attack. (Rc is a measure of hardness; it refers to a Rockwell hardness level in the C range. Hardness and its method of measurement are explained in Section VI. A). Optimum hardness for the best strength of the 440C would be 58 Rc.

Standard steel dies are normally made from a 5% carbon, air-hardening material, designated A2. Premium steel dies are made from D2 or D3 steel. Ductility is not a critical factor in the selection of die steels, and therefore premium steel, although more expensive, is usually the wisest choice. Because of its greater ability to resist wear, its life will be several times that of a standard steel die for the same application.

Where an extremely abrasive material is being compacted, it may be advantageous to specify carbide-lined dies. Although the initial cost is much higher, the increased production life usually more than justifies the expenditure. Bear in mind, when making the decision, that these dies require more careful handling. Improper insertion techniques or dropping on a concrete floor may wipe out part or all of your investment.

Carbide is not a panacea to all die-wear problems. Several other negative aspects must be considered before selection. Carbide is a sintered material and as such it is more porous than tool steel. These microscopic pores can minutely add to a tablet ejection problem. They also form an excellent lapping surface that can wear away the punch tips more rapidly. This may in some instances create a false economy. The die life may be extended many times, but the cost savings in the dies by the selection of carbide can be more than offset by the possibility of shortened punch life. Carbide should be specified only when sufficient production history has been established for the particular product using premium steel dies as a basis.

Heat treatment of the tools in manufacturing is, of course, extremely important. The life of the tooling can be severely reduced by improper procedures. Excess carbon can be introduced or lost from the surface of the tool at the elevated temperatures required. Introducing carbon can create a brittle outer structure that can start cracks in the punch cup edges. The loss of carbon will leave the tool with a soft outer surface that will rapidly wear away in use, together with any delicate engraving. The usual heat-treatment systems employed for pharmaceutical tooling are (1) molten salt baths, (2) electrically heated ovens where the steel is heated and quenched under a vacuum, and (3) electrically heated ovens where the carbon balance of the furnace atmosphere is carefully controlled.

The degree of hardness employed in the tool must be correlated to the application. As a general rule, an increase in hardness increases wear resistance but decreases ductility and toughness, all within the limits of the particular steel involved.

The higher-speed compressing machines should employ punches with a shank and head hardness of at least 54/56 Rc, preferably 58/59. This may be too hard to provide the needed ductility for a fragile punch tip. To overcome this problem, a selective heat-treatment procedure is employed known as tip drawing. This involves the timed immersion of the punch tips in molten lead held to a critical temperature. The punch tip hardness is thereby drawn down to the required level without affecting the rest of the tool.

Proper heat treatment of the tools is one of the important areas where great dependence must be made on the reliability of the vendor. There is no good nondestructive metallurgical test available that will assure you that the incoming tools have received the correct treatment for the application.

The Rockwell hardness check is an indication but in no way is it the complete story. Tools with the correct specified hardness could still have problems. For instance:

1. During the heat-treatment stage of the punch, it has approximately 0.012 in. of excess material over all its surfaces, with the exception of the punch cup. This material will be removed in subsequent grinding operations. The punch cup, however, will receive only a light polishing. Consequently, any carbon exchange, with its detrimental effect as mentioned previously, will be removed with the grinding stock on any measurable surface, but not in the most delicate part of the punch.
2. An adverse grain structure can be created by improper overheating of the steel in the austenizing step.
3. To achieve the optimum metallurgical structure for the steels involved, it is important that both the initial and tempering temperatures be properly established. Various combinations can often be employed to achieve the same hardness, but with varying effects on the toughness of the tool.

B. Tooling Tolerances and Clearances

This subject can be divided into two categories. The first consists of those dimensional variations permitted the manufacturer for the most economical construction of the tooling and machine, commensurate with the required tablet quality; and second, the permissible wear on the tool before it need be discarded.

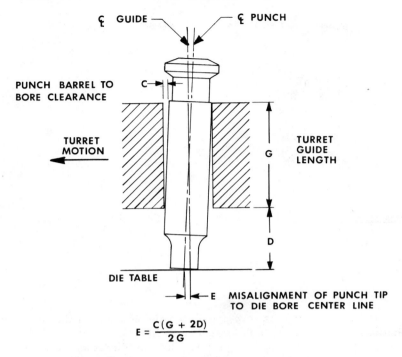

Figure 7. Punch-to-die misalignment.

The former can be further separated into the tolerances that affect the machine operation and the flight and centering of the tooling and those that affect the actual tablet being compacted.

Figure 7 depicts a typical station of upper punch and die in a rotary tablet press. The upper punch has the minimum nominal clearance to its guiding surface in the turret that is commensurate with the lubrication film requirements. The involved machining tolerance would permit this clearance to vary from 0.00175 to 0.00275 in.

The die should be a snug fit in the die pocket to minimize its center-line shift due to the radial pressure of the die locking screw. This shift, up to 0.00025 in., is due to the required manufacturing tolerances on the die outside diameter and the turret die pocket. The combination of these two adverse effects can permit the punch tip to strike the die surface as it enters the bore.

The degree of interference is reduced by the punch tip-to-die bore clearance, which will range from approximately 0.001 in. to 0.005 in., dependent on the tablet size. It can be increased by the concentricity tolerance between the punch tip-to-barrel and die bore-to-die outside diameter, which can add up to 0.0005 in. to the effect. The sum of all the tolerances and clearances involved could add up to as much as 0.005 in. overlap of the punch tip as it tries to enter the die bore. This could even be true on a new machine. Although the probability of all these

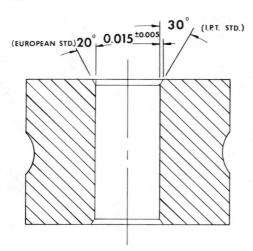

Figure 8. Die chamfer.

tolerances being in the adverse mode is very small, the die must accept the punch tip under all conditions or a smash-up in the machine would be inevitable.

The die bore must have an entry angle or chamfer that will direct an offset tip into the bore. The accepted American standard of a 30° angle on this chamfer (Fig. 8) does an effective job, so the negative effect on the punch tip life is small. However, the European standard of 20° should be considered to further reduce the deflection forces involved.

Wear on the guiding surfaces, turret guide, and punch barrel will add to the interference problem. Older machines should be checked periodically for excessive upper punch "play" to avert unnecessary wear on an expensive set of tools. To measure the play, drop the punch tip down until it is just above the die surface. Using a dial indicator, measure the total amount of tip movement in the direction of travel of the punch. It should not exceed 0.010 to 0.012 in.

The bore in the die should be straight and square with the die faces. A barreled die (Fig. 1) is very detrimental to good tablet production, in that the tablet would be formed at one diameter and then constricted as it leaves the die on ejection. This can cause excessively heavy ejection pressures and/or fracture of the tablet. Bell mouthing is not as serious (within limits); in fact, it can be of aid in air relief and ejection.

The dimensions that most seriously affect the geometry and compaction of the finished tablet are the punch length from the bottom of the cup to the head flat and, to a lesser degree, the die bore diameter. In any one set of tooling, these dimensions should be held as uniform as possible.

The American Pharmaceutical Association, Industrial Pharmaceutical Technology (IPT) Section Committee on Specifications, in cooperation with the leading tooling manufacturers, has established the maximum dimensional variations permissible. Study of their published material is recommended in conjunction with this chapter. The tolerances involved permit proper mechanical tooling performance in the tablet press and a good-quality tablet at a reasonable cost for the tools.

The dimensions we will be concerned with in the following exercise are: Bottom of cup to head flat ± 0.001 in. and the die bore -0.0000 + 0.0005 in.

The effect of these allowable dimensional differences between the tools in any one set will depend greatly on the size of the tablet being produced. To illustrate this, we will compare a small, thin tablet and a relatively larger tablet as follows:

Tablet A: 1/4-in. diameter x 0.090-in. thick, flat faced (FF)
          1.75:1 compaction ratio
Tablet B: 7/16-in. diameter x 0.200-in. thick (FF)
          1.75:1 compaction ratio

The term "compaction ratio" as employed here refers to the volume of the uncompressed granulation at the weight adjustment point to the volume of the finished tablet. This will vary with different granulations and will be affected by the speed and filling efficiency of the tablet press.

The tolerance on the die bore (+0.0005 - 0.0000 in.) will permit a 0.40% total volume change for tablet A but only 0.23% variation in tablet B, the larger-diameter tablet.

The most adverse tolerance combinations of the punches would be to match a short lower with a short upper punch (-0.001 in. each) and a long lower and upper (+0.001 in. each). These extremes would result in a 0.002 in. variation in the uncompressed fill depth and a 0.004 in. variation in the compacted tablet thickness.

The ±0.001 in. tolerance on the lower punch working length can affect the die fill of the thinner tablet, A, by ±0.68%, and the thicker tablet, B, by ±0.28%. The resultant weight variation could be cumulative with the variation due to die bore diameter. The compression ratio will be affected by both the upper and lower punch working lengths and is independent of the die bore variation. The percentage change due to the 0.004-in. difference in tablet thickness that could occur between any two press stations is partially offset by their respective die fill (the short lower accepts more material than the long lower punch). But again this density variation would be more serious with the thinner tablet: tablet A, 3.18%, and tablet B, 1.43%.

It can be concluded from the above that a possibly significant variation in tablet geometry could be caused by the industry-accepted standards for the punch length tolerances, the effect being more pronounced with thinner tablets.

The calculations are based on the tooling being matched in their most adverse relationship. The probability of this occurring in actual practice and the real need for increased accuracy for the product involved must be considered before specifying tighter (and more costly) tooling tolerances. It may be desirable in some situations to actually match the punches for length in each station of the turret (i.e., a short lower with a long upper, and vice versa). This would have the major corrective effect on the variation of the tablet density without resorting to more expensive tool construction.

C. Check List

The following information would aid in expediting a tooling order and also permit possible constructive criticism by the vendor.

1. Size and shape of tablet.
2. Design drawing (or drawing number if repeat order).

3. Hob number if a repeat order.
4. Any problems experienced with the previous tooling (or if a new product, any anticipated difficulties: e.g., heavy compaction required, tendency for air entrapment, etc.).
5. Number of tools required (are overruns accepted?).
6. Tableting machine to be employed (manufacturer and number of stations). Is it a standard or a special model? If the latter, a tool drawing or sample tool(s) are required.
7. Steel to be used and required hardness.
8. Any special features required (e.g., chrome plating, special keying, fluting, non-IPT specifications, etc.).
9. Is the striking of a new face design or sample station required?
10. When the tools will be needed.
11. Any special shipping instructions.

V. Hobbing

This is the procedure in which a hardened steel form (hob), having a mirror image of the required punch face, is pressed with heavy tonnage into a soft steel punch blank.

The procedure of preparing the hob is as follows:

1. A mutually accepted and approved drawing at approximately 10:1 magnification is photographed and reproduced on a dimensionally stable film, usually a polyester.
2. The film is used to make a contact print on a photosensitized plate.
3. The plate is chemically etched to produce a relieved outline of the required engraving.
4. The plate is then used as a template on an engraving machine (pantograph).
5. Employing a cutter very accurately ground to the required draft and tip radius, the pantograph operator reproduces the design to the required size on the face of the soft hob blank (Fig. 4).
6. The hob is then checked for dimensional accuracy, heat-treated to produce the proper hardness, and polished.
7. When requested, a sample striking made from the hob will be furnished the customer for approval.

The life of the hob is limited by the number of punches produced, the degree of pressure required to bring up the engraving detail, and the punch steel employed. The original cost of the hob is borne by the customer, but all maintenance and replacement costs are absorbed by the manufacturer.

VI. Use and Care of the Tooling

A. Incoming and Routine Inspection

Pharmaceutical punches and dies are precision tools that require dozens of different machining operations to complete. The manufacturer performs inspection checks after each operation to ensure that the final product will be to specification. On completion, the tool is given a full 100% inspection before shipment.

In spite of all the checks and double checks, mistakes and errors can be made and, therefore, pharmaceutical companies should have an incoming inspection procedure to check the vendor's product. It is suggested that at least a spot check of critical dimensions be made on all tools received to ensure good tablet production capability.

The basic equipment required for an inspection facility is:

1. A clean, well-lighted area with a wood- or Masonite-covered benchtop
2. Surface plate (approximately 12 x 12 in.)
3. Dial indicator (0.0005-in. increments, 0.500 travel) with stand
4. Accurate (hardened and ground) V block
5. Micrometers 0-1 and 1-2 in.
6. Set of length standards or JO blocks
7. Set of ball and telescope gages to measure die bores
8. Illuminated magnifying glass.

This list can be expanded to the limit of any budget with equipment such as optical comparators, air gages for die bores, Magnaflux equipment, digital-readout height gages, a steel hardness-checking device, and a toolmaker's microscope. Although these devices are all quite useful and will speed up and/or expand the quality assurances, the return on the investment becomes more marginal. The basic equipment outlined, however, will permit confirmation of the essential measurements.

The dial indicator is used to check the overall length of the punch and the length of the punch to the bottom of the cup. It would be set up using the length standards or JO blocks (dimensionally precise hardened steel blocks that are combined to produce the desired dimension). It is also used for checking the punch tip to barrel and the die bore concentricity by rotating the punch or die in the V block (Fig. 9).

The micrometers are used to check the barrel, tip, head, and neck diameters of the punch and the height and outside diameter of the die.

The die bore would be checked with the ball or telescope gages or plug gages can be employed.

A magnifying glass can be used to detect possible rough spots in the punch face embossing. However, if a precise dimensional check of the logo is needed, it would require the use of a toolmaker's microscope.

An optical comparator is often used for the dimensional measurement since it is much faster than the microscope. This could be used in conjunction with an overlay, an accurately drawn outline of the design on glass or dimensionally stable plastic film. Caution must be used with an overlay system to avoid measurement errors. The embossing ridges composing the design are all radiused. As a consequence, the reflected light from the punch face that produces the image is dependent on its angle of incidence as it bounces off these curved surfaces. Both the comparator and the microscope are affected. However, the available depth perception on the microscope permits a much better judgment of the correct measuring points. If a comparator is employed, it should have the light source as parallel as possible with the viewing line of sight to minimize the possibility of error. ("Through the lens" lighting is best.)

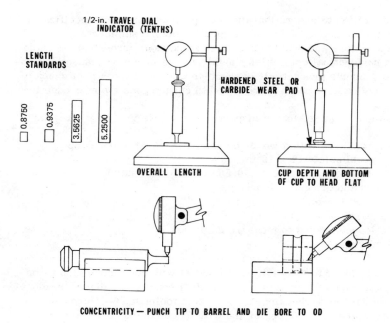

Figure 9.   Punch and die inspection equipment.

    The most popular device for measuring the steel hardness is a Rockwell Hardness Checker. This unit forces a diamond stylus into the steel with a fixed pressure. The amount of penetration is related to the hardness and appears on a dial indicator on the machine.

    The normal Rockwell range for the steels used in pharmaceutical tooling is the C scale. It will be specified as a double number, which indicates the accepted tolerance (e.g., a punch barrel hardness would be specified as 56/58 Rc). Since the accepted practice is to round off the reading to the closest whole number, the actual acceptance level for this hardness would be 55.5/58.5 Rc. The slight ridge around the indentations caused by this measurement device must be stoned flush before using the tool.

    When measuring, it is important to note that anything but an absolutely firm or rigid support of the test piece will introduce an error in the reading. Measurement on a curved surface such as a punch barrel or tip creates an error due to the unequal resistance of the metal flow at the penetration point. The smaller the diameter, the greater the deviation from the true hardness. The manufacturer of the instrument supplies a compensation chart for correcting the reading. Three readings should be taken: the first is discarded and the second and third are averaged.

    Magnaflux equipment is used to check for minute cracks or flaws that are not readily apparent. These faults are not usually present in new tools, but can appear in the life cycle of the tool as it fatigues. This equipment is not too useful as an incoming checking device, but is helpful when running routine checks on used tools.

Each time a set of tooling is removed from the machine, it should be immediately checked for signs of cam wear before the tablet machine is set up for its next production run. Badly worn or "galled" areas on the punch heads would indicate rough spots on the cams and/or pressure roll faces which, if not corrected, will cause unnecessary abuse to the next set of tooling.

The tools should be checked for other visual indications and dimensional variations calling for rework or replacement (e.g., curled cup edges, worn logo design, die bore "rings"). Periodic length checks on the critical cup bottom-to-head flat dimension should be made to see if length resizing is required (see Sec. VI.E).

B. Handling and Storage of Tooling

The hard steel structure of tooling often creates a feeling of industructibility to the uninitiated. This, of course, is not true, as attested by the number of tools that are ruined by careless handling and storage. The cup edges on the punches are especially delicate. Contact of these areas with another punch or the press turret when inserting or removing the tools can cause them to crack or chip. A slight crack can result in chipping during the production run, with a possible serious contamination of the latter.

A good procedure to follow is to make punch handling boxes (Fig. 10). The box should be large enough to hold a full set of tools or of a size that meets "in-plant" weight limits. A wooden or metal tray with a perforated wooden top to accept the punches works quite well. The dies, which are much less subject to damage, can be handled in a smaller tray.

When removing the punches from the tablet press, each punch should be wiped and dropped into a hole in the tray top as it is removed. Do not accumulate and clean these as a group, since possible rolling on a cart top can damage the tips. The trays should be brought to a cleaning and inspection area, where the tools can be thoroughly cleaned, inspected for abnormal wear, and a rustproof oil applied.

If rework or replacement is indicated, this should be inaugurated. Rough areas on the punch heads would indicate that some attention should be given to the press cams before resuming the operation of the machine. If the tools are acceptable for their next production run, they can be returned to the handling boxes; or, to save the cost of the number of boxes required for storage, a more compact procedure is to return the tools to their protective cardboard sleeves and store in metal file drawers. Never store any tools unless they have been adequately cleaned and have a good application of rust-preventive oil.

Rust is very detrimental to the tool. Obviously, rust and its accompanying pitting on the punch cup could result in picking and obliteration of any delicate engraving. However, corrosion on the remainder of the tool surface can result in a problem that is just as serious. It can adversely affect the fatigue resistance of the tool. Although the general loss of section due to corrosion is negligible, the stress concentration effect of the corrosion pits formed can result in punches failing at the key insert or at the punch neck.

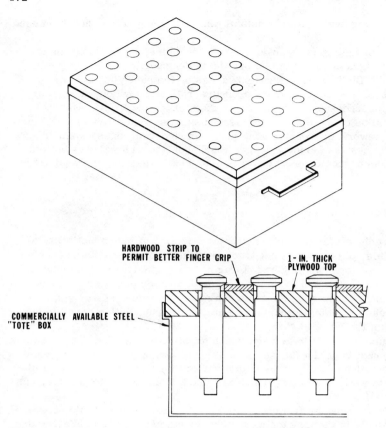

Figure 10. Punch handling box.

C. Tool and Die Control

A good tooling program should include an accurate recording of the history of each set of tools employed. The advantage of this, once established, is that future tooling requirements can be better forecast. The information is of further value for possible upgrading of the life of new tool sets (e.g., better steel for the application and/or heat treatment). It is also a good check on the reliability of the vendor since, as mentioned previously, some tooling quality must be accepted "on faith." The information that should be included in the record is shown on a typical 5- x 8-in. file card (Fig. 11).

The tools should be kept in sets. An inexpensive electric pencil can be used to put a code number on the neck of the punch to avoid mix-ups.

D. Punch Lubrication

A good film of lubricant on the punch contact areas of the turret would theoretically eliminate any possibility of metal abrasion, and would therefore prolong indefinitely

Product: _GUMBUT_____ NDA# _XYZ_____ Hob # _1592_

Tool: UP LP Die Size/Shape: _3/8 STD. CONC._ Steel: _S-5_ Rc BBL/Tip: _56/52_

Vendor: _BEST MFG._____ P.O.# _6295___ Date: _7/17/75_ Qty: _61_

Date	No. Tablets Produced	Press Employed	Condition and/or Needs	Set Ready for Reuse
10/18/75	73 M	RP MII	—	10/12 GM
1/7/76	18 M	"	REPOLISH FACE (ONE DROPPED)	1/9 GM
2/20/76	54 M	"	RESIZE LENGTH	2/25 GM
5/4/76	60 M	"	MONOGRAM WORN – DISCARD —	GM

Spares on Hand: _X 10/18/75_

    5   1/9/76

Figure 11. Tool record card.

this factor in the wear life of the tool. Unfortunately, this protective barrier between the metal surfaces cannot always be maintained. Free-flowing oils will "heal" worn spots in the film; however, their very ability to flow permits possible product contamination and requires constant replenishment. Greases, which are more apt to stay in place, flow and "heal" only when the film is broken to the degree where metal-to-metal contact is made, which in turn causes sufficient frictional heat to melt the grease.

The lubricant should meet several requirements: (1) it must have the film strength to resist the contact pressures involved; (2) it should not be easily contaminated by the dust from the granulation such as occurs with sugar and mineral oil; (3) it must adhere well to the metal surfaces to minimize any tendency to run off; and (4) it should be "edible" when used on the upper punches, where the possibility of product contamination exists.

Upper punch barrels and heads present the greatest problem. Approved (edible) lubricants have adequate film strength to work reasonably well in the punch barrel guide and upper cam area. However, they must be applied very sparingly. The possibility exists of forming black specks, which are a combination of lubricant, dust, and worn-off metal. These can drop into the product. The relatively poor film strength of these lubricants will break down in the head/cam contact area unless the punches remain free in their guides.

Normal practice is to apply a few drops of light mineral oil (approximately 10W) in the palm of the hand and rub sparingly on the punch barrel before inserting it in the turret. Grease would be applied to the punch heads using a small paint brush at periodic intervals during the production run. (The brush should be examined regularly and discarded if there are any indications of loose bristles.) The frequency of application would be dependent on the operating conditions (i.e., press speed, dust conditions, and round or irregularly shaped tools). Because irregularly shaped tools cannot rotate to better distribute the available lubricant, they will require considerably more attention than will round tools.

Teflon, which is gaining in popularity, reduces the possibility of the formation of the black specks. However, it does not always withstand the extra demand placed on the lubricant at the higher machine speeds that are available today.

Since the normally used Teflon is not miscible with oil (the combination will form a binding substance), it is imperative that all traces of oil be removed from the guides before applying. Teflon powder mixed with a volatile solvent would be brushed or sprayed on the punch barrel before insertion in the turret. This material does not usually have sufficient strength to enable its use on the cam tracks; therefore, grease must be employed on the punch heads. Careful application of the grease would be required to prevent it from coming in contact with the barrel lubricant.

The use of plastic dust cups on the upper punch tips is strongly recommended to trap possible falling particles. When employing unkeyed punches in turrets that have keyways, a further precaution is to employ inserts to fill these unused channels.

The lubrication of the lower punches presents a different problem than that of the uppers. In this case it is a matter of the product contaminating the lubricant. Material sifting through the clearance between the lower punch tip and die bore drops down along the punch barrel to the lower cam track. This sifted material rapidly blots up the applied lubricant, causing the need for more frequent replenishment. The demand on the lubricant film is usually much higher than with the upper punch, owing to the heavier ejection and punch pulldown forces that are encountered.

Oil spray mist systems, with their coalescing nozzles aimed at the ejection cam surfaces, can be employed. High film-strength grease applied periodically during the production run is also effective. A light oil would be applied to the barrels.

The more recently designed presses employ stripper seals at the top of the lower punch guides. These prevent the sifted tableting material from reaching the cam area and, therefore, greatly reduce the lubrication problem.

The cutting or grinding action employed to machine the turret, cams, or tools leaves microscopic sharp ridges that can puncture the best lubrication film. It is advisable when starting up a new press or installing any new "wear" components that the press be operated under very light loading, with more than normal lubrication, until these sharp surfaces are lapped down. This greatly reduces the demand on the lubrication and permits the use of the poorer film-strength approved lubricants.

Good dust control is important to the proper lubrication of a tablet press. The vacuum nozzles furnished as standard on the machine are usually adequate. However, improvements based on the actual operating conditions and granulation employed often can be made. Care must be exercised to avoid pulling granulation out of the die cavity prior to compaction by too much or misdirected air flow.

E. Refinishing

The good working life of the tooling can be extended to a degree by the careful reworking of certain critical areas.

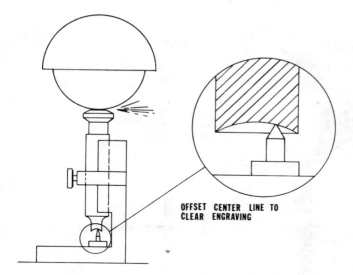

OFFSET CENTER LINE TO
CLEAR ENGRAVING

Figure 12. Punch length sizing on a surface grinder.

The erosion inherent in the compacting process can start small pits in the punch face. Unless smoothed out in time, these areas will enlarge and get rougher, resulting in granulation adherence or picking. Judicious application of a fine diamond paste with a small, soft, rotary-end bristle brush will usually be very effective.

Plain cupped punches can be reground with a wheel dressed to the required radius; however, this requires more extensive equipment (i.e., chucking lathe and tool post grinder). A chucking lathe can also be employed to correct curled-in punch cup edges. A fine abrasive stone would be applied to the curled edge as the punch rotates. Care must be exercised in this operation to avoid contacting any embossing present.

The punch head, which is subject to cam and pressure roll wear, should be carefully checked each time the tools are removed from the machine. Any rough areas should be smoothed with a fine-grit emery cloth, or the angles can be reground. The marks need not be removed entirely. In fact, with irregularly shaped tools, which do not rotate in their turret guides, the angular wear flats created convert the original line contact with the cam to an area contact. The latter decreases the unit contact pressure, resulting in a decelerated wear rate (providing that they are smoothed).

It is usually advisable to periodically check the critical length of the punch (the dimension from the bottom of the cup to the head flat). This length can be resized to uniformity within the set, when required, through use of a simple fixture, shown in Figure 12, used in conjunction with a small surface grinder. The V block holds the punch in a vertical position. The center of the cup rests on a pointed brass or nylon plug. (If embossing is present in the cup center, it will be necessary to offset the plug.)

The tools should all be at uniform temperature before any measurements are made. This could become critical when sizing the length, owing to the coefficient

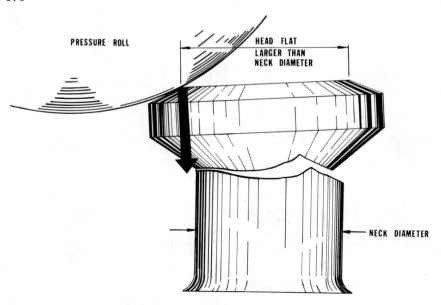

Figure 13. Punch head.

of expansion of the steel. This factor is 6.3×10^{-6} in.$^{-1}$ $^\circ$F^{-1}. For example, if the tools were cleaned in a hot bath, it is conceivable that the last out could be 30° F warmer than the first ones cleaned. This 30° temperature difference would cause a 5 1/4-in. long punch to grow in length by 0.001 in. If sized at this length, it would become too short when it cooled down (0.0000063 in. x 5.25 in. x 30° F = 0.00099 in.).

Before grinding, check all the punches to find the shortest. Set this one up first and bring the grinding wheel down so that it barely touches and just begins to spark. Then grind all of the other punches to this length.

One word of caution: The diameter of the head flat must not exceed the neck diameter of the punch or the compression roll force on the punch head may cause the punch head to break off as the tablet is formed (Fig. 13). If the head flat gets too large, the outside head angle will require regrinding. However, care must be exercised not to get the heads too thin for fear of breakage in use.

Because of the cyclic pressure to which the punch is subject in its operation to compact the tablet, fatigue due to the constant flexing may cause premature failure. It is advisable when the more fragile punch cup shapes are employed to periodically stress-relieve the tools. This is a simple operation that involves baking the tools in an oven for several hours at a temperature approximately 30 to 50° F below their original tempering temperature. This value for the particular set of tools involved can be obtained from the supplier.

The reworking of the dies is limited to the enlarging of the bore to the "die ring" diameter. The "ring" is an eroded band in the die bore located in the final compaction area of the tablet. This worn section permits a tablet to be formed that is larger in diameter than the mouth of the bore that it must pass in ejection.

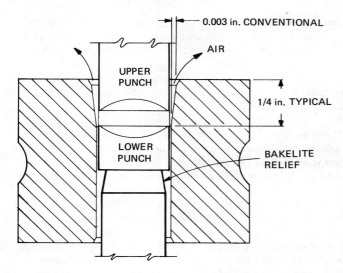

Figure 14.   Tapered die bore and Bakelite relief.

   Polishing will not be effective in this case. It will require enlargement of the
entire bore to the diameter of the worn area. This can be accomplished through
use of a honing machine. However, a wooden dowel rod wrapped with fine emery
cloth used in the chuck of a drill press will suffice. Obviously, there is a limit
to how far the bore can be enlarged, since excessive sifting and tablet "flash"
will result.

VII.   Problem Solving

A.   Special Tooling Features

Problems that arise when employing a more difficult granulation can sometimes
be alleviated or eliminated by design changes in the tooling.
   The tendency of the tablet to "cap" or delaminate as it is ejected can be reduced by tapering the die bore (Fig. 14). This not only permits better air es-
capement during compression, but also permits the tablet to expand at a more
gradual rate as it leaves the die bore. It also has an advantage in that it reduces
the required ejection force.
   Its disadvantage is that it raises the initial cost of the die and prohibits "turning over" the die for extended die life, since a taper on the lower end of the die
would permit excessive escape ("sifting") of the granulation if deep-fill cams are
employed.
   If material has a tendency to adhere to the die bore wall, causing the lower
punch tip to bind, a Bakelite relief would be helpful. This is a method of obtaining a sharp lower edge on the tip straight, which tends to scrape the die bore
clean as the punch lowers (Fig. 14).

Chrome plating can be used to alleviate a tendency of product adherence to the punch face or die bore. The plating, as employed on pharmaceutical tooling, is referred to as hard chrome, differing from the normal decorative plating in that a thickness of only 0.0001 to 0.0002 in. is applied directly to the steel surface. This is to assure the best bonding. Although some additional wear and slight corrosion resistance is also gained by this form of plating, the possible adverse effects must be considered before selection.

If the entrapped hydrogen, a normal consequence of plating, is not completely baked out by the plater (not always possible), the resultant hydrogen embrittlement can cause premature punch cup failure. Further, the added chrome layer does not have the same flexural aspect as the parent steel and therefore could start cracks that can progress to punch cup failure or possibly spall (flake) off and contaminate the product.

The dust of some materials tends to combine with the lubrication and cause binding of the punches in their turret guides. This can be helped by machining vertical grooves in the punch barrels to reduce their contact area and to give them a self-cleaning action as they rotate with round tools. This is called fluting. This is not recommended except as a last resort, because it can cause product contamination if used on upper punch barrels and excess lower cam lubrication problems due to the sifted granulation if used on the lowers. It is far better to increase the exhaust system on the press, try for more compatible barrel lubrication, or run the product on one of the new-design presses that employ seals on the lower punch guides.

Worn upper punch turret guides can cause excessive contact of the punch tip with the die chamfer as it enters the die. This causes the edges of the cup to curl in, creating a problem as the tablet separates from the upper punch face. Although this hooked edge can be stoned out, it leaves a slight radius on the outside of the cup lip. This radius permits a firm ridge or "flash" on the tablet to be formed that is difficult to remove in the dedusting operation. It would be wiser to specify a smaller upper punch tip diameter, which would create a larger tip-to-bore clearance. The flash would not be any smaller, but it would be considerably softer and more apt to be completely removed in the cleaning operation.

Two or more tablets can be made at each station of the press through use of multiple-insert tooling (Fig. 15A). This can greatly increase the production output of the machine. However, it has several negative aspects that must be considered before investing in this higher-cost tooling: (1) since the punch length would be composed of two components, the length variation due to the required tolerance of both could be cumulative and thereby add to the nonuniformity of the tablets; (2) since the die bores do not all have exactly the same relationship to the powder feeding area, the die fill uniformity may be affected; (3) the setup of the press is more involved and time consuming; and (4) since it will probably require a slower turret rpm the increase in the press output rate will not be directly in proportion to the number of inserts/stations.

Core rod tooling (Fig. 15B) can be employed on most standard presses to make tablets that have a hole through their center (Fig. 15). Although this tablet configuration has an advantage where the need for more tablet surface area is indicated, it does require a considerably lower press output speed and much more expensive tooling.

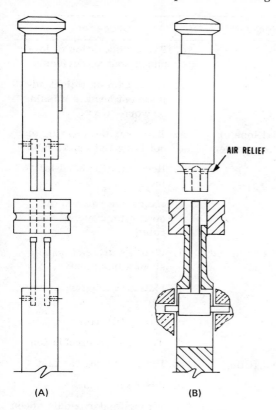

AIR RELIEF

(A)   (B)

Figure 15. (A) Multiple-insert tooling, (B) core rod tooling.

B. Compressing Problems

Compressing problems may be caused by the granulation, the tablet press, or the compaction tooling. This chapter was to be concerned only with the latter; however, since many problems are interrelated, it was felt that sufficient interest and help would be gained by including the following troubleshooting list (starred items indicate features not available on all model machines).

Problem	Possible causes	Check for
A. Nonuniform tablet weight	1. Erratic punch flight	a. Freedom of punch barrels in guides (must be clean and well lubricated)
		b. Excess machine vibration
		c. Worn or loose weight adjustment ramp

Problem	Possible cause	Check for
		*d. Proper operation of lower punch control devices
		*e. Limit cam on weight adjustment head is missing or worn
	2. Material loss or gain after proper die fill	*a. Tail over die missing or not lying flat on die table
		*b. Recirculation band leaking
		c. Excessive vacuum or nozzle improperly located
	3. Feeders "starved" or "choked"	a. Wrong setting of hopper spout adjustment
		b. Material bridging in hopper
		c. Wrong fill cam
		d. Too much recirculation
	4. Dies not filling	a. Press running too fast
		b. See A3 and A5
		*c. Wrong feeder paddle speed or shape
	5. Lower punch starts pulling down without material coverage	a. Inadequate recirculation
		b. Recirculation scraper missing or bent
	6. Bad scrape-off	a. Scraper blade bent, worn, or bad spring action
	7. Nonuniform punch length	a. Punch cup bottom to head flats to be ±0.001 in., per IPT standards
	8. Die(s) projecting above die table	a. Clean die pocket or check die dimension
B. Nonuniform tablet thickness	1. Nonuniform tablet weight	a. See A above
	2. Pressure roll bounce	a. Overload release improperly set

Problem	Possible cause	Check for
		b. Operation near maximum density point of granulation (within allowable tablet tolerances, increase thickness and/or reduce weight)
		c. Pressure roll freedom and face condition
		*d. Air entrapment in hydraulic overload system
		e. Worn roll carrier pivot pins
	3. Nonuniform punch lengths	a. Punch cup bottom to head flats to be ±0.001 in., per IPT standards
C. Nonuniform density (friability)	1. Uniform tablet weight and thickness	a. See above.
		b. See "capping" (H)
	2. Unequal granule distribution in die cavities	a. Stratification or separation in hopper
		*b. Excess recirculation (causes classification of granulation since only the finer mesh material escapes the rotary feeders)
D. Excess machine vibration	1. Worn drive belt	
	2. Mismatched punch lengths	See A-7
	3. Operating near maximum density point of granulation	a. Increase tablet thickness and/or reduce weight within allowable tablet tolerances
	4. Heavy ejection pressure	a. Worn ejection cam
		b. Need for more lube in granulation or tapered dies
		c. Barreled dies
	5. Improper pressure-release setting	a. Increase to limit of tools

Problem	Possible cause	Check for
E. Excess punch head and cam wear	1. Binding punches	a. Dirty punch guides
		b. Inadequate and improper lubrication
		c. Inadequate exhaust
	2. Rough spots on surfaces from previous operation	a. Not polishing off rough spots caused by normal wear or accidents
F. Dirt in product (black specks)		a. Need for more frequent cleaning
		b. Excess or wrong lubrication
		c. Proper punch dust cups and keyway fillers
		d. Feeder components rubbing
		e. Punch-to-die binding
G. Excessive material loss	1. Incorrect feeder fit to die table	a. Feeder bases incorrectly set (too high or not level)
		*b. Feeder pan bottoms worn due to previous incorrect setting (relap if necessary)
	*2. Incorrect action on recirculation band	a. Gaps between bottom edge and die table
		b. Binding in mounting screw
		c. Too little holddown spring pressure
	3. Die table scraper action insufficient	a. Scraper blade worn or binding
		b. Outboard edge permitting material to escape
	4. Loss out of die prior to upper punch entry	*a. Tail over die not lying flat on die table
	5. Loss at compression point	a. Compressing too high in the die
		b. Excessive or misdirected suction on exhaust nozzle

Problem	Possible cause	Check for
	6. Excessive "sift-ting"	a. Excessive lower tip-to-die bore clearance
		b. Excessive fines in the granulation
		c. Tapered dies installed upside down
H. "Capping"	1. Air entrapment	a. Compress higher in the die
		b. Reduce press speed
		*c. Employ precompression
		d. Reduce quantity of fines in the granulation
		e. Reduce cup depth on punches
		f. Taper dies
	2. Excess pressure	a. Reduce weight and/or increase thickness within allowable tolerances
	3. "Ringed" or barreled die bore	a. Reverse dies
		b. Hone or lap bores
		c. Compress higher in the die
	4. Too rapid expansion	a. Taper dies
I. Punch face "picking"	1. Excess moisture	a. Moisture content of granulation
		b. Room humidity condition
	2. Punch face condition	a. Punch face pits and/or improper draft on embossing (try repolishing)
		b. Try chrome-plating the punch faces
	3. Insufficient compaction force	a. Increase weight and/or reduce thickness within allowable tolerances

VIII. Summary

Careful consideration and implementation of the many factors involved in a good workable tooling program will reap benefits in many ways.

A well-thought-out design that satisfies the needs of production, packaging, and marketing, coupled with the manufacture of the tools to the exacting specifications required, are necessary to produce the highest quality product at the lowest overall cost.

The number of tablets that these tools will produce during their usable life and the resultant tooling cost per tablet will be a function of their design, the steel and hardness selected, and the quality of the maintenance and handling program employed.

The time required to implement the tooling for a new tablet design will be a function of the correctness and completeness of the information supplied to the tooling manufacturer.

Tooling suppliers have gained a wealth of experience in dealing with many compressing problems through the years. Do not hesitate to draw on this information if the need arises. They will be pleased to help where they can in the solution of any tablet compressing problem.

Author Index

Where authors' names are cited, numbers in parentheses are reference numbers, and indicate that an author's work is referred to although his name is not cited in the text. Underlined numbers give the page on which the complete reference is cited.

Subject Index